Introduction to Neuropharmacology

To: Joel Elkes

Introduction to Neuropharmacology

Philip B. Bradley BSc(Hons), PhD, DSc, FIBiol
Emeritus Professor of Pharmacology, University of Birmingham, UK

WRIGHT

London   Boston   Singapore   Sydney   Toronto   Wellington

WRIGHT

is an imprint of Butterworth Scientific

Part of Reed International P.L.C.

First published 1989

© **Butterworth & Co. (Publishers) Ltd, 1989**

British Library Cataloguing in Publication Data

Bradley, P. B. (Philip Benjamin), *1919–*
   Introduction to neuropharmacology.
   1. Neuropsychopharmacology
   I. Title
   615′.78

   ISBN 0-7236-1271-4

Library of Congress Cataloging-in-Publication Data

Bradley, P. B.
   Introduction to neuropharmacology

   Bibliography: p.
   Includes index.
   1. Neuropharmacology. I. Title. [DNLM: 1.
   Nervous System–drug effects. QV 76.5 B811i]
   RM315.B655   1989   615′.78   88-26290
   ISBN 0-7236-1271-4

Typeset by SB Datagraphics Ltd, Colchester, Essex.
(An Ician Communications Group company)
Printed and bound by Hartnoll Ltd, Bodmin, Cornwall

Preface

This book is intended for students of medicine, dentistry, pharmacy, the neuro-sciences and other biological disciplines. It is hoped that it may also be of value to those working in related disciplines such as psychiatry, and to the interested layman. The book bridges the gap between pharmacology and therapeutics as far as the nervous system is concerned, since the emphasis is on the mechanisms of action of drugs which are important for their clinical uses, although other drugs, such as drugs of abuse, are also discussed.

The idea for the book arose through many years of teaching pharmacology to medical, dental and science students and being constantly asked, 'Where can I read more?' There are, of course, many excellent general textbooks of pharmacology but few of these deal in detail with the mechanisms of action of drugs on the nervous system, especially on the brain, and those which do tend to be very large and expensive. This book aims to provide the necessary detail concisely and inexpensively.

Neuropharmacology is a relatively new discipline and is still advancing rapidly. Thus, new drugs with new applications are constantly appearing and concepts which are valid today may be invalid tomorrow. Nevertheless, it is hoped that most of the ideas and concepts referred to in this book will stand the test of time, although inevitably some material will need to be revised.

I should like to thank my former colleagues in the Department of Pharmacology, University of Birmingham, with whom I had many discussions over the years and who have therefore contributed indirectly to this book. I am grateful to Mrs Karen Helliwell who prepared most of the illustrations, to Mr Pete Nobbs for the photographs and, finally, to my wife who read the text.

Philip B. Bradley
Birmingham
September 1988

Introduction

Mankind has always sought to help those who suffer from disease and, of the curative methods used, one of the oldest and most successful has been treatment with drugs. This is especially true of drugs acting on the nervous system. In fact, the earliest historical records indicate that man has long had some useful folk knowledge of drugs to heal, to soothe the spirits and to relieve pain. Thus, the ancient Greeks were aware of the properties of naturally occurring salicylates: for example, Hippocrates recommended the juice of the poplar tree for the treatment of eye diseases and extracts of the leaves of the willow for the relief of pain in childbirth; both of these plants contain natural salicylates, the forerunners of aspirin. Most of the drugs used by the early civilizations were herbal remedies, i.e. extracts of plants, very often mixtures of a number of different plants and usually containing large amounts of inactive material as well as the active constituents. Some were of animal origin, or were inorganic. Knowledge of the uses to which these 'folk remedies' could be put was acquired by a process of 'trial and error', i.e. empirically rather than by any rational process and, of course, it did not include any understanding of the biological actions of the drugs, nor of their chemistry.

This kind of folk medicine continued into the nineteenth century, when the scientific revolution, and developments in chemistry in particular, brought about remarkable changes. Through the use of chemical analysis it became possible to separate the various constituents of the crude herbal extracts; then each constituent could be tested separately for biological activity, and finally the chemical nature of the active component or components could be determined. A further step, having determined the chemical structure of the active component, was to synthesize it and then make analogues of the original drug. These analogues might be more active, i.e. possess increased potency, or produce fewer side-effects, or even be cheaper to make.

Important though the contributions of both organic and analytical chemistry were at this stage, the testing of the individual constituents for their actions on living systems represented the birth of the science of pharmacology. Thus, pharmacology is concerned with the study of the biological actions of drugs. One could, therefore, define a drug as a substance with biological actions. However, this raises the question, can all substances, which are biologically active, be called drugs? As many drugs are used exclusively for their therapeutic effects, one possibility would be to define a drug as a substance used for the treatment, diagnosis or prevention of disease. However, this definition is too restricted for pharmacology as there are many drugs which are used experimentally but which have no therapeutic application. Furthermore, it must be recognized that drugs are now used for purposes other than therapy and experimental pharmacology. Thus, drugs are used for social (e.g. oral contraceptives) and antisocial (drug abuse) purposes, as well as for their psychological effects (psychotomimetic drugs) and even, in the wider context, for political (e.g. anti-riot agents) and military (chemical warfare) applications. Therefore a wider definition than one simply based on drug therapy is required, especially as pharmacologists are concerned with all aspects of the actions of drugs, whether therapeutically useful or not. A drug may therefore be defined as 'a chemical substance which, by interacting with living tissues, changes their function'. This definition has the advantage of including endogenous substances which may be used as drugs. It also serves to emphasize differences, which are sometimes confused, between physiology and pharmacology. Physiology is concerned with the actions of endogenous substances in the normal quantities in which they occur in the body, whereas pharmacology deals with their actions when they are administered in 'non-physiological' amounts.

Contents

Part 1

General principles

Chapter 1

Characteristics of drug action

There are two important features concerning the biological action of drugs. The first is that most drugs produce their effects in very small doses, i.e. in very low concentrations in the tissues. Thus, if it were possible to calculate the number of molecules of a drug present in a tissue, and to try to relate this to the surface area of the cells on which the drug was presumably acting, then it would be found that there were not sufficient molecules of the drug present to cover even a fraction of the total cell surface. How then does the drug modify the function of the cells?

The second feature is that the majority of drugs are highly specific in terms of their chemical structure. Thus, altering the structure of a drug may result in a reduction in, or a complete loss of, biological activity and there are many examples of stereoselectivity where only one isomer or enantiomorph is pharmacologically active. To explain these two features of the actions of drugs, the existence of a specialized region of the cell membrane, or 'receptor', is postulated and it is with this that the drug interacts. The receptor concept is usually attributed to a German chemist, Paul Erhlich (1900), who proposed the term 'receptive substance' for the chemical groups in the tissue which produced a biological response by combining with complementary groups of 'foreign' molecules, i.e. drugs. A similar idea was put forward by the English physiologist Langley (1878), to explain the actions of pilocarpine and atropine on salivary secretion.

The high potency of drugs can therefore be explained in terms of an interaction between the molecules of the drug and a specialized region of the cell membrane, the receptor, which mediates the response of the cell. The chemical specificity of drugs is explained in terms of a chemical relationship between the drug molecule and the receptor. The receptor concept is of fundamental importance to pharmacology, which would have no rational basis without it.

The biological action of a drug is therefore explained in terms of an interaction with specific receptors for that drug. This interaction is thought to be a physico-chemical reaction which depends on the molecules of the drug being attracted to a corresponding or complementary molecular structure of the receptor. In order to explain this in more detail, drugs can be considered to possess three properties: selectivity, affinity and intrinsic activity.

Selectivity

This relates to the specificity of a drug for a particular receptor. A drug which is selective, and not all drugs are, will interact only with its own receptors and not

3

those for other drugs or other types of drug. In this way a drug will produce effects in tissues or organs where its receptors are present and not where they are absent, and we can explain why drugs act only at certain sites in terms of the presence of its specific receptors and the selectivity of the drug for those receptors. A very simple analogy for this is that of the lock (receptor) and key (drug), but a better analogy is illustrated diagrammatically in Figure 1.1a, where the drug is seen to have the correct 'shape' to fit the receptor.

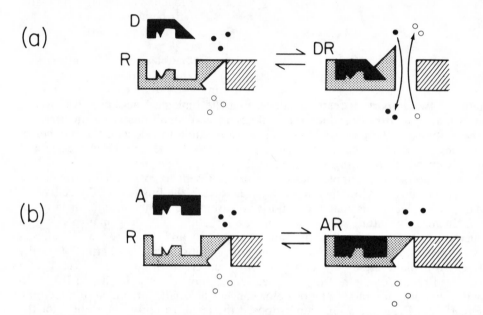

Figure 1.1 Diagrammatic representation of drug–receptor interaction. (a) Drug D has the correct shape to fit the receptor R, forming a drug–receptor complex DR and this results in a conformational change in the receptor and the opening of a pore in the adjacent membrane. Drug D is therefore an agonist. In (b) drug A also has the correct shape to fit the receptor, forming a drug–receptor complex AR, but in this case there is no conformational change, i.e. no response. Drug A is therefore an antagonist

Affinity

Apart from the drug having the right shape or chemical structure to fit the receptor, there must also be some force or forces attracting the molecules of the drug to the surface of the receptor in order to form a drug–receptor complex, which initiates the biological response. This attraction of the drug for the receptor is known as the 'affinity' of the drug and, because most drug–receptor interactions are reversible, the forces involved are normally weak chemical bonds, of which there are three main types, as follows:

1. *Ionic bonds* represent the electrostatic attraction between oppositely charged ions. Drug molecules are often large and contain many potential cationic and anionic groups of all kinds, capable of forming ionic bonds with oppositely charged groups on the receptor. The proteins and nucleic acids of the receptor will also possess potential cationic and anionic groups. In addition, many drugs are ionized in solution and will therefore be charged. Ionic bonds dissociate

readily, so the drug–receptor interactions in which they are involved will be reversible. The bond strength is of the order of 21 kJ mol^{-1} (5 kcal mol^{-1}) and the force of attraction (F) between the ionic groups diminishes as the square of the distance (r) between them, i.e. $F \propto 1/r^2$.

2. *Hydrogen bonds* represent a special kind of ionic bond. Many hydrogen atoms, present on or near the surface of a molecule—particularly a large molecule— possess a partial positive charge and can therefore form ionic bonds with negatively charged atoms, such as oxygen or nitrogen. Hydrogen bonds are usually weaker than ionic bonds, the bond strength being of the order of 8– 21 kJ mol^{-1} (2–5 kcal mol^{-1}) and inversely proportional to the fourth power of the distance between the drug and the receptor, i.e. $F \propto 1/r^4$.

3. *van der Waals'* bonds or dipole bonds, are formed by the weak attraction between dipoles or induced dipoles, arising from the distortion of the orbits of outer electrons of atoms when the latter are in close proximity to one another. They are weak, the bond strength being of the order of 2 kJ mol^{-1} (0.5 kcal mol^{-1}), and decrease in strength even more rapidly with increasing separation, i.e. $F \propto 1/r^7$.

It is probable that all three types of reversible bond, i.e. ionic, hydrogen and van der Waals', have a role in drug–receptor interactions. Thus, ionic bonding may be important initially in attracting the molecules of the drug to the surface of the receptor, but as the two come closer together, hydrogen and van der Waals' forces may come into play. The affinity of a drug for its receptor may therefore depend upon the presence of a number of bonds of different types. In addition, van der Waals' bonds, although relatively weak, when summed up over a large number of individual atoms may result in considerable binding strength. Furthermore, the combination of a number of bonds of different types over the surface of the drug molecule and its receptor probably helps to determine the degree of 'fit' which is achieved, and also helps to determine the degree of selectivity of the drug. This is illustrated for the cholinergic receptor in Figure 4.6 (see Chapter 4).

There is a fourth type of chemical bond which needs to be considered as it does occur in pharmacology, although rarely. This is the covalent bond which is formed when two atoms share a pair of electrons. It is the bond which holds together the atoms of organic molecules and is relatively strong, with a bond strength of the order of 420 kJ mol^{-1} (100 kcal mol^{-1}). Because of the high binding energy, covalent bonds are irreversible at normal temperatures. Thus, when they occur in pharmacology, long-lasting effects are produced.

The affinity of drugs for their receptors can now be measured, using radio-labelled compounds, *in vitro*.

Intrinsic activity

This is the ability of a drug to produce a biological response once it has become attached to the receptor. It is necessary to invoke the concept of intrinsic activity because drugs exist which show selectivity and affinity for receptors but do not evoke a response. Thus intrinsic activity, which is a measure of the biological effectiveness of a drug, is independent of affinity, which represents the ability of the drug to form a stable complex with the receptor. Intrinsic activity therefore represents the mechanism by which the binding of a drug to the receptor is translated into a pharmacological response. It is the least well understood aspect of drug action at the present time (but see Chapter 3). It is generally accepted that some kind of conformational change in the macromolecules forming the receptor complex occurs and this results in a response. This change may alter the properties of the cell membrane, i.e. a change in the passive permeability to ions (Figure 1.1a), or in an active transport mechanism, or it may be linked to the activation of an enzyme, leading to the formation of a 'second messenger'.

The kinetics of drug–receptor interactions

If the interaction between the drug molecule (D) and the receptor (R) to form a drug–receptor complex (DR),

$$D + R \rightarrow DR$$

involves a simple chemical reaction, then it should obey the laws of chemistry, in particular the Law of Mass Action which states that the rate at which a reaction proceeds is proportional to the active masses of the reacting substances. For substances in solution, the active mass is determined by the solar concentration. Thus, the reaction can be expressed in the following form:

$$[X] + [R] \rightleftharpoons [XR] \tag{1.1}$$

where [X] is the molar concentration of the drug
   [R] is the concentration of free or 'unoccupied' receptors, and
   [XR] is the concentration of drug–receptor complexes or 'occupied' receptors.

Because this reaction is reversible, i.e. it will proceed in both directions, then at equilibrium:

$$\frac{[X][R]}{[XR]} = \text{a constant } K_D \tag{1.2}$$

K_D is defined as the Dissociation constant and $1/K_D$ is the Association constant.
   If there is a finite number of receptors, R_t, then $[R_t]$ will be the total concentration of receptors, and

$$[R_t] = [R] + [XR]$$

$$\text{or } [R] = [R_t] - [XR]$$

and substituting for [R] in Equation 1.2

$$\frac{[X]([R_t] - [XR])}{[XR]} = K_D \tag{1.3}$$

or

$$\frac{[X][R_t] - [X][XR]}{[XR]} = K_D$$

and

$$\frac{[X][R_t]}{[XR]} - [X] = K_D$$

or

$$\frac{[X][R_t]}{[XR]} = K_D + [X]$$

or

$$\frac{[R_t]}{[XR]} = \frac{K_D + [X]}{[X]}$$

and inverting

$$\frac{[XR]}{[R_t]} = \frac{[X]}{K_D + [X]} \tag{1.4}$$

The ratio $[XR]/[R_t]$ represents the fraction of receptors occupied by the drug.
  Rearranging Equation 1.4:

$$[XR] = \frac{[R_t][X]}{K_D + [X]} \tag{1.5}$$

In Equation 1.5, $[R_t]$ and K_D are constants so there is a relationship between
[XR], the number of receptors occupied by the drug and [X], the concentration of
the drug. Plotting [XR] against [X] gives a hyperbolic function (Figure 1.2a) in
which $[XR] = 0$ when $[X] = 0$, and [XR] approaches $[R_t]$ when [X] is very large.
However, if [XR] is plotted against the logarithm of [X] (Figure 1.2b), a sigmoid
curve results and this is very similar to the dose–response curve obtained experimentally with many drugs.

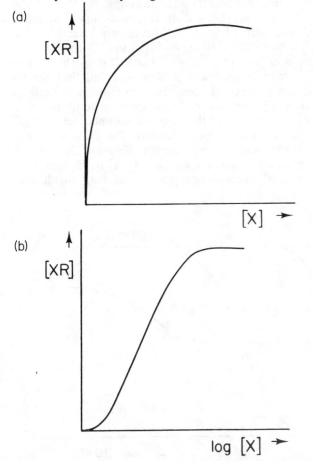

(a)

[XR]

[X]

(b)

[XR]

log [X]

Figure 1.2 Graphs obtained by plotting (a) [XR] against [X] and (b) [XR] against log [X] in equation 1.5
in the text, based on the assumption that the drug–receptor interaction obeys the laws of
thermodynamics

Dose–response relationships

Most drug–receptor interactions are reversible and produce graded responses. Thus, the magnitude of the response varies with the concentration of the drug and as the amount of drug present is increased, so the size of the response increases. This graded relationship between dose and response is expressed in terms of a dose–response (D/R) curve (see Figure 1.3), in which the amplitude of the response is plotted against the log of the concentration of the drug. Dose–response curves are most readily obtained using isolated tissues, e.g. muscle, or an isolated organ. The preparation is suspended in an organ bath which enables various parameters to be kept constant, e.g. temperature, oxygenation, ionic composition of the medium, etc. The organ bath also provides for the response, e.g. contraction of the muscle, to be recorded continuously. Various concentrations of the drug can then be introduced sequentially into the medium bathing the tissue and the size of the response measured at each concentration, the drug being 'washed out' each time with fresh medium so that the response returns to, or near to, control level. This is the classic bioassay technique which is unique to experimental pharmacology.

As can be seen in Figure 1.3, the typical log dose–response curve, obtained experimentally in bioassay studies is sigmoid in shape and closely resembles that seen in Figure 1.2b which was derived theoretically from Equation 1.5 above. Thus, we may conclude that many drug–receptor interactions do in fact obey the Law of Mass Action. However, in doing so it is necessary to bear in mind that certain assumptions have been made. These are (1) that the response amplitude is proportional to receptor occupancy, (2) that one molecule of drug combines with one receptor, and (3) that a negligible fraction of the drug is combined, i.e. that [X] remains constant, or $[X] = [X_t]$, the total drug concentration. The close similarity between the experimentally and theoretically derived curves (Figures 1.2b and 1.3) suggests that assumption (1) is probably correct and, since [XR] in Equation 1.5 represents, by definition, the number of receptors occupied by the drug, this has led

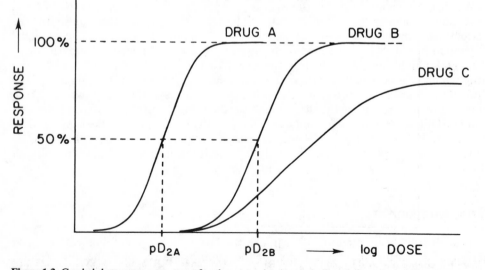

Figure 1.3 Graded dose–response curves for three agonist drugs, A, B and C, acting at the same receptors but with different potencies and maximum effects (see text)

to one of the theories of drug action, namely the 'Occupation Theory'. This theory simply states that the size of the response is related to the number of receptors occupied by the drug. However, it is known that the reaction in 1.1 on p. 6 proceeds simultaneously in both directions, so that some drug–receptor complexes are dissociating as others are being formed, and that an equilibrium is reached for any particular value of [X]. This consideration has led to the proposal of a 'Rate Theory' of drug action, such that the size of the response is determined by the rate of occupation of receptors by the drug. These two theories are in fact very similar and together provide predictions which explain many drug–receptor interactions.

Agonists

A drug which produces a response is known as an agonist and agonists possess all three of the properties described above, i.e. selectivity, affinity and intrinsic activity. However, the extent to which they possess these three properties may vary. Thus, all three drugs for which the D/R curves are shown in Figure 1.3 are agonists. The maximum responses produced by drugs A and B are similar: therefore they have similar intrinsic activity. However, for a given response y, a larger dose of drug B is required, compared with drug A; thus, drug A is more potent than drug B, having a greater affinity for the receptors. Drugs B and C have similar affinities, but drug C has a lower intrinsic activity than B or A (i.e. a smaller maximum response). Also, although drugs B and C have similar affinities, the slope of the D/R curve for drug C is less than that for drug B. This means that for a given increase in dose, there will be a smaller change in the response for drug C than for B. This kind of difference may be important in some clinical situations, for example where the margin between the therapeutic and toxic effects of a drug is small, so that a drug with a shallow D/R curve (e.g. drug C) might be preferable to one with a steep slope. Thus, it can be seen that the potency of agonist drugs depends both on their affinity and also on their intrinsic activity.

When the concentration of the agonist is such that the response is half of the maximum response (see Figure 1.3), then $[X] = K_D$. Thus, the value for the dissociation constant can be determined from the agonist D/R curve. The value for [X] which produces half the maximum response is usually expressed numerically as the pD_2, which can be defined as the negative $\log_{10}$ of the concentration of the drug which produces half maximum response and is a measure of the potency of the drug. Other ways of expressing the potency of agonists are EC_{50}, which is the effective concentration of the drug which produces 50% of the maximum response, and MED, the Median Effective Dose. One practical advantage of the sigmoid D/R curve is that it is linear over the greater part of the range of drug concentrations. It can therefore be plotted experimentally by obtaining just a few points (minimum three) and drawing a straight line through them.

Drug antagonism

It has already been mentioned that drugs exist which do not possess intrinsic activity. Such drugs show selectivity for the appropriate receptor and also affinity. However, once having become attached to the receptor, the drug molecule is unable to produce any conformational change in the receptor membrane, i.e. it does not initiate a response. This is illustrated diagrammatically in Figure 1.1b, in which drug A has the correct shape to fit the receptor but not to induce a conformational change so that the pore in the membrane remains closed and no response occurs. Although drug A has no action of its own, by virtue of the fact that it is occupying the receptor, it will prevent access to the receptor of an agonist drug, if the two are present simultaneously. Thus, drug A will block or antagonize the actions of an agonist drug and is known as an antagonist. Because the agonist and antagonist are competing for the same receptor, this type of action is known as competitive antagonism. Competitive antagonism is illustrated by the D/R curves in Figure 1.4a. The left-hand curve (bold line) is the D/R curve for the agonist on its own, i.e. with no antagonist present, while the curves to the right (thinner lines) represent the D/R curves for the agonist in the presence of two different concentrations of antagonist, $[A_2]$ being greater than $[A_1]$. Thus, the effect of introducing the antagonist is not to alter the shape of the D/R curve for the agonist, but to shift it to the right in a parallel fashion, so reducing the effective potency of the agonist. Increasing concentrations of the antagonist therefore progressively shift the D/R curve for the agonist to the right so that the end result is a family of parallel curves: this is characteristic of competitive antagonism. Note that the agonist can still achieve the same maximum response irrespective of the concentration of the antagonist, and therefore the antagonism is surmountable.

The kinetics of the reaction between antagonists and receptors will be similar to those for agonists. Thus, if K_A is the dissociation constant for the antagonist, at equilibrium:

$$\frac{[A][R]}{[AR]} = K_A \qquad (1.6)$$

where [A] is the molar concentration of the antagonist
      [R] is the concentration of free receptors, and
      [AR] is the concentration of antagonist–receptor complexes.

Cf. Equation 1.2.

However, in the case of antagonists we do not measure a response but the effect on the agonist D/R curve and, in fact, the degree of shift to the right of the agonist D/R curve is proportional to the concentration of the antagonist. Thus, the potency of the antagonist can be expressed in terms of the increased concentration of agonist its presence requires in order to produce a given level of response. This is the pA_2 for the antagonist, defined as the $\log_{10}$ concentration of the antagonist which causes a doubling of the concentration of the agonist in order to produce the same response which the agonist produced in the absence of the antagonist. Thus, in Figure 1.4a, if $[y] = 2[x]$, then the $pA_2 = \log_{10}[A_1]$. The pA_2 value is important: it can be used not only to compare the potencies of different antagonists, but high values of pA_2 indicate a high specificity of antagonism and conversely low values of pA_2 suggest unspecific antagonism. The value of the pA_2 should be the same for the same antagonist tested with different agonists acting on the same receptor. Similarly, if the same combination of antagonist and agonist produces the same pA_2 value in different test systems, then the receptors in these systems are likely to be the same. Schild plots are often used in this kind of study (see below).

Not all antagonisms between drugs are competitive and another type of antagonism is illustrated in Figure 1.4b. Again the bold line represents the D/R

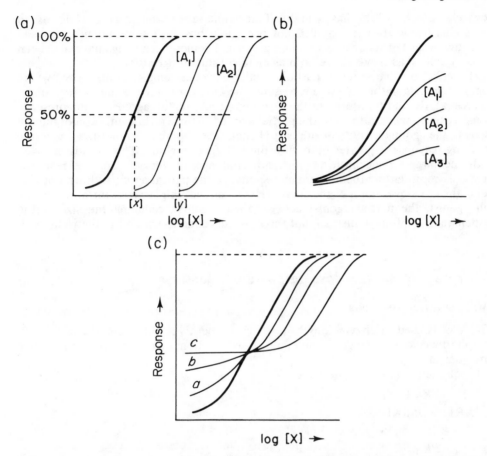

Figure 1.4 Dose–response curves for an agonist drug in the presence of (a) a competitive antagonist, (b) a non-competitive antagonist and (c) a partial agonist. In each case the bold line represents the D/R curve for the agonist alone. In (a) and (b), $[A_1]$, $[A_2]$ and $[A_3]$ represent increasing concentrations of the antagonist, as do a, b and c in (c). In (a) $[x]$ and $[y]$ represent the concentrations of the agonist producing the same response, in the absence and presence of the antagonist, respectively

curve for the agonist on its own. Introducing the antagonist ($[A_1]$) does not shift the D/R curve for the agonist appreciably to the right, but has the effect of reducing the size of the maximum response which can be achieved, irrespective of the concentration of the agonist. Further increases in the concentration of the antagonist ($[A_2]$ and $[A_3]$) reduce the maximum response still further. This type of antagonism is known as non-competitive antagonism and, in this case, the antagonism is insurmountable. Non-competitive antagonism occurs when the antagonist forms strong bonds with the receptors so that the rate of dissociation of antagonist–receptor complexes is very slow.

Partial agonists

Yet another kind of antagonism is seen when an agonist with high intrinsic activity (i.e. high maximum response) is combined with a weaker agonist (low intrinsic activity) but one which has a high affinity. The latter will be able to act as an antagonist to the stronger agonist, but because it possesses some intrinsic activity (although weak) of its own, it is called a partial agonist. Such drugs have also been called 'dualists' as they behave both as agonists and antagonists.

The effect of combining a partial agonist with a stronger agonist is shown in Figure 1.4c. Again the bold line represents the D/R curve for the full agonist alone. Curves (a), (b) and (c) represent the D/R curves for the full agonist in the presence of increasing concentrations of the partial agonist. At a low concentration of the full agonist, the agonist activity of the partial agonist is apparent, so that the size of the resulting response is greater than with the full agonist alone. This is most marked with the largest concentration of the partial agonist (curve (c)), the response produced representing the maximum response of the partial agonist, this point also being the cross-over point of the curves. However, with higher concentrations of the full agonist, the partial agonist acts as an antagonist, reducing the size of the responses to the full agonist, so that the D/R curves are displaced to the right.

Other ways of plotting dose–response relationships

The Lineweaver–Burk plot

This plot is used in enzymology to test for competitive inhibition. It can be used in pharmacology in agonist–antagonist interactions to test for competitive antagonism.

If equation 1.5 above is inverted:

$$\frac{1}{[XR]} = \frac{K_D + [X]}{[R_t][X]}$$

or

$$\frac{1}{[XR]} = \frac{K_D}{[R_t]} \cdot \frac{1}{[X]} + \frac{1}{[R_t]} \tag{1.7}$$

Since K_D and R_t are constants, Equation 1.7 provides a linear relationship between the reciprocal of [XR] and the reciprocal of [X]. Thus, when the reciprocal of the amplitude of the response is plotted against the reciprocal of the dose of the agonist, a straight line is obtained (see Figure 1.5a). This type of graph is also known as a double reciprocal plot. The intercept of the graph with the ordinate is the reciprocal of the maximum response and is a measure of the intrinsic activity of the drug. As the graph is a straight line, this point can be determined by projection, i.e. without having to measure the maximum response experimentally. Secondly, if the graph is projected back to intercept with the abscissa, i.e. for negative values of 1/[X], this intercept represents the negative reciprocal of the dissociation constant, i.e. $-1/K_D$ and is a measure of the affinity of the drug. A competitive antagonist will change the slope of the D/R curve but the intercept with the ordinate will remain the same (i.e. no change in maximum response, see Figure 1.5a). With a non-competitive antagonist, however, not only will the slope change but so will the intercept with the ordinate (Figure 1.5b). In this case if the graphs are projected back, they will have a common intercept with the abscissa. The main use of Lineweaver–Burk plots is, in fact, to determine whether antagonism is competitive or not and this can be done with very few experimental measurements being required to construct the graphs.

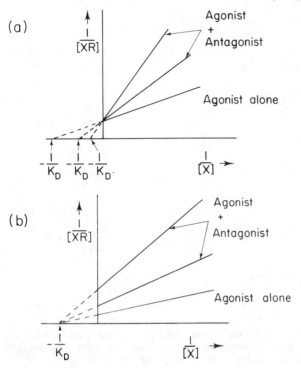

Figure 1.5 Lineweaver–Burk or double reciprocal plots of dose–response curves for an agonist alone and in the presence of two different concentrations of an antagonist. In each case the reciprocal of the response is plotted against the reciprocal of the concentration of the agonist. (a) represents competitive antagonism and (b) non-competitive antagonism (see text for further details)

The Schild plot

This is a useful method for estimating the pA_2 of an antagonist and, again, of determining whether the antagonism is competitive. First, a series of conventional D/R curves is plotted for various concentrations of the antagonist, as in Figure 1.4a. Then a value for x is obtained for each antagonist concentration, such that, for equal effects:

$$x = \frac{\text{concentration of agonist in presence of antagonist}}{\text{concentration of agonist without antagonist}}$$

The logarithm of $(x - 1)$ is then plotted against the negative logarithm of the concentration of the antagonist, i.e. $-\log [A]$ (Figure 1.6). The graph should be a straight line with a slope of unity or near to unity, if the antagonism is competitive, and the intercept with the abscissa represents the pA_2 of the competitive antagonist. Obviously, if the slope does not approximate to unity or the points do not lie on a straight line, the antagonism is not competitive.

The Scatchard plot

This is used in studies of the binding of drugs to tissue fractions. The high-affinity binding of radiolabelled agonists and antagonists to receptors can be measured *in*

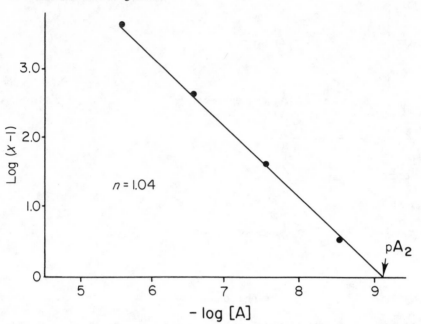

Figure 1.6 Schild plot. The value of log $(x - 1)$ is plotted against $-\log[A]$, which is the negative log of the molar concentration of the antagonist. If the regression line has a slope of unity or near to unity, the antagonism is competitive. The intercept with the abscissa gives the pA_2 for the antagonist

vitro. This can be done either by introducing the radioactive material (ligand) into the intact tissue, i.e. *in vivo*, and then measuring the amount of radioactivity after various stages of fractionation of the tissue, or it can be done by extracting the receptor sites first and then introducing the labelled ligand.

The Scatchard plot is obtained by rearranging Equation 1.3, i.e.:

$$\frac{[X]([R_t] - [XR])}{[XR]} = K_D$$

or

$$\frac{[X]}{[XR]} = \frac{[K_D]}{[R_t] - [XR]}$$

and inverting

$$\frac{[XR]}{[X]} = \frac{[R_t] - [XR]}{K_D}$$

In this case [XR] represents the concentration of the bound ligand and [X] the concentration of the unbound or free ligand. Plotting the ratio of bound:free ligand (i.e. [XR]:[X]) against the concentration of the bound ligand [XR], gives a straight line (Figure 1.7). The slope of this line is $1/K_D$ and the intercept with the abscissa is a measure of $[R_t]$, so that it is possible to determine the number of binding sites (B_{max}).

A Scatchard plot which produces a simple straight line indicates the existence of a single binding site. A plot which departs significantly from linearity may indicate

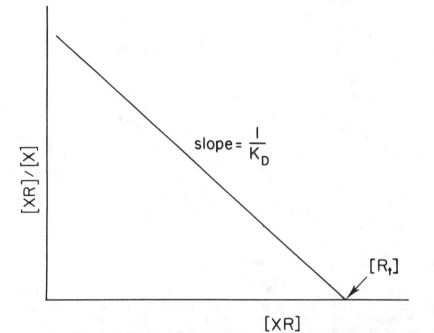

Figure 1.7 Scatchard plot. Plotting the ratio of bound:free ligand ($[XR]$:$[X]$) against the concentration of bound ligand ($[XR]$), gives a straight line if there is a single binding site, with a slope of $1/K_D$, the intercept with the abscissa representing a measure of $[R_t]$ (or B_{max})

that there is more than one binding site with different dissociation constants, and the interpretation of the slopes and intercepts becomes complicated.

Using these techniques a number of binding sites for drugs have been found which appear to be identifiable with specific receptors. However, caution needs to be exercised in interpreting the data from radioligand binding studies. For example, the fact that the tissues have to be subjected to homogenization and, in some cases, solubilization with detergents before the radioactivity can be measured means that one cannot be certain that the properties of the binding site *in vitro* are identical to the properties of the receptor *in vivo*. Furthermore, the presence of a binding site does not necessarily indicate the existence of a pharmacological receptor, i.e. not all binding sites are receptors. Such sites are sometimes referred to as 'acceptors'.

Spare receptors

It follows from the fact that not all agonist drugs acting on the same receptors produce the same maximum response (cf. drugs A and C in Figure 1.3), that the maximum response does not necessarily occur when all the receptors are occupied, i.e. for maximum response $[XR] \neq R_t$. Indeed, it is now generally accepted that the maximum response to an agonist occurs when only a fraction of the total number of receptors is occupied, and the receptors remaining unoccupied are called 'spare receptors'. This might seem to imply that the Law of Mass Action no longer applies. However, if $[R_t]$ is redefined as the total number of receptors which need to be

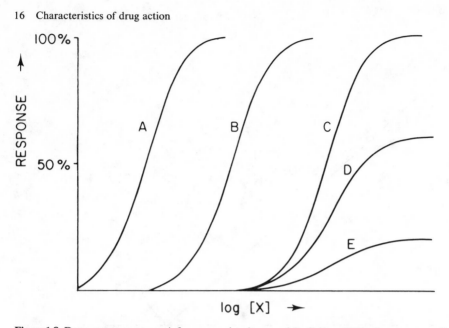

Figure 1.8 Dose–response curves A for an agonist alone, and B, C, D and E in the presence of increasing concentrations of an irreversible antagonist. The fact that the agonist can still produce the same maximum response, even with the antagonist occupying an increasing proportion of receptors (curves B and C) indicates the presence of 'spare' receptors. However, with high concentrations of the antagonist (curves D and E), the number of receptors available, including the spare receptors, is insufficient to maintain the response at its original maximum

occupied to produce the amplitude of maximum response, instead of the total number of receptors present in the tissue, then all is well. In this way the difference in the amplitude of the maximum responses produced by drugs A and C in Figure 1.3 can be explained as being due to the difference in the intrinsic activity of the drugs rather than differences in the numbers of receptors occupied.

The existence of spare receptors can be demonstrated experimentally by plotting D/R curves for an agonist in the presence of increasing concentrations of an irreversible (non-competitive) antagonist (Figure 1.8). As the antagonist binds irreversibly to the receptors, it will prevent the binding of the agonist to a proportion of the receptors. With small concentrations of the antagonist this proportion will be small and the agonist, in high concentrations, can still produce a maximum response (curves B and C) because the number of receptors available, i.e. not occupied by the antagonist, is still in excess of the number needed to produce the maximum response. However, increasing the concentration of the antagonist further, a point is reached when the number of 'spare' receptors is insufficient to produce the full response and curves D and E are the result.

Chapter 2

Factors affecting responses to drugs

In the previous chapter it was assumed that the drug was already at its site of action in order to produce its effects. However, most drugs are administered at a considerable distance from their desired site of action and various factors, other than those considered in Chapter 1, i.e. absorption, distribution, metabolism and excretion, may affect the responses that the drug produces at its target organ or tissue. Thus, whereas most of this book is concerned with the effects of drugs on the body, it is necessary to consider as well, at least briefly, the effects that the body may have on drugs.

Absorption

The physicochemical factors which control the absorption of drugs are important because they determine whether or not a drug reaches its site of action. A drug may have to penetrate many cellular membranes before it reaches the receptors on which it is to act. Most drugs are administered orally and must therefore be absorbed from the gastrointestinal tract (GIT). If they are to act on the central nervous system (CNS), they must also penetrate the blood–brain barrier. Both the gastrointestinal tract and the brain are surrounded by layers of cells which control the uptake of substances, whether nutrients or drugs. This cell membrane consists of a bimolecular layer of lipid, sandwiched between two protein layers. The molecules of lipid have hydrophobic tails and hydrophilic heads and, in an aqueous medium, they tend to aggregate with the hydrophobic tails coalescing and the hydrophilic heads forming a polar surface. This kind of aggregation provides the stable structure for most biological membranes. In some regions of the membrane, proteins penetrate the lipid and may extend all the way through it, forming small pores (Figure 2.1). Other protein molecules may connect both surfaces of the membrane and act as transport or carrier mechanisms. Hydrophilic molecules, like water itself and water-soluble substances which are sufficiently small, together with small ions like chloride and potassium, can pass freely through the pores. The lipid nature of the membrane will enable drugs which are lipid soluble to pass through it while lipid-insoluble drugs will not. Thus, lipid solubility is important for drugs which are given orally and also for drugs acting on the CNS, irrespective of the route of administration. The lipid solubility of a drug is, of course, determined by its chemical structure; thus, the structure of a drug is important not only for its action on receptors but also determines the way in which it is absorbed.

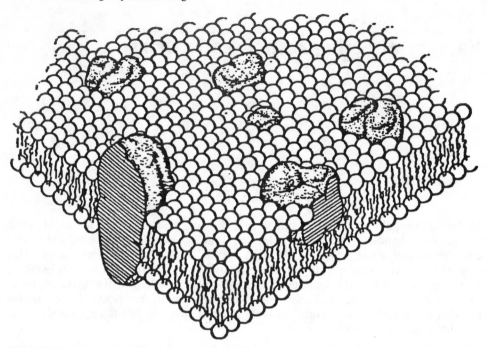

Figure 2.1 Schematic three-dimensional representation of a cell membrane showing the bimolecular lipid layer with the polar heads of the lipids at the surface, together with protein molecules which penetrate through the whole membrane (modified from Singer and Nicolson, 1972)

The passage of drugs through biological membranes

Drugs and nutrients can pass through membranes by either passive or active processes. Passive transport, such as diffusion, does not require metabolic energy but active transport does.

Passive diffusion

Drugs which are non-electrolytes and are lipid soluble will dissolve in the cell membrane and cross by diffusion, provided that there is a concentration gradient between the two surfaces of the membrane. In this case there will be movement of drug molecules from a region of higher concentration to one of lower concentration, i.e. the drug moves down the concentration gradient. Thus, substances with a high lipid–water partition coefficient will be absorbed more readily. In the case of drugs which are organic electrolytes, the extent of penetration of the cell membrane will depend upon the degree of ionization of the drug in an aqueous medium. A drug which is only poorly ionized, i.e. a weak acid or weak base, will exist to a greater extent in the unionized, lipid-soluble form and will therefore be absorbed, whereas a drug which is fully ionized will be present only as ions and will not be absorbed.

The degree to which a substance is ionized in solution is determined by its ionization constant, pK_a, which is the pH at which the substance is 50% ionized. It follows therefore, that if the pH on the two sides of the cell membrane is different, this will affect the distribution of a weak electrolyte. Because the membrane will be permeable only to the unionized form, this form of the substance will reach the same concentration on both sides of the membrane at equilibrium. However, the amount of the ionized form present on both sides will depend on the pH according to the Henderson–Hasselbalch equation:

$$pK_a = pH + \log\frac{\text{(concentration of unionized form)}}{\text{(concentration of ionized form)}}, \text{ for an acid,}$$

and

$$pK_a = pH + \log\frac{\text{(concentration of ionized form)}}{\text{(concentration of unionized form)}}, \text{ for a base.}$$

The higher the pH of the medium (i.e. the more alkaline), the greater will be the degree of ionization of acid drugs and the less the ionization of basic drugs, but with a low pH the opposite will be true. This means that when the pH of the aqueous phase on the two sides of the membrane is different, acidic drugs will be in greater concentration on the side with a higher pH (alkaline) and basic drugs will be in greater concentration on the side with a lower pH (acidic). Therefore weak acids present in the lumen of the stomach, which has a low pH, will be rapidly absorbed into the blood (neutral pH) and a weak base present in the blood stream will be excreted into the lumen of the GIT (Figure 2.2). Aspirin, which is a weak acid, is therefore well absorbed from the stomach in man, whereas drugs which are weak bases are not.

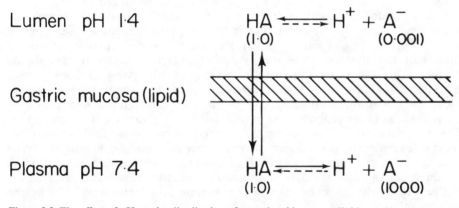

Figure 2.2 The effect of pH on the distribution of a weak acid across a lipid membrane, e.g. gastric mucosa, which is permeable only to the unionized form of the drug (HA). The relative concentrations of the unionized drug (HA) and the ionized form (A⁻) at steady state are shown in parenthesis

Filtration through pores

The lipid membrane of cells contains small pores, as already mentioned, through which some drugs may pass by diffusion. This process will depend primarily on molecular size but may also be influenced by the presence of electrical charges on the molecule. Furthermore, if there is a difference in hydrostatic or osmotic pressure across the membrane, there will be bulk flow of water through the pores and this will carry with it solutes of sufficiently small molecular size.

Facilitated diffusion

Some substances diffuse through membranes more rapidly than would be expected from their lipid solubility or molecular size. This phenomenon is thought to be attributable to the presence of a carrier mechanism in the cell membrane. Thus, the molecules or ions in solution form loose complexes with carrier macromolecules at the surface of the membrane; these complexes are then transported across the membrane after which the substance is released from the carrier at the opposite side of the membrane. A characteristic of this kind of carrier-facilitated diffusion is that it does not appear to be dependent upon the metabolic energy of the cell. In addition, it can be selective, in that each carrier may combine with only one substance or a limited range of substances. Facilitated diffusion is important for the absorption of sugars and amino acids from the intestine. Its relevance as a mechanism for the absorption of drugs is doubtful, however.

Active transport

This is a process by which substances pass across a biological membrane against an electrochemical concentration gradient and which depends on the utilization of energy provided by the metabolic activity of the cell. There may be movement of a solute against a concentration gradient or, if it is electrically charged, against a potential gradient, or a combination of the two. Because metabolic energy is required, active transport can be blocked by metabolic inhibitors. It can also be inhibited competitively by the presence of another substance which utilizes the same transport mechanism. Either of these effects can be produced by drugs.

As with facilitated transport, active transport is thought to involve carriers, the main difference being the need for metabolic energy in the latter case. Thus, a molecular structure (e.g. a carrier protein) inside the surface of the membrane combines with the substance to be transported and carries it across the membrane to release it on the other side. Active transport processes have two main characteristics, the first being some degree of selectivity which depends on the chemical structure of the substance being transported, although this selectivity may not be so great as to prevent substances with similar structure from competing for the carrier mechanism. In this way drugs may produce competitive inhibition of the transport of an endogenous substance. Secondly, because a finite quantity of carrier is available at any one time, the carrier-facilitated transport can become saturated. One of the best examples of active transport involving metabolic energy, which is also influenced by drugs, is the extrusion of sodium ions from nerve cells by the 'sodium pump'.

Distribution

After a drug has reached the systemic circulation it may be carried in free solution in the plasma, in which case it can be readily transported to its site of action, unless there are other membranes to be crossed, e.g. the blood–brain barrier (see below). However, a drug which is lipid soluble will tend to bind to macromolecules in the body, of which the most likely are the plasma proteins. The binding of drugs to plasma proteins is of considerable importance for their actions because only the unbound or 'free' drug can act on receptors. This is because the drug–protein complex is too large to pass through cell membranes. Plasma protein, therefore, has the effect of reducing the concentration available at the receptors, i.e. of reducing the response. The binding is reversible and there will be a dynamic equilibrium between the bound and unbound forms of the drug. Although binding to plasma proteins reduces the effective concentration of free drug, it also provides a source of free drug to replace that removed by excretion and metabolism. Binding can therefore prolong the duration of action of a drug as well as influencing the size of the response. The main protein involved in the binding of drugs is serum albumin but globulins and haematoxylin can also play a part.

Plasma proteins are not the only site for the binding of drugs which are highly lipid soluble. Fat, which is a major constituent of the body, accounting for about 10% of body weight in normal individuals and up to 30% in obese subjects, will sequester lipid-soluble drugs. Anaesthetic drugs, for example, will readily penetrate fat depots from which they will be slowly released. Again, this can affect the duration of action.

The presence of a second drug may displace a 'bound' drug, thus increasing the 'free' concentration and this can lead to the development of toxic effects.

Volume of distribution

For a drug to be effective it must reach and maintain an adequate concentration at its site of action. The volume of distribution (V) is the theoretical volume that would accommodate all the drug in the body if its concentration throughout the body were the same as that in the plasma. Thus:

$$V = \frac{\text{amount of drug injected}}{\text{plasma concentration}}$$

The volume of distribution can be measured by injecting a known amount of the drug intravenously and then determining its concentration in the plasma after an appropriate time interval. If the drug were confined to the plasma, then V would be equal to the plasma volume (about 3 litres in an adult) and, conversely, if the drug were distributed throughout the body water, V would be about 42 litres. A knowledge of the volume of distribution enables calculation of the dose which will achieve the correct therapeutic concentration at its site of action.

Bioavailability

This term is used to describe the proportion of drug administered which reaches the systemic circulation unchanged. It is important for drugs which are given orally, where a number of factors can affect the bioavailability, for example the membranes of the alimentary canal (already referred to). Another important factor for some drugs is the 'first pass' effect. This is attributable to metabolism taking place in the liver as a result of absorption of drugs through that part of the epithelium of the GIT which is drained by veins of the hepatoportal system. For drugs that are susceptible to hepatic metabolism, a substantial proportion of the orally administered dose may be metabolized before it reaches its site of action.

The blood–brain barrier

The barrier separating the bloodstream from the brain differs from other cell membranes and this is of importance for drugs acting on the CNS. The boundary between blood plasma and the tissues of the CNS is less permeable to water-soluble substances than that between plasma and other tissues. There is therefore no aqueous diffusion across the blood–brain barrier. The reason for this is that the blood capillaries in the CNS are continuous, with tight junctions between the endothelial cells, whereas in other tissues the capillary junctions are separated by slits which allow the penetration of substances which are hydrophilic, e.g. dissociated acids, bases and proteins. As well as the tight junctions, most of the external surface of the capillary walls in the brain is covered by glial cells (astrocytes) and these form an additional barrier to aqueous diffusion. However, the barrier is not absolute and lipid-soluble substances, which can penetrate cell membranes, readily enter the brain. There is also active transport of substances into the brain and this includes metabolic substrates as well as the precursors for neurotransmitters. These transport mechanisms also operate for drugs which are related chemically to the endogenous substances.

The probable consequence of the relative impermeability of the cerebral capillary endothelium is to make the transfer of material into the brain a more selective process than it is for other tissues. Thus selective active transport, as well as the 'tight' capillary junctions, contributes to the properties of the blood–brain barrier, which are therefore not due to any one phenomenon. One important feature of the blood–brain barrier is that its properties may be altered in disease states.

Metabolism

The metabolic conversion of drugs in the body can lead to a decrease or increase in activity. Active drugs may be inactivated by processes such as oxidation, reduction and hydrolysis. The metabolism of drugs occurs mostly in the liver, although the walls of the GI tract, the lungs and the kidney are also important sites. The products of degradative metabolism of drugs are usually more readily excreted as they are more water soluble and also more readily ionized than the parent compound.

Some drugs are metabolized by normal metabolic processes, i.e. by enzymes which have natural substrates in the body. This is especially true of drugs which are endogenous substances or are closely related to such substances, and it may be necessary to inhibit the action of the metabolizing enzymes when the drug is being administered in order to produce an effect. However, most drugs are metabolized by enzymes which are located intracellularly in the liver. The hepatic endoplasmic reticulum contains these microsomal enzymes, the main function of which appears to be the metabolism of substances which are foreign to the body. As the microsomal enzymes are closely associated with lipoprotein membranes, only lipid-soluble drugs which can penetrate the endoplasmic reticulum will have access to the enzymes and will be metabolized. The principal reaction catalysed by the enzymes is oxidation, which requires molecular oxygen and reduced nicotinamide adenine dinucleotide ($NADH_2$) as coenzyme. The source of oxygen is cytochrome P-450, which is localized intracellularly in the endoplasmic reticulum, and is widely involved in the oxidation of drugs. Cytochromes consist of porphyrin rings containing iron which can be readily converted from ferric to ferrous, and vice versa: thus, the cytochromes can function as electron carriers.

The activity of the drug-metabolizing enzymes of the hepatic endoplasmic reticulum is influenced by a number of factors, such as the presence of other drugs, age, sex, etc. In man, a number of drugs inhibit the metabolism of other drugs: for example, ethanol inhibits the metabolism of barbiturates when both are present in the body. Drugs can also increase their rate of metabolism, or that of other drugs, by induction of the metabolizing enzymes. This is mainly due to the increased synthesis of cytochrome P-450.

The metabolic reduction of drugs is less common than oxidation. Reduction is also catalysed by microsomal enzymes. For example, the gaseous anaesthetic halothane is dehalogenated to trifluoroethane, which then undergoes microsomal oxidation. The hydrolysis of esters is brought about by esterases which are present in the blood, liver, kidneys and other tissues. Probably the most important esterases are the cholinesterases which are discussed in Chapter 4.

Another way in which drugs can be inactivated is by conjugation. The most common type of conjugation is with glucuronic acid, which is present in the body (being derived from glucose) and readily forms conjugates with hydroxyl, carboxyl, amino and sulphydryl groups, which may be present on the drug molecule or introduced during metabolism. Conjugation is a synthetic process, requiring in most cases the participation of enzymes and a source of energy, which is usually provided by adenosine triphosphate (ATP). As with metabolism, the end products of conjugation are usually more water soluble and less lipid soluble than the original drugs and, therefore, are more readily excreted by the kidneys. The main site of conjugation is the liver.

It is possible to utilize the metabolic processes of the body in order to produce an active compound from a pro-drug, which may be inactive or relatively inactive.

Excretion

The second major process through which the activity of drugs is terminated is excretion. This can occur with the unchanged drugs, or with their metabolites. The principal route for excretion is through the kidneys, but secretion into the bile or through the lungs or skin may also be important, for example with volatile anaesthetics and ethanol. Metabolites which are more highly ionized than the parent drug at physiological pH, and those which are more water soluble, will generally be excreted more readily. The major mechanisms of excretion by the kidney are glomerular filtration and secretion into the lumen of the proximal tubules by active transport and passive diffusion. A drug will be filtered if its molecular size is not excessively large and thus, the free plasma fraction of most drugs is rapidly filtered through the glomerulus. The fraction of drug which may be bound to plasma proteins will not be excreted. Passive reabsorption of the drug from the proximal tubules may occur, particularly if it is lipid soluble.

The active secretion of drugs in the proximal tubules is carrier-mediated by the same processes that transport endogenous anionic and cationic substances across the tubular cells. As a result, competition for the carrier mechanism may occur and this can lead to the presence of one drug delaying the excretion of another.

Passive diffusion can occur through both the proximal and distal tubules. Lipid-soluble drugs may diffuse in either direction, depending upon the concentration gradient and the pH of the blood and renal tubular fluid. Thus, the pH of the urine may be important and can be altered to increase the excretion of a drug.

The excretion of drugs by the kidneys may be influenced by the following factors:

1. The pK_a of the drug – this is important for weak electrolytes;
2. The lipid solubility of the unionized drug, and
3. The rate of flow of urine – fast flow will reduce the tendency for passive reabsorption from the tubules.

Chapter 3

The principles of synaptic transmission

The term 'synapse' was first proposed by Sherrington for the transverse membranes that separate two neurones in regions of close juxtaposition. Sherrington further proposed that transmission across synapses differs from conduction along nerves, in that it (1) is one-way and (2) involves a delay. In fact, synapses are now known to possess two further properties: (3) they fatigue readily and (4) they are the site of action for many drugs. The term synapse is also often used to describe the junction between a motor nerve and a muscle or gland. Strictly speaking, such junctions should be termed 'neuro-effector' junctions and the term synapse should be restricted to junctions between neurones.

In the mammalian nervous system, transmission at synapses is mediated chemically, i.e. by the release of a neurotransmitter. Thus, while the transfer of information from one part of a nerve cell to another is electrical (e.g. by propagated action potentials), the transfer of information from one neurone to another is a chemical event, i.e. via a neurotransmitter which is released from one neurone and acts on the other. However, in certain invertebrates and lower vertebrates, there are junctions which appear only to operate electrically, i.e. transmission is produced by local circuit currents; such junctions have been termed 'ephapses'.

The neurone

Nerve cells, especially those in the brain, although they all possess the same basic components, i.e. cell body, axon and dendrites (Figure 3.1), vary considerably in form. Thus, the axon may be very long (motor nerve) or short (interneurone), or it may divide into two (sensory neurones). In the same way, synaptic junctions can vary considerably. Near their endings the axons may branch many times and, if myelinated, lose their myelin sheath. At synapses, the fine naked branches may end in small swellings or synaptic knobs, which make contact with the cell body of another neurone (axo–somatic synapse), or with the dendrites (axo–dendritic) or the axon hillock (axo–axonal) (Figure 3.2). In the brain, a single nerve fibre may synapse with many other neurones, and may itself have presynaptic terminals from a number of other neurones impinging on it; the system of interconnections can therefore be extremely complex.

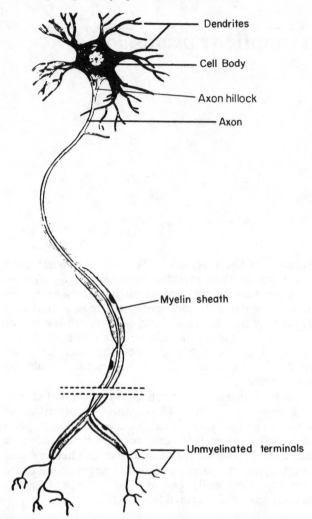

Dendrites

Cell Body

Axon hillock

Axon

Myelin sheath

Unmyelinated terminals

Figure 3.1 Schematic drawing of a nerve cell showing some of the structures referred to in the text

Synaptic transmission

In the peripheral nervous system synaptic transmission is mainly excitatory, i.e. nerve impulses from presynaptic terminals are transmitted across the synapse and excite the postsynaptic neurone, thus initiating action potentials in the postsynaptic neurone. This principle also applies to neuro-effector junctions, although inhibition can occur. In the central nervous system (CNS), however, impulses in presynaptic terminals may result in either excitation or inhibition of the postsynaptic neurone. Thus, both excitatory and inhibitory synapses are present in the brain and spinal cord.

The neurotransmitter is present in the presynaptic nerve terminals where it may be stored in synaptic vesicles ready for release and where, in many cases, it is also

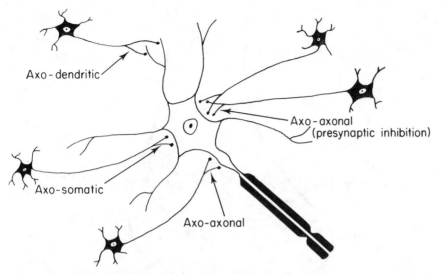

Axo-dendritic

Axo-axonal
(presynaptic inhibition)

Axo-somatic

Axo-axonal

Figure 3.2 Diagram of the various types of junctions between presynaptic nerve terminals and the cell body, dendrites or axons of the postsynaptic cell (modified from Bowman and Rand, 1980)

synthesized, the enzymes involved in the synthesis being associated with the mitochondria (see Figure 3.3). The transmitter is released from the nerve terminals as the result of the arrival of action potentials, the release being dependent upon the influx of calcium ions (Ca^{2+}). The released transmitter diffuses across the synaptic gap to stimulate a receptor on the postsynaptic neurone and this action results in a response in the postsynaptic cell. Many substances have been proposed as synaptic transmitters or neurotransmitters, the best-known being acetylcholine (ACh), noradrenaline, dopamine, 5-hydroxytryptamine (5-HT, serotonin), certain amino acids such as glutamic and aspartic acids, γ-aminobutyric acid and glycine, and also many peptides. However, the transmitter role of many of these substances is confined to the central nervous system (see Chapter 10) and the principal neurotransmitters at peripheral junctions are acetylcholine, noradrenaline and dopamine, although there is evidence that 5-hydroxytryptamine, together with substances like histamine and adenosine, may be neurotransmitters peripherally, in addition to their other roles, e.g. as hormones.

Excitatory transmission

When an excitatory transmitter is released, it diffuses across the synaptic gap to the postsynaptic receptor which is a specialized region of the membrane of the postsynaptic neurone (Figure 3.3). The action of the transmitter on the receptor is to cause an increase in the permeability of the postsynaptic membrane to small ions (Na^+, K^+ and Ca^{2+}), which results in a decrease in the membrane potential, i.e. there is a local depolarization. This depolarization, which is of brief duration, is known as an excitatory postsynaptic potential (or EPSP). Such responses differ from the all-or-none responses of nerve fibres in a number of ways: (1) they are graded; (2) they have a refractory period and therefore successive responses can summate; (3) they are non-propagated and decay quickly. However, if the EPSP is sufficiently large in amplitude or extends over a large enough area of the

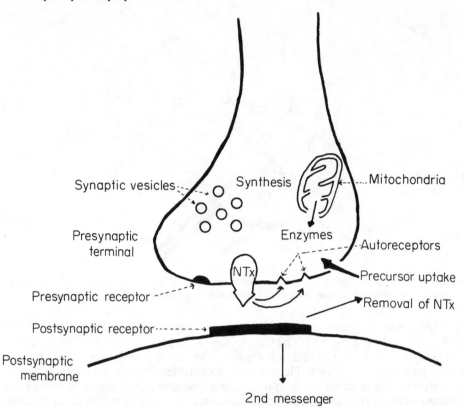

Figure 3.3 Diagrammatic representation of a typical synapse showing the principal structures involved in the process of synaptic transmission. NTx, neurotransmitter

postsynaptic membrane, or summates with other EPSPs, the threshold for excitation of the postsynaptic cell may be reached and a propagated action potential results. This will, of course, obey the 'all-or-none' law. Meanwhile, inactivating mechanisms will have removed the transmitter and the postsynaptic membrane will have repolarized.

Inhibitory transmission

An inhibitory transmitter has the opposite action to an excitatory transmitter and causes local hyperpolarization of the postsynaptic membrane, producing an inhibitory postsynaptic potential (IPSP). Again, the action of the neurotransmitter is to increase the permeability of the postsynaptic membrane but, in this case, the increase in permeability is selective for potassium and chloride ions, the increased efflux of these ions being responsible for the hyperpolarization. This type of response is also graded. Inhibitory synapses can prevent the membrane of the postsynaptic neurone from being depolarized by other events, e.g. by excitatory neurotransmitters. Another type of inhibitory synapse is found in the CNS. In this case the junction is between two presynaptic terminals (i.e. axo–axonal, Figure 3.2). Thus, in Figure 3.4, A is a presynaptic excitatory terminal, stimulation of which

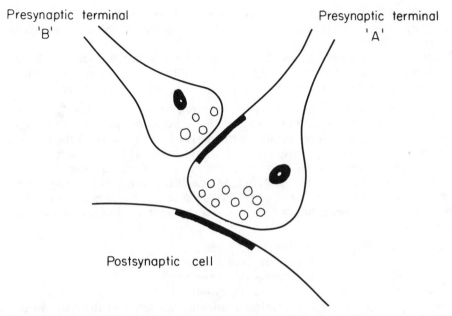

Presynaptic terminal
'B'

Presynaptic terminal
'A'

Postsynaptic cell

Figure 3.4 Axo–axonal junction between two presynaptic terminals, showing how presynaptic inhibition occurs

evokes an EPSP on the postsynaptic neurone. However, stimulation of B, while it has no direct effect on the postsynaptic cell, reduces the release of transmitter from A, thus reducing the size of the EPSP produced by A. The mechanism for this is detailed in Chapter 10 (see also Figure 10.16).

Criteria for synaptic transmitters

At various times, many substances have been proposed as synaptic transmitters and more may well be suggested in the future. Before a neurotransmitter role for a substance can be finally accepted, it should fulfil certain criteria, although in the CNS it is sometimes difficult to obtain adequate evidence. The criteria are basically as follows:

1. The substance should be present in the presynaptic nerve terminals and should be released on stimulation of the nerve. Thus, the enzymes responsible for the synthesis of the transmitter substance should be present in the nerve terminal, together with an uptake system for the precursor of the transmitter (Figure 3.3). Alternatively, the transmitter may be synthesized elsewhere, e.g. in the cell body, and transported to the terminal region. The freshly synthesized transmitter is usually stored in synaptic vesicles, which can vary in form with different transmitters, and may contain other substances which are released together with the neurotransmitter.
2. The putative transmitter substance should produce the same effect on the postsynaptic receptor as the endogenous transmitter. Thus, the same response should be obtained with local application of the putative transmitter, e.g. by

local microinjection or by microiontophoresis, as is seen with stimulation of the presynaptic nerve. Furthermore, both responses should be similarly blocked by antagonist drugs.

3. There should be mechanisms present at the synapse for the removal of the transmitter after it has acted. This can be by the action of enzymes which inactivate the transmitter or its removal by other processes, e.g. re-uptake.

The details of the processes involved in synaptic transmission vary from one transmitter to another and are therefore best discussed as the individual transmitters are considered. Most drugs acting on the nervous system produce their effects by modifying or interfering with synaptic transmission although there are, of course, exceptions, and drugs which affect the activity of the nervous system in other ways are discussed in Chapter 9. In many cases the receptors for drugs acting on the nervous system are also the receptors for neurotransmitters. Nevertheless, effects on synaptic transmission can be produced at different sites and in different ways, for example:

1. Presynaptic: effects on   (a) uptake of precursor;
                               (b) synthesis of transmitter;
                               (c) storage of transmitter;
                               (d) release of transmitter.
2. Postsynaptic: effects on   (a) agonists mimicking the action of the transmitter;
                               (b) antagonists blocking the action of the transmitter and agonist drugs;
                               (c) removal of the transmitter.

Actions at all of these sites will be considered in discussing the actions of the various drugs.

Receptor–response mechanisms

So far, it has been assumed that activation of the postsynaptic receptor results in a conformational change in the membrane which alters its permeability to ions. Thus, the opening of a pore (ionophore) in the membrane of the postsynaptic cell (see Figure 1.1) allows the passage of ions, e.g. sodium ions, to which the membrane was previously impermeable. This type of mechanism, mediating the response of the postsynaptic cell, is present at nicotinic receptors for acetylcholine (Chapter 5). Ionophores for other ions, such as chloride ions, are associated with inhibitory transmission in the CNS (see Chapter 10). However, the receptors for some neurotransmitters, particularly the catecholamines, are linked not to ionophores but to enzymes which are located within the membrane of the postsynaptic cell. These enzymes act as transducers for the action of the neurotransmitter (first messenger) from the outside of the cell to the inside and hence produce 'second messengers'.

Second messengers

The enzyme adenylate cyclase is present in the plasma membrane of most cells and, in the presence of magnesium ions, it catalyses the conversion of adenosine triphosphate (ATP) to $3',5'$ cyclic adenosine monophosphate (cyclic AMP). Cyclic AMP activates specific protein kinases by causing phosphorylation and these, in

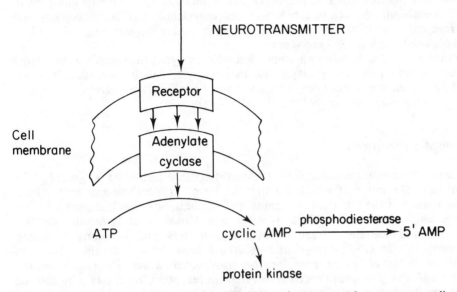

NEUROTRANSMITTER

Cell
membrane

Receptor

Adenylate
cyclase

ATP   cyclic AMP $\xrightarrow{\text{phosphodiesterase}}$ 5' AMP

protein kinase

Figure 3.5 Diagrammatic representation of cyclic AMP acting as a second messenger to mediate the postsynaptic action of a neurotransmitter

turn, phosphorylate proteins. This process, which utilizes ATP, is important in carbohydrate metabolism and the conversion of ATP to cyclic AMP by activation of the enzyme, adenylate cyclase, can be stimulated by adrenaline and glucagon acting on hormonal receptors. A similar process appears to occur at the receptors for certain neurotransmitters, e.g. β-adrenoceptors, some receptors for 5-hydroxytryptamine, histamine H_2 receptors and dopamine D_1 receptors. At these sites the adenylate cyclase is stimulated through activation of the receptors by the neurotransmitter or an agonist drug, and catalyses the conversion of ATP to cyclic AMP (Figure 3.5). However, at some receptors (e.g. α-adrenoceptors), stimulation of the receptor causes inhibition of the activity of adenylate cyclase and hence a decrease in the intracellular concentration of cyclic AMP. Some receptors, e.g. muscarinic receptors for acetylcholine, are linked to the enzyme guanylate cyclase; this enzyme converts guanosine triphosphate (GTP) to cyclic guanosine monophosphate (cyclic GMP) which acts as a second messenger in an analogous way to cyclic AMP. Whereas cyclic AMP is found throughout the nervous system, cyclic GMP shows a regional localization, although the significance of this is not known at present.

It is thought that the phosphorylation of membrane proteins through the mediation of the second messengers, i.e. cyclic AMP and GMP, can result, in some cases, in changes in membrane permeability to specific ions and in others, to activation of further enzyme systems which then mediate the biological response. Both cyclic AMP and GMP are inactivated by hydrolysis, a process which involves phosphodiesterase enzymes. The activity of the second messengers, and hence the response of the postsynaptic cell, can be influenced by drugs acting on the enzymes involved, i.e. adenylate cyclase, guanylate cyclase and phosphodiesterase.

Another type of second messenger is represented by the breakdown of phosphatidylinositol, a reaction which is mediated by the enzyme phospholipase C, which is located in cell membranes. This reaction leads to the opening of calcium channels in the cell membrane. Muscarinic receptors for acetylcholine, β-adrenoceptors and some receptors for histamine and 5-hydroxytryptamine appear to be linked to phospholipase C as a second messenger.

Calcium ions, which have an important role in synaptic transmission, being involved in both pre- and postsynaptic mechanisms, can be regarded in some respects as a second messenger, in that they can affect the activity of protein kinases and regulate the metabolism of cyclic AMP.

Presynaptic receptors

The release of neurotransmitter from presynaptic nerve terminals is controlled by calcium ions, the influx of which through the terminal membrane directly stimulates the release of the transmitter. Removal of calcium, or its replacement by other ions, e.g. magnesium (Mg^{2+}), blocks transmission. However, other mechanisms are known to influence the release of neurotransmitters and at many synapses, particularly in the CNS, presynaptic receptors have been identified. Thus, in addition to the specific receptor for the transmitter which is present on the membrane of the postsynaptic cell (postsynaptic receptor), receptors may also be present on the presynaptic terminals (presynaptic receptors) which release the neurotransmitter (Figure 3.3).

Presynaptic receptors are of two types. Those which are specific for the transmitter which is released from the terminals on which they are situated are known as 'autoreceptors'. Their function appears to be to regulate the release of the transmitter and, in most cases, activation of the presynaptic receptors causes a reduction in the release of transmitter. Thus, some of the neurotransmitter which is released from the nerve terminals into the synaptic gap, reaches the autoreceptors, activation of which causes a reduction in the further release of the transmitter. The second type of presynaptic receptor is specific, not for the transmitter which is released by the terminals on which it is present, but for a different neurotransmitter. Thus, the release of a particular neurotransmitter can be regulated by the presence of other neurotransmitters which may be released from the terminals of other neurones. Systems of this type can therefore provide mechanisms for interactions between different neurotransmitter systems.

Part 2

The peripheral nervous system

Chapter 4

The somatic motor system

The peripheral nervous system can be divided into two parts: the somatic system which controls the activity of voluntary or striated muscle, and the autonomic nervous system which controls the activity of smooth muscle of the blood vessels and viscera, as well as other internal organs such as the heart, glands, etc. Different substances mediate transmission at the various synapses and neuro-effector junctions of the peripheral nervous system and the general scheme is illustrated in Figure 4.1. This diagram will be referred to again in other chapters.

The somatic system

This is the motor system of the body and the neurones involved are the motor neurones. The cell bodies of these neurones are present in the motor nuclei of the cranial nerves of the brain stem and in the anterior horn of the spinal cord. Their axons form the motor fibres which innervate the voluntary muscles. These fibres are often long, they are large in diameter, at least compared with other nerves and they are myelinated, so that they are fast conducting. There are no synapses outside the central nervous system (CNS), so the only peripheral junction is the neuro-effector junction with the muscle cell, the neuromuscular junction (Figure 4.2). Here the transmitter is acetylcholine.

The neuromuscular junction

The short latency and brief contraction of striated muscle in response to a single nerve impulse led many investigators to doubt the possibility of a chemical transmitter operating at the neuromuscular junction. However, Henry Dale and his colleagues were able to demonstrate that acetylcholine (ACh) was released when somatic motor nerves were stimulated. They also showed that the release of acetylcholine was not due to contraction of the muscle, because it still occurred when the muscle was paralysed with curare but not when the muscle was denervated. Furthermore, locally applied acetylcholine mimicked the effects of nerve stimulation in causing contraction.

Acetylcholine is synthesized in motor nerve terminals from the precursor, choline, and acetyl coenzyme A, by the transfer of an acetyl group in the presence of a specific enzyme, choline acetyltransferase (Figure 4.3a). Choline and coenzyme A are widely distributed and are found in most tissues of the body, choline being an

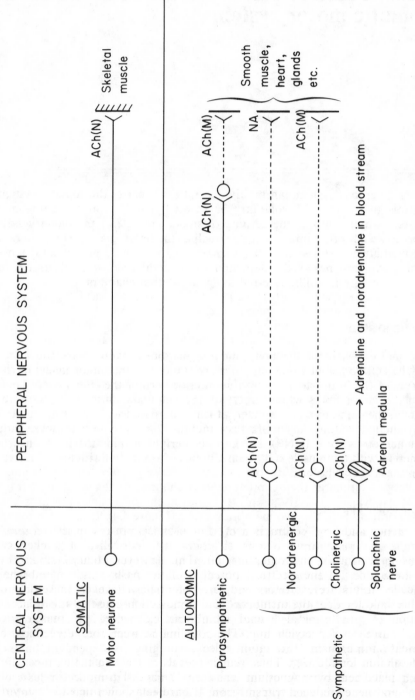

Figure 4.1 Diagram showing the principal pathways of the peripheral nervous system, indicating the transmitters involved at the different synapses and neuro-effector junctions. In the autonomic system, preganglionic fibres are represented by solid lines and postganglionic fibres by interrupted lines. ACh(N), cholinergic nicotinic receptors; ACh(M), cholinergic muscarinic receptors; NA, noradrenaline. Note that the chromaffin cells of the adrenal medulla release a mixture of adrenaline and noradrenaline into the bloodstream (see Chapter 8)

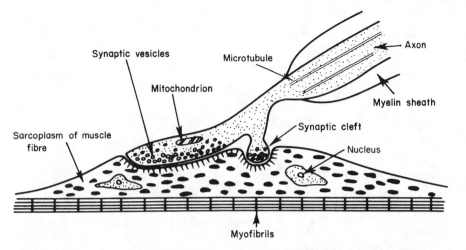

Figure 4.2 Diagrammatic representation of a section through the neuromuscular junction showing the structures referred to in the text (modified from Birks, Huxley and Katz, 1960)

essential constituent of diet. The choline in plasma is conveyed into the nerve by a high-affinity active transport process. There is also a low-affinity transport mechanism for choline but this is present in most cell membranes and is probably concerned with the uptake of choline for the synthesis of phospholipids. Choline acetyltransferase is present only in cholinergic neurones. It is synthesized in the cell body and passes down the axon by a process of axoplasmic flow, which involves neurofilaments or microtubules, (Figure 4.2), to the terminal region. Some synthesis of acetylcholine occurs throughout the cell but most takes place in the cytoplasm of the terminals. Acetyl coenzyme A is formed in the mitochondria of the terminal (Figure 4.2).

The acetylcholine is stored in the nerve terminals in synaptic vesicles which are spherical and 30–60 nm in diameter. The vesicles are synthesized initially in the cell body and pass to the terminals by axoplasmic flow. However, in the nerve terminals the vesicles may be recycled. With the arrival of nerve impulses at the terminal region, the vesicles discharge their content of acetylcholine into the synaptic cleft by a process of exocytosis. This is simply the movement of vesicles towards the terminal membrane where the two membranes fuse (Figure 4.4). It has been found that in the resting state, i.e. when no nerve impulses are present in the terminal region, there is small random release of vesicles resulting in 'quanta' or 'packets' of acetylcholine appearing in the synaptic cleft. This in turn produces small but detectable fluctuations in the electrical potential of the postsynaptic membrane, which are called miniature excitatory endplate potentials. However, these do not reach the threshold level for the membrane and so no action potential is produced. Depolarization of the terminal axonal membrane by nerve impulses greatly accelerates the release of acetylcholine. The coupling between the nerve impulse and the release mechanisms (excitation–release coupling) is dependent on the presence of calcium ions (Ca^{2+}). Thus, reduced levels of Ca^{2+} in the extracellular fluid, or its replacement by magnesium ions (Mg^{2+}), results in reduced release of acetylcholine and hence reduced transmission. It has been shown that Ca^{2+} enters the axoplasm of the nerve terminal when depolarization occurs and that the amount

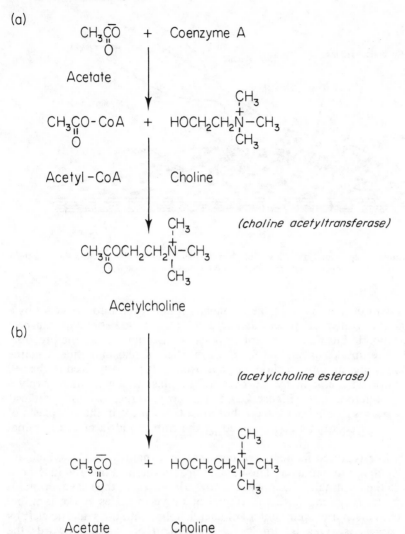

Figure 4.3 The synthesis (a) and hydrolysis (b) of acetylcholine. The enzymes involved are shown in italics

of acetylcholine released by a nerve impulse is a function of free Ca^{2+} concentration. The quantity of acetylcholine released also increases if the frequency of nerve stimulation is increased. Only about 80% of the acetylcholine present in the nerve terminals is available for release by nerve impulses, this being the so-called 'releasable' pool. The remaining 20% forms a 'non-releasable' pool.

The released acetylcholine, after it has diffused across the synaptic cleft, acts to produce a conformational change in the postjunctional membrane of the motor endplate, causing a local increase in permeability to cations, especially Na^+ and K^+, and this results in depolarization of the membrane of the muscle cell. This depolarization is of very brief duration, being terminated within a few milliseconds

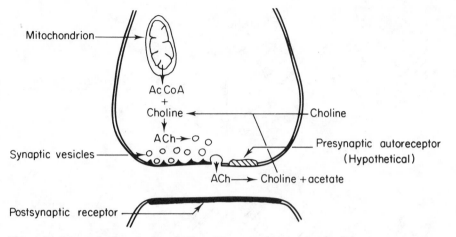

Figure 4.4 Schematic diagram of a cholinergic synapse (see text for details)

by the rapid hydrolysis of acetylcholine. The hydrolysis (Figure 4.3b), which produces choline and acetate (as well as water), is mediated by the enzyme acetylcholinesterase (AChE), which has a very high level of catalytic activity. At the neuromuscular junction, most of the acetylcholinesterase is localized to the postsynaptic membrane but some is also present in the presynaptic terminals where it probably has the function of regulating the storage of acetylcholine. However, there is evidence that acetylcholine receptors may be present on the prejunctional membrane, i.e. that there are presynaptic autoreceptors for acetylcholine at the neuromuscular junction. These autoreceptors, activated by the transmitter already released, may provide a positive feedback control system, which serves to maintain the availability of acetylcholine, particularly when the demand is high, for instance when there are many nerve impulses in the presynaptic fibre. In other words, the autoreceptors may have a mobilizing function, shifting the stored or reserve acetylcholine into a readily releasable pool (Figure 4.4).

Approximately half the choline formed by enzymatic hydrolysis of acetylcholine is transported back into the presynaptic nerve terminals by a high-affinity sodium-dependent active transport system and is used in the synthesis of fresh acetylcholine. There is a limited amount of choline in motor nerve terminals and the active transport system appears to be the principal mechanism for regulating the synthesis of acetylcholine. Thus, blocking the uptake of choline (see Chapter 5) can block transmission at the neuromuscular junction. The enzyme acetylcholinesterase, which hydrolyses acetylcholine, is also known as 'true' or specific cholinesterase. It occurs in nervous tissue and in striated muscle but is also present in other tissues, such as non-cholinergic nerves and red blood cells, where its function is not known. There is another enzyme, pseudo- (or non-specific) cholinesterase, which is present in a large number of tissues, such as plasma, intestine, skin, etc. In the intestine the enzyme is thought to control the actions of acetylcholine as a local hormone, maintaining tone. In other tissues its function is unknown. The different types of cholinesterase are distinguished by the substrates on which they act. Thus, both true cholinesterase and pseudocholinesterase catalyse the hydrolysis of acetylcholine, but only true cholinesterase acts on acetyl-β-methylcholine, and only pseudocholinesterase acts on benzoylcholine and succinylcholine. There is, in fact, more than one

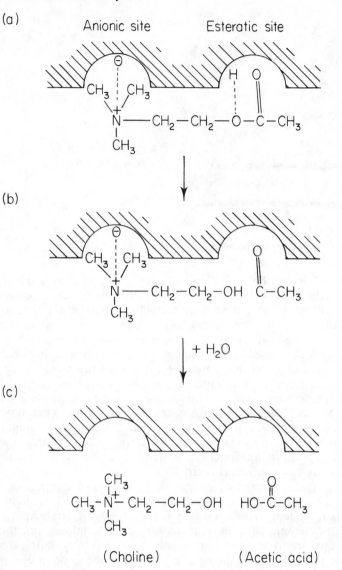

(a)

Anionic site　　　Esteratic site

Acetylcholinesterase

(b)

(c)

(Choline)　　　　　(Acetic acid)

Figure 4.5 Stages in the hydrolysis of acetylcholine by acetylcholinesterase: (a) binding of the acetylcholine molecule to the active site on the enzyme; (b) the first stage in the hydrolysis, liberating choline, and (c) the second stage, yielding acetic acid and the reactivated enzyme

type of pseudocholinesterase, of which butyrylcholinesterase is the most important in mammals.

Acetylcholinesterase has two binding sites: an anionic site to which the cationic head of the acetylcholine molecule is attracted, and an esteratic site which accepts the ester group of the acetylcholine molecule (Figure 4.5a). The esteratic site has both basic (anionic) and acidic (cationic) groups which bind, respectively, the carbon and carbonyl atoms of acetylcholine. Studies of the molecular structure of

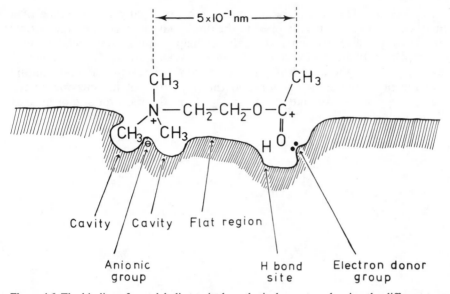

Figure 4.6 The binding of acetylcholine to its hypothetical receptor, showing the different types of chemical bonds involved

this enzyme have provided good evidence that, at the esteratic site, the hydroxyl group of serine and the imidazole nitrogen of histidine provide the basic group, while the hydroxyl groups of tyrosine may provide the cationic groups. The esteratic site on the enzyme seems to be primarily concerned with the hydrolysis of acetylcholine. Once the enzyme–substrate complex has been formed, the hydrolysis is believed to take place in two stages. First the acetylcholine molecule is pulled apart and choline is liberated (Figure 4.5b). At this stage, for a brief period, the enzyme is acetylated. However, in the second stage, the enzyme reacts with water to yield acetic acid and the reactivated enzyme (Figure 4.5c). Pseudocholinesterase also possesses two binding sites (which is why this enzyme can also catalyse the hydrolysis of acetylcholine), whereas other cholinesterases possess only an esteratic site. However, pseudocholinesterase differs from acetylcholinesterase in that the binding site corresponding to the anionic site of acetylcholinesterase forms a dipolar rather than an anionic bond.

The receptor for acetylcholine at the neuromuscular junction has probably been subjected to more extensive study than any other receptor. This is partly due to the fact that a number of naturally occurring toxins (e.g. snake venoms, see Chapter 5) bind very tightly to the receptor and these, if made radioactive, can be used as chemical labels for the receptor. Secondly, it has been possible to make a large number of substances, chemically related to acetylcholine, and these have been used for structure–activity studies. The results of these various studies have suggested that certain spatial and physicochemical criteria must be met for agonist and antagonist drugs to interact with the acetylcholine receptor. In the case of the receptor at the neuromuscular junction, there are two sites at which binding between the drug molecule and the receptor occurs (Figure 4.6). These are an anionic site which forms an ionic bond with the cationic quaternary nitrogen of the acetylcholine molecule, and an ester site where hydrogen bonding with the carbonyl oxygen atom occurs. The spatial requirements are principally the presence of a minimum of two methyl groups attached to the quaternary nitrogen and the critical length of the alkyl chain, which is thought to help stabilize the acetylcholine–receptor complex through the existence of van der Waals' forces (see Chapter 1). The similarity between the known requirements for the acetylcholine postsynaptic receptor at the neuromuscular junction and the properties of the enzyme acetyl-cholinesterase suggest that the latter may in fact form the receptor site or at least part of it.

Chapter 5

Drugs affecting neuromuscular transmission

The actions of acetylcholine (Figure 5.1a) at the neuromuscular junction can be mimicked by the drug nicotine (Figure 5.1b), whereas at neuro-effector junctions at the terminals of the postganglionic fibres of the parasympathetic branch of the autonomic nervous system, the actions of acetylcholine are mimicked by the drug muscarine (see Chapter 7). Thus, two types of receptors for acetylcholine exist: 'nicotinic' and 'muscarinic'. In addition to the neuromuscular junction, the cholinergic synapses in both sympathetic and parasympathetic ganglia are nicotinic (see Chapter 6). It is best to consider the actions of drugs at the neuromuscular junction according to whether they act at prejunctional sites or postsynaptically.

(a) 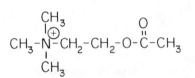   (b)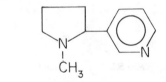

Figure 5.1 The chemical structure of (a) acetylcholine and (b) nicotine

Drugs acting prejunctionally

Effects on synthesis

No drugs are known which affect cholinergic transmission by a specific action on the synthesis of acetylcholine, i.e. by blocking the enzyme choline acetyltransferase, although drugs with such an action could well be useful. Substances which affect the activity of this enzyme are known but they have other effects as well. However, the synthesis of acetylcholine can be influenced indirectly by drugs which block the active transport mechanism for the uptake of choline into presynaptic nerve terminals.

Hemicholinium (Figure 5.2a) *and triethylcholine* (Figure 5.2b)

Both of these drugs resemble acetylcholine in structure and it is thought that they compete with choline for the transport system and so reduce the amount of choline available in the terminal for acetylation to acetylcholine. Thus, the block in neuromuscular transmission produced by hemicholinium develops slowly, as the stores of acetylcholine in the terminals are depleted. The block can be overcome by providing an excess of choline. These drugs have no therapeutic applications but are useful tools in experimental pharmacology. There is some similarity between the effects of hemicholinium on neuromuscular transmission and the symptoms of myasthenia gravis (see below). Both the low-affinity and high-affinity uptake systems for choline are blocked by these drugs but the high-affinity system, being concerned with the synthesis of acetylcholine in the motor nerve terminals, is the most sensitive.

(a)

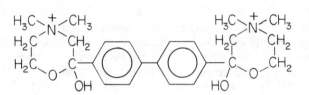

(b)

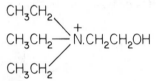

Figure 5.2 The chemical structure of (a) hemicholinium (HC-3) and (b) triethylcholine

Effects on release

The release of acetylcholine from nerve terminals can be affected in a number of ways. The fact that the release is calcium dependent (see Chapter 4) means that substitution of other ions can influence the release of acetylcholine. Thus, the presence of magnesium ions depresses transmission, as does simply reducing the extracellular concentration of calcium ions (Ca^{2+}). These effects are more marked on the evoked release of acetylcholine than on spontaneous release. A high concentration of potassium ions (K^+) will increase the release of acetylcholine by depolarizing the terminal membrane. Compounds which sequester calcium, e.g. chelators, will depress transmission.

There are a number of venoms and toxins which have very potent actions on neuromuscular transmission, affecting the storage and release of acetylcholine. These are discussed in a separate section (see below). Some antibiotics, e.g. streptomycin, neomycin and kanamycin, and also tetracyclines, in large doses can produce neuromuscular block. This can be an unwanted side-effect which can be important in patients in whom transmission is already impaired through other causes, e.g. by drugs or disease. The failure of transmission due to antibiotics resembles that due to low Ca^{2+}. However, this does not appear to be the mechanism through which all antibiotics affect neuromuscular transmission. Streptomycin, for example, appears to have a postjunctional action and prejunctionally is thought to depress the mobilization of acetylcholine. Some compounds, e.g. tetraethyl-ammonium, guanidine and 4-aminopyridine, facilitate the release of acetylcholine from nerve endings indirectly, by acting on the nerve to increase the duration of the action potential. 4-Aminopyridine has an anticurare action.

Local anaesthetics (see Chapter 9), given by intra-arterial injection, prevent or reduce the release of acetylcholine at the neuromuscular junction. However, as these drugs block axonal conduction this is likely to be an indirect effect, especially as the fine non-myelinated terminals of the motor nerves will be particularly sensitive to this action. Local anaesthetics also have some postjunctional blocking action due to stabilization of the postjunctional membrane. In normal use, local anaesthetics are unlikely to produce any effects on neuromuscular transmission; however, the use of large doses needs to be avoided in patients in whom transmission is already impaired.

Certain α-agonists, such as adrenaline and noradrenaline (see Chapter 8), have a weak facilitatory action on neuromuscular transmission. This effect, which is seen as an increase in the evoked release of acetylcholine, is probably an indirect action which increases the availability of Ca^{2+} to activate the release mechanism. The facilitatory effect is not normally apparent unless transmission is already depressed, e.g. by partial curarization, junctional fatigue or myasthenia gravis (see below).

Drugs which act postsynaptically

The principal group of drugs with postsynaptic actions at the neuromuscular junction is the 'neuromuscular-blocking drugs'. These can be classified into two main types according to their mechanism of action. The first are the non-depolarizing acetylcholine antagonists, which simply antagonize the actions of acetylcholine at the receptor and are, in most cases, competitive antagonists. Thus, the antagonism they produce, or the block in transmission, can be overcome by increasing the amount of acetylcholine available at the receptor. The way in which this can be done will be discussed later. The second group consists of agonists which block transmission by a prolonged depolarizing action. However, the distinction between these two types of action is not always completely clear, and there is a phenomenon known as 'dual' or 'mixed' block.

Non-depolarizing blocking drugs

D-Tubocurarine (Figure 5.3a)

This is the dextro-isomer of curare which is the best-known example of a non-depolarizing blocking drug. Curare, which is the generic term for the crude plant extract, was used as an arrow poison by the South American Indians who paralysed their prey with curare-tipped arrows. However, D-tubocurarine is a pure alkaloid which possesses the most potent blocking activity. The main clinical use for D-tubocurarine has been as a muscle relaxant, as an adjunct to surgical anaesthesia. In doses larger than those needed to block neuromuscular transmission, D-tubocurarine blocks transmission at autonomic ganglia and this results in a fall in blood pressure.

(a)

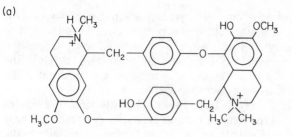

(b)

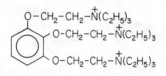

(c)

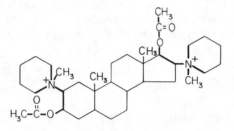

(d)

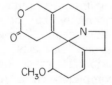

(e)

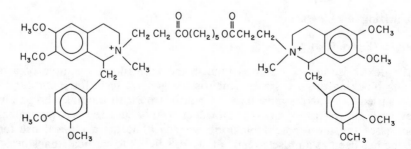

Figure 5.3 The chemical structures of some non-depolarizing neuromuscular blocking drugs:
(a) D-tubocurarine, (b) gallamine, (c) pancuronium, (d) dihydro-β-erythroidine and (e) atracurium

By a similar action it also depresses the secretion of adrenaline from the adrenal medulla and this too will contribute to the fall in blood pressure. Tubocurarine also releases histamine from mast cells, causing hypotension and bronchospasm, and it is therefore contra-indicated in patients suffering from bronchial asthma and other allergic conditions.

The block in neuromuscular transmission produced by D-tubocurarine is a classic example of competitive antagonism which may be overcome by increasing the availability of acetylcholine at the junction, e.g. by the use of anticholinesterase drugs (see below). D-Tubocurarine is poorly absorbed from the GI tract, which accounts for the fact that the S. American Indians were not affected by eating meat from animals which were poisoned with curare.

Gallamine (Figure 5.3b)

This was the first of a number of synthetic non-depolarizing neuromuscular blocking drugs. The action of gallamine is similar to that of D-tubocurarine with about one-fifth of the potency and a slightly shorter duration of action. Gallamine has less tendency than tubocurarine to release histamine and to block autonomic ganglia.

Pancuronium (Figure 5.3c)

This has a steroid structure to which two fragments of the acetylcholine molecule are attached; however, it has no steroid-like activity. It is as potent as D-tubocurarine, with the same duration of action and a slightly slower onset. Like gallamine, it does not release histamine or block autonomic ganglia in doses which produce neuromuscular block. However, both gallamine and pancuronium possess some atropine-like activity and appear to block selectively muscarinic receptors in the heart, while not affecting the muscarinic receptors at other parasympathetic nerve terminals. This action, which reduces the influence of the vagus nerve on the heart, can lead to the development of tachycardia and hypertension. D-Tubocurarine, in doses which produce neuromuscular block, does not have this action. Both gallamine and pancuronium block the uptake of noradrenaline in sympathetic nerve terminals and may also cause the release of noradrenaline. These actions tend to increase their cardiovascular effects.

Dihydro-β-erythroidine (Figure 5.3d)

This drug, with a curare-like action, is also a plant extract. It is not used as a muscle relaxant, however. Erythroidine and its derivatives are well absorbed after oral administration and also cross the blood–brain barrier. This may explain why extracts of plants containing erythroidines have not been used as arrow poisons.

Atracurium (Figure 5.3e)

This is a relatively new drug with a moderate duration of action (15–35 min). It can cause histamine release but is less potent than D-tubocurarine in this respect. Atracurium is unstable at physiological pH and breaks down spontaneously into inactive metabolites; it is also broken down by esterases in the plasma. Because atracurium does not depend upon the liver or kidneys for its elimination, it can be used where renal or hepatic function is impaired.

Depolarizing blocking drugs

Nicotinic agonists, if applied in sufficiently large concentrations and for a sufficient length of time, will block transmission at the neuromuscular junction by producing a persistent depolarization. Acetylcholine itself should, of course, be capable of producing this effect, but under normal circumstances its hydrolysis by cholinesterase is so rapid that the effect is transient unless the cholinesterase is inhibited (see below). However, drugs which are resistant to, or only metabolized slowly by, cholinesterases will be effective. The principal group of drugs with this type of action consists of the methonium compounds, of which decamethonium and suxamethonium are the best known.

Decamethonium (Figure 5.4a)

This contains two quaternary nitrogen atoms, linked by a polymethylene chain with ten carbon atoms. The separation of the nitrogen atoms appears to be optimal for a blocking action at the neuromuscular junction (cf. ganglion blockers, Chapter 6), and is similar to the distance between the quaternary nitrogen atoms in the tubocurarine molecule (Figure 5.3a). It is thought that this distance may correspond to the separation between adjacent acetylcholine receptors at the neuro-effector junction. Decamethonium does not release histamine or block autonomic ganglia. It is not metabolized by cholinesterase and its effect is therefore long lasting. Because of this, together with the fact that there is no way of reversing the effects of decamethonium, it is not used clinically to produce muscular relaxation (see below).

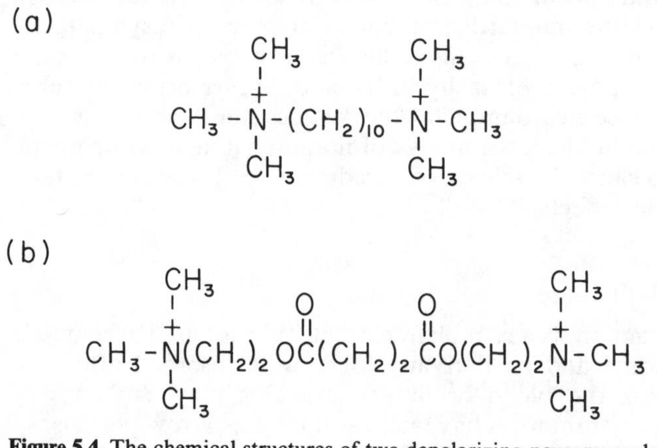

(a)

$$CH_3 - \overset{\overset{\displaystyle CH_3}{|}}{\underset{\underset{\displaystyle CH_3}{|}}{\overset{+}{N}}} - (CH_2)_{10} - \overset{\overset{\displaystyle CH_3}{|}}{\underset{\underset{\displaystyle CH_3}{|}}{\overset{+}{N}}} - CH_3$$

(b)

$$CH_3 - \overset{\overset{\displaystyle CH_3}{|}}{\underset{\underset{\displaystyle CH_3}{|}}{\overset{+}{N}}}(CH_2)_2 \; O\overset{\overset{\displaystyle O}{\|}}{C}(CH_2)_2 \; \overset{\overset{\displaystyle O}{\|}}{C}O(CH_2)_2 \; \overset{\overset{\displaystyle CH_3}{|}}{\underset{\underset{\displaystyle CH_3}{|}}{\overset{+}{N}}} - CH_3$$

Figure 5.4 The chemical structures of two depolarizing neuromuscular blocking drugs: (a) decamethonium; (b) suxamethonium (succinylcholine)

Suxamethonium (succinylcholine; Figure 5.4b)

This drug resembles two atoms of acetylcholine joined end to end, thus producing the optimum distance (for neuromuscular block) between the two quaternary nitrogen atoms (see Figure 5.4b). It has a similar mode of action to that of decamethonium but the blockade is short lived, lasting for only a few minutes. This short duration of action is due to the fact that, although suxamethonium is not hydrolysed by acetylcholinesterase, it is broken down by butyrylcholinesterase which is present in plasma. Suxamethonium does not liberate histamine but it has weak muscarinic and ganglion-stimulant actions which can result in the development of undesirable cardiovascular effects, e.g. tachycardia, mild hypertension and cardiac arrhythmias.

Because the depolarizing blockers are agonists at acetylcholine receptors, they cause stimulation initially and this is followed by prolonged depolarization of the receptor which, in the depolarized state, cannot be activated by acetylcholine or by other agonists. There are, however, some species differences in the actions of the depolarizing blockers (these are discussed in the next section).

Dual blockade

This is produced by drugs which behave as partial agonists in some species. For example, in most muscles in man and cat, decamethonium and suxamethonium produce neuromuscular blockade by depolarization, as described above. However, in some slowly contracting muscles of the cat and in other species, e.g. dog, monkey, guinea-pig and rabbit, these two drugs produce a 'dual' block. When the drug is first injected the muscles twitch due to the agonist action and then become depolarized, as expected, but after a while it is found that the block can be antagonized by the use of an anticholinesterase. As this is not possible with a pure depolarizing block, it is assumed that the blockade has changed from a depolarizing to a non-depolarizing block, similar to that produced by curare. Although this phenomenon has been demonstrated mainly by the use of isolated muscle preparations from experimental animals, it appears to have some relevance to man in patients suffering from myasthenia gravis, in which depolarizing blocking drugs produce a dual blockade (see 'Clinical uses of drugs affecting neuromuscular transmission', below).

Drugs which prolong the actions of acetylcholine

The mechanisms involved in the hydrolysis of acetylcholine at the postsynaptic receptor of the neuromuscular junction have been described in Chapter 4. Drugs which inhibit the action of acetylcholinesterase (AChE), thus preventing the hydrolysis of acetylcholine, will cause its accumulation in the body, so prolonging and intensifying its actions at effector sites, e.g. the neuromuscular junction. All the drugs in this category, the anticholinesterases, or cholinesterase inhibitors, produce their effect by combining with the enzyme, so that its active site is no longer able to hydrolyse acetylcholine. The drugs are of two types, 'reversible' and 'irreversible'.

Reversible inhibitors of cholinesterase

Physostigmine (Figure 5.5a)

This is a naturally occurring inhibitor of cholinesterase. It is a substituted carbamyl ester which is hydrolysed, albeit slowly, by cholinesterases. As physostigmine is a tertiary amine its degree of ionization will depend on the pH of the medium. It is

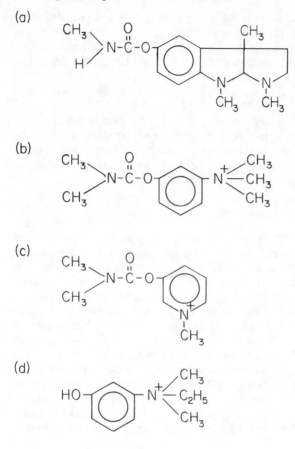

Figure 5.5 The chemical structures of reversible inhibitors of cholinesterase: (a) physostigmine, (b) neostigmine, (c) pyridostigmine and (d) edrophonium

well absorbed from the gut and also crosses the blood–brain barrier readily, so producing effects in the CNS. Physostigmine blocks access to the enzyme by acetylcholine and hence retards its hydrolysis. The slow breakdown of the inhibitor by cholinesterase is probably responsible for the reversibility of the action as very little is released from the enzyme unchanged. Physostigmine therefore acts as competitive substrate for the enzyme.

Neostigmine **(Figure 5.5b)**

This is a synthetic drug and is a quaternary ammonium compound. It is therefore completely ionized in aqueous solution and, consequently, it does not cross the blood–brain barrier and has only peripheral actions. However, it is also poorly absorbed from the gut. Because of the absence of central effects, neostigmine is the preferred drug in the treatment of myasthenia gravis (see 'Clinical uses of drugs affecting neuromuscular transmission', below).

Pyridostigmine (Figure 5.5c)

This is another synthetic drug and is a quaternary nitrogen compound, resembling neostigmine in its actions, except that they are longer lasting.

Edrophonium (Figure 5.5d)

This drug inhibits acetylcholinesterase reversibly by combining with only the anionic site. Its onset of action is rapid and its duration of action very short.

All these drugs, if given in sufficiently large doses, will inhibit cholinesterase at other sites in the body, e.g. at ganglia and at muscarinic receptors. Some of these actions are made use of clinically (see below). The molecule of physostigmine contains a urethane group (Figure 5.5a) and, in fact, the animal anaesthetic urethane (ethyl carbamate) possesses some anticholinesterase activity, as do a number of other drugs, e.g. decamethonium.

Irreversible inhibitors of cholinesterase

These are mainly organic esters of phosphoric acids and have been known for some time. They were first used as insecticides, and some still are, but their high level of toxicity led to their development in chemical warfare as 'nerve gases'. A large number of these compounds have been produced and some of their structures are shown in Figure 5.6.

(a)

(b)

(c)

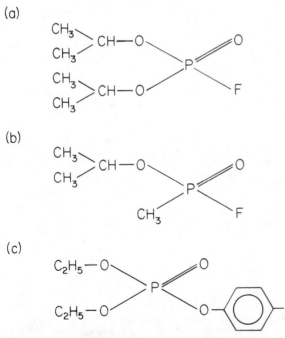

Figure 5.6 The chemical structures of three different types of organophosphorous compound: (a) di-isopropylfluorophosphate (DFP, dyflos), which has been used clinically, (b) sarin, a nerve gas and (c) paraoxon, an insecticide

Most organophosphorous compounds do not possess a quaternary nitrogen atom and react only with the esteratic site of cholinesterase. The inhibition occurs in two stages. First, the inhibitor and the enzyme combine to form a complex which can be readily dissociated, e.g. by dilution of the inhibitor, or by the presence of an excess of acetylcholine (Stage 1, Figure 5.7). In the second stage, a stable linkage is formed

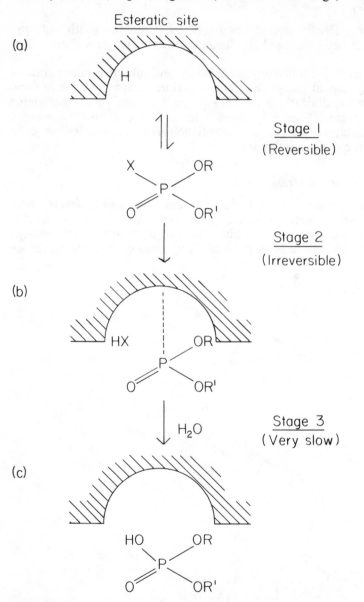

Figure 5.7 Stages in the inhibition of cholinesterase by organophosphorous compounds: (a) represents the active enzyme interacting reversibly with the inhibitor (Stage 1); (b) is the phosphorylated, inactive enzyme formed by the development of a stable link between the esteratic site on the enzyme and the phosphorus moiety of the inhibitor (Stage 2); (c) represents the reactivated enzyme produced by very slow hydrolysis of the phosphorylated enzyme

between the esteratic site on the enzyme and the phosphorus moiety of the inhibitor (Stage 2). This process is comparable to that which occurs with acetylcholine (see Chapter 4) but the phosphorylated enzyme, unlike the acetylated enzyme, is very stable and hydrolyses extremely slowly, sometimes taking several months for the enzyme to be reactivated (Stage 3). Thus, the term 'irreversible', as applied to the organophosphorous inhibitors of cholinesterase, is relative.

The reversible inhibitors, neostigmine and physostigmine, are fairly selective for cholinesterases, but the organophosphorous inhibitors are less specific and also inhibit carboxylic esterases such as trypsin, chymotrypsin and lipases. They are mostly effective against both types of cholinesterase.

As already indicated, the hydrolysis of the phosphorylated enzyme complex is extremely slow. However, there are some drugs which are capable of reactivating cholinesterase, the most important of which are the oximes. One example is pralidoxime (Figure 5.8a) which possesses a quaternary nitrogen atom which will be attracted to the anionic site on the enzyme (Figure 5.8b). The free oxime group of

(a)

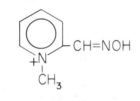

Pralidoxime

(b)

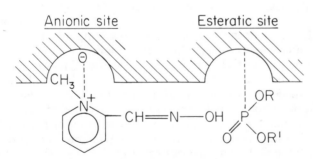

Figure 5.8 (a) The chemical structure of pralidoxime; (b) the interaction between pralidoxime and cholinesterase to regenerate the active enzyme

pralidoxime is then at the correct distance to attract the phosphorus bound to the esteratic site. The reactivator–inhibitor complex then 'lifts' off the enzyme. The reactivators are effective only if given immediately before or soon after exposure to the inhibitor. The reason for this is that the phosphorylated enzyme appears to undergo a process of 'ageing', as a result of which it becomes more resistant to the action of the reactivator. The rate at which the ageing process takes place varies with different organophosphorous compounds. It is thought to be due to the removal of an alkoxyl group by hydrolysis. The toxic symptoms associated with poisoning by organophosphorous inhibitors of cholinesterase are those associated with overactivity of the parasympathetic system (see Chapter 7), together with fasciculations of skeletal muscle. Death is caused by respiratory failure due to paralysis of the respiratory centre of the brain and neuromuscular blockade of the muscles controlling respiration. Treatment with atropine (see Chapter 7) will relieve the parasympathetic effects and to some extent the action on the respiratory centre. It is possible to provide some protection against the lethal effects of organophosphorous compounds by first administering a reversible inhibitor such as physostigmine. This combines with a fraction of the enzyme, protecting it from the action of the organophosphorous inhibitor. Atropine and the oximes are also used for prophylaxis.

Prolonged exposure to small concentrations of organophosphorous compounds, e.g. insecticides, can give rise to neurotoxic effects. These consist of peripheral neuritis, followed by motor incoordination; paralysis develops as a result of demyelination of nerves in the CNS and anterior horn cells of the spinal cord. All the compounds which produce this effect are inhibitors of butyrylcholinesterase, the enzyme present in the Schwann cells and oligodendrites which are responsible for the production of myelin.

Clinical uses of drugs affecting neuromuscular transmission

The neuromuscular blocking drugs are used as an adjunct to general anaesthesia where muscular relaxation or paralysis is desirable. Both the non-depolarizing and the depolarizing blockers have been used for this purpose. The first of these drugs to be used was tubocurarine but it has largely been replaced by the synthetic compounds gallamine and pancuronium, which have fewer side-effects. Although the effect of these drugs is relatively long lasting, e.g. 30 min for tubocurarine, it can readily be reversed by introducing a stimulant drug such as neostigmine; however, atropine must also be given in order to avoid stimulating muscarinic receptors, for example those in the heart. The actions of the depolarizing blockers such as suxamethonium cannot, of course, be reversed by neostigmine, but they are, in any case, of shorter duration, approximately 5 min. Thus, because of its rapid onset of action and short duration, suxamethonium is the drug of choice for intubation (the insertion of an endotracheal tube for the administration of gaseous anaesthetic and/or control of respiration). Prolonged or repeated administration of suxamethonium can lead to the development of a dual block. To test whether or not this is the case, a short-acting anticholinesterase drug such as edrophonium may be given. If dual blockade is present there will be a transient relief of the block, in which case neostigmine (plus atropine) can be administered. As suxamethonium is metabolized mainly by pseudocholinesterase, its action will be prolonged in individuals in which there is an abnormal genetically related variant of this enzyme.

Neuromuscular blocking drugs have been used to relieve painful muscle spasms, e.g. in tetanus. They are also useful in preventing violent convulsions from occurring when electroconvulsive therapy is administered to psychiatric patients.

Apart from their use in reversing the actions of non-depolarizing neuromuscular blocking drugs, the anticholinesterases are used to relieve the symptoms of myasthenia gravis. This is a chronic disease in which there is a progressive weakness of the skeletal muscles, which increases with use, although partial recovery may occur with rest. The condition may be localized to a small group of muscles, e.g. those of the face, or it may be widespread and involve the respiratory muscles. The muscles of myasthenic patients behave as though they were paralysed with curare, or had been treated with hemicholinium. Thus the muscle fibre responds normally to direct electrical stimulation, but stimulation of the motor nerve results in a rapid fall in the amplitude of the evoked muscle twitches. As the symptoms of myasthenia can be relieved by the administration of anticholinesterase drugs, i.e. by increasing the amount of acetylcholine available at the neuromuscular junction, and can be mimicked by hemicholinium, it was thought at one time that there was simply an impaired synthesis of acetylcholine. However, it is now known that this is not the case. Myasthenia gravis is sometimes associated with tumours of the thymus gland and removal of the gland in these cases also improves the symptoms of myasthenia. There is now abundant evidence that myasthenia gravis is, in fact, an autoimmune disease and that antibodies to the acetylcholine receptor protein, which have been found in the plasma of myasthenic patients, are probably responsible for the symptoms. Nevertheless, drugs which increase the amount of acetylcholine available are still used for treatment and are effective. Neostigmine is preferred to physostigmine as it does not possess central actions, and edrophonium, being ultra short-acting, is useful in diagnosis. Pyridostigmine, although less potent than neostigmine, is also used for treatment as it has a longer duration of action. Excessive doses of these drugs can cause a depolarizing block or 'cholinergic crisis', the symptoms of which are muscle fasciculation, pallor, sweating, small pupils and excessive salivation, all signs of excessive nicotinic and muscarinic cholinergic activity. Corticosteroids are also used in the treatment of myasthenia gravis and the immunosuppressant drug azathioprine is effective in some cases. Marked clinical improvement, although only temporary, has been obtained with plasmaphaeresis (exchanging plasma with that from a normal donor). The indirectly acting sympathomimetic amine ephedrine has some beneficial effect in myasthenia and was at one time used in treatment. Its action may be related to the facilitatory effect of α-adrenoceptor agonists on depressed neuromuscular transmission.

Venoms and toxins that affect neuromuscular transmission

A number of very potent agents, either derived from micro-organisms or present in the venoms of snakes or spiders, have effects on transmission at the neuromuscular junction or on motor nerves. Probably the best-known of these is botulinum toxin.

Botulinum toxin

The anaerobic bacterium *Clostridium botulinum* produces a highly toxic substance, botulinum toxin, which results in the clinical syndrome 'botulism'. The organism, which is active when ingested by mouth, can infect foods, particularly meat and vegetables, and poisoning arises from the consumption of canned foods which have been inadequately sterilized during the canning process and which have been consumed without subsequent cooking. The toxin produces muscular paralysis by preventing the release of acetylcholine from nerve terminals. Transmission in motor nerves is unaffected and there is no depletion of acetylcholine in the terminals; nor is the responsiveness of the postsynaptic receptor altered. The action of the toxin is thought to be related to the entry of Ca^{2+} into the terminal, which activates the release mechanism for acetylcholine. The effects of poisoning with botulinum toxin are usually fatal due to paralysis of the muscles controlling respiration and the fact that the action of the toxin is very long lasting, i.e. several weeks or months. There is no known antidote but the chances of recovery are increased if artificial respiration is given.

Tetanus toxin

This toxin is produced by the bacterium *Clostridium tetani* which is present in soil. Poisoning usually occurs through the infection of wounds with material containing spores of the bacterium. The main action of this toxin is central and it interferes with inhibitory mechanisms in the spinal cord giving rise to the characteristic tonic spasms of striated muscle. The action is probably due to a blockade of the release of inhibitory amino acid transmitters. Tonic spasm of the masticatory muscles results in 'lockjaw', a fairly common symptom. Death due to poisoning by tetanus toxin results from paralysis of the respiratory muscles. Tetanus toxin also has some action at the neuromuscular junction, causing a block of the release of acetylcholine, similar to that produced by botulinum toxin.

Venom of the black widow spider (*Latrodectus mactans tredecimguttatus*)

This causes disruption of synaptic vesicles containing acetylcholine and hence depletion of the nerve terminals of the transmitter. Paralysis therefore follows spasm due to the initial explosive release of acetylcholine. It is thought that the venom affects the process of recycling of synaptic vesicles. Thus, after fusing with the terminal membrane, and the release of their content of acetylcholine, the vesicles are unable to re-form.

β-Bungarotoxin

This is present in the venom of snakes of the genus *Bungarus,* e.g. *Bungarus multicinctus* (the Taiwan banded krait), and has an action similar to that of black widow spider venom, causing depletion of synaptic vesicles. Some other poisonous spiders possess venoms with a similar action. These venoms are not selective for cholinergic nerve terminals and other nerve endings, e.g. adrenergic, may be affected.

α-Bungarotoxin

This is present in the same venom in which β-bungarotoxin is found. However, it has a completely different action, binding to postsynaptic nicotinic acetylcholine receptors with a very high affinity. The binding is irreversible and transmission is therefore blocked. Both α- and β-bungarotoxin are polypeptides, of which there are multiple forms.

None of the toxins and venoms described above have any clinical uses. However, a knowledge of their actions may be important when dealing with poisoning by these substances and some, notably α-bungarotoxin, have been used extensively to study acetylcholine receptors.

Toxins and venoms that act on motor nerves

These affect transmission in nerves. For example, tetrodotoxin, which is found in the puffer fish (a delicacy in the far East), selectively blocks sodium channels in nerve and muscle membranes. It therefore prevents the increase in sodium conductance which accompanies depolarization; it does not affect potassium conductance. Tetrodotoxin blocks the conduction of action potentials without altering the resting membrane potential. Saxitoxin, which is found in certain shellfish such as the Alaskan butter clam, but which originates in unicellular dinoflagellates on which the clams feed, has an action similar to that of tetrodotoxin but also affects neuromuscular transmission. Tetrodotoxin has been used extensively in studies of the mechanisms of nerve conduction. Batrochotoxin, which is found in the skin of the S. American arrow-poison frog (*Phyllobates aurotaenia*), has the opposite action to tetrodotoxin and saxitoxin, causing the sodium channels to remain permanently open. There is an initial excitation but the persisting depolarization results in the blocking of the conduction of action potentials, together with a fall in membrane potential.

Chapter 6

The autonomic nervous system

The autonomic nervous system consists of those nervous elements (i.e. neurones, ganglia and plexuses) that regulate the involuntary or automatic functions of the body. Thus, the nerves of the autonomic system innervate visceral smooth muscle, the heart, blood vessels and glands, as well as smooth muscle in structures such as the pupil and ciliary muscle of the eye and the pilomotor muscles of the skin. The glands innervated by this system include those associated with the digestive, respiratory and urinogenital systems, together with those of the head and skin. However, this does not include endocrine glands and certain exocrine glands which are under hormonal control. Most of the principles concerning the pharmacology of the peripheral autonomic system and its effector organs are those which apply to the somatic nervous system (i.e. motor nerves and striated muscle), which is under voluntary control. There are, however, some important differences. If somatic nerves are cut, their effector muscles become paralysed and eventually atrophy, whereas the smooth muscle and glands of the autonomic system do not atrophy and show some independent activity after their nerves have been cut.

The autonomic nervous system consists of a central portion within the CNS and a peripheral portion outside the brain and spinal cord. The main centres of the brain which are involved in the regulation of autonomic activity are situated in the hypothalamus and medulla oblongata. Efferent fibres from the hypothalamus form synapses with groups of cell bodies of medullary neurones and also with neurones in the lateral horn of the spinal cord. These medullary and spinal neurones send out axons that leave the CNS to synapse with cell bodies of final neurones, the efferent axons of which innervate smooth muscle and glandular tissue. The cell bodies of the final neurones usually occur in clusters which are called ganglia. Thus, the medullary and spinal neurones are preganglionic and their efferent fibres are the preganglionic fibres, whereas the neurones that comprise the ganglia are postganglionic and their efferent fibres, which innervate the effector organs, are the postganglionic fibres.

The motor fibres of the somatic system (see Chapter 4) are all myelinated and are 1–12 μm in diameter. The preganglionic fibres of the autonomic system are also myelinated but are usually smaller in diameter (i.e. 1–3 μm). Postganglionic fibres are non-myelinated and generally less than 1 μm in diameter.

Although many autonomic functions occur without conscious thought and are under hypothalamic and/or medullary control, it is clear that higher centres in the brain (e.g. the cerebral cortex) can influence autonomic activity. Thus, nervous tension or emotional stress is often associated with autonomic stimulation, i.e. sweating, raised blood pressure and heart rate, pupillary dilatation, and so on.

The subdivisions of the autonomic nervous system

The sympathetic system

This consists of preganglionic fibres arising from the thoracic and lumbar regions of the spinal cord, together with the peripheral ganglia in which they synapse, and the associated postganglionic axons (Figure 6.1). The cell bodies of the preganglionic neurones are located in the spinal cord from the first thoracic segment to the second or third lumbar. The preganglionic fibres pass from the spinal cord with the anterior roots and leave the vertebral column with the segmental spinal nerves. They branch off from the spinal nerves as myelinated trunks (white rami) and join the chain of sympathetic ganglia, which are situated on either side of the vertebral column (Figure 6.1). The sympathetic chains extend from the cervical to the sacral

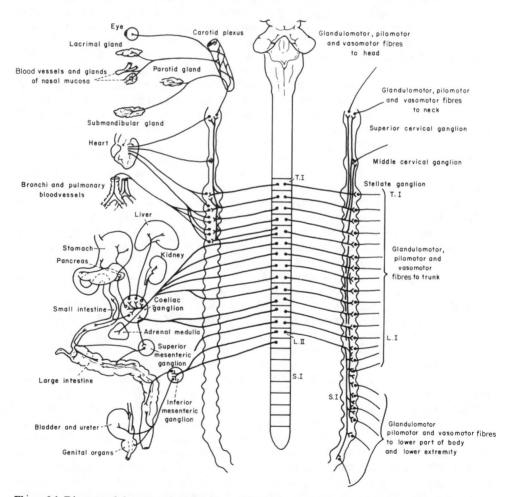

Figure 6.1 Diagram of the sympathetic division of the autonomic nervous system, showing the relationship of the autonomic ganglia to the spinal cord, the course of the pre- and postganglionic fibres, and the organs innervated (modified from Anson, 1966)

vertebrae, but the white rami from the spinal nerves to the sympathetic chains are confined to the thoracolumbar segments from which there is a sympathetic outflow. Preganglionic axons entering the sympathetic ganglia in the white rami terminate in one of three ways:

1. Many preganglionic fibres terminate in their own ganglia to make synaptic contact with secondary neurones (postganglionic), the axons of which then form grey rami that pass back to the somatic nerve and are thereby distributed to the structures innervated. As already indicated, these postganglionic fibres are non-myelinated.
2. Some preganglionic axons entering the sympathetic chains do not form synapses but pass straight through and make synaptic connections with postganglionic sympathetic neurones in ganglia and plexuses in the abdominal cavity. These are the prevertebral sympathetic ganglia, which are unpaired and comprise the coeliac and the superior and inferior mesenteric ganglia. They are mainly concerned with intestinal movements.
3. Some preganglionic fibres emerging from the tenth and eleventh thoracic segments of the spinal cord run in the greater splanchnic nerve to terminate on chromaffin cells in the adrenal medulla. The adrenal chromaffin cells are analogous to sympathetic ganglion cells.

The course of the pre- and postganglionic fibres of the sympathetic system, together with the organs innervated by this system, is shown in Figure 6.1.

The parasympathetic system

The preganglionic fibres of the parasympathetic system do not synapse with ganglia close to the vertebral column. Instead, they synapse with ganglia which are very close to, or often in, the effector organ (Figure 6.2). The cell bodies of the ganglion cells are often diffusely distributed within a tissue, for example in the gastrointestinal tract where they lie in the myenteric (Auerbach's) plexus and thus no discrete ganglia, such as occur in the sympathetic system, are visible. The postganglionic fibres arising from parasympathetic ganglia are very short, branched processes and, like sympathetic postganglionic fibres, are non-myelinated.

The parasympathetic nerves to all but the pelvic organs travel with some of the cranial nerves, the IIIrd (oculomotor), the VIIth (facial), the IXth (glossopharyngeal) and the Xth (vagus) (see Figure 6.2). Of these nerves, the vagus has the widest distribution, supplying all the smooth muscle in the thoracic and abdominal organs. Pelvic organs (uterus, terminal portion of the colon, rectum, bladder and external genitalia) receive their parasympathetic nerve supply from the second, third and fourth sacral segments of the spinal cord (Figure 6.2).

Transmission at autonomic ganglia (Figure 6.3)

Acetylcholine is the transmitter released from the presynaptic nerve terminals in both sympathetic and parasympathetic ganglia (see Figure 4.1). The action of acetylcholine on the postsynaptic receptors on the ganglion cells is mimicked by nicotine and not by muscarine, and therefore transmission in ganglia is regarded as 'nicotinic'. In many ways it resembles transmission at the neuromuscular junction; however, ganglionic transmission is true synaptic transmission as it is between

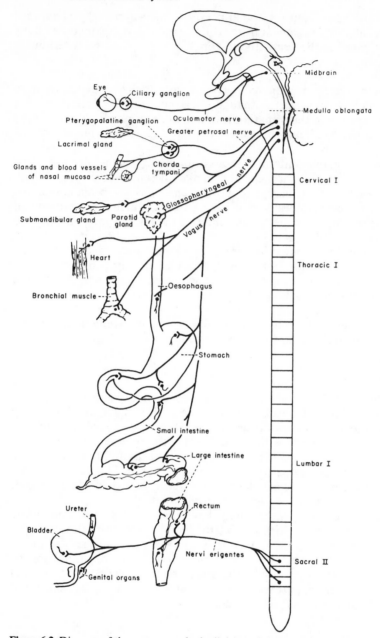

Figure 6.2 Diagram of the parasympathetic division of the autonomic nervous system, showing the course of the preganglionic fibres and the relationship of the parasympathetic ganglia, together with the postganglionic fibres, to the organs innervated (modified from Anson, 1966)

neurones and no effector organ is involved. The presynaptic mechanisms appear to be very similar to those at the neuromuscular junction. Thus, there is evidence for the storage of acetylcholine in vesicles and its quantal release from preganglionic nerve terminals, the acetylcholine which is released being that most recently synthesized. As with other cholinergic junctions, the release of transmitter is enhanced by Ca^{2+} and depressed by Mg^{2+}.

One important difference between autonomic ganglia and the neuromuscular junction, however, is in the distribution of acetylcholinesterase. Whereas at the neuromuscular junction most of the enzyme is concentrated close to the postsynaptic receptor (muscle endplate) where it will be well placed to hydrolyse the acetylcholine after it has induced a muscle twitch, and very little is present in the terminals, in autonomic ganglia most of the cholinesterase is present in the presynaptic fibre and very little is present on the surface of the ganglion cells. From this it must be concluded that enzymatic hydrolysis of acetylcholine is not an important mechanism for terminating transmitter action in ganglia. This conclusion is supported by the finding that inhibition of cholinesterase by anticholinesterase drugs produces less striking effects on ganglionic transmission than on other cholinergic systems, e.g. the neuromuscular junction. Thus, the termination of the transmitter action of acetylcholine in autonomic ganglia may be partly by enzymic action and partly by diffusion. The functional significance of the presence of cholinesterase at presynaptic sites is not clear. Part of the enzyme is intracellular and some is on the surface of the preganglionic fibres. This latter site supports the presence of presynaptic receptors for acetylcholine. Such receptors have been demonstrated on ganglia in the frog but not in mammals.

Perhaps the most important difference between autonomic ganglia and the neuromuscular junction, and one which is important for transmission and the actions of drugs, is morphological. The junctional sites on striated muscle occupy small discrete areas of the surface of the individual muscle fibres and are relatively isolated from those on adjacent fibres. In the superior cervical ganglion on the other hand, approximately 100 000 cells are packed into the space of a few millimetres and both pre- and postganglionic fibres form complicated ramifications. This difference in structure may account for the differences in potency shown by the methonium compounds of differing chain length, acting as 'ganglionic' and neuromuscular blockers (see below). This suggests that there is a different orientation of the acetylcholine receptors in the two structures, and this difference has been utilized in the development of drugs to act selectively at ganglia.

Junctions in ganglia also differ from the neuromuscular junction in their electrical properties. Thus, the ganglionic postsynaptic potential is more complex than the motor endplate potential. Whereas the latter is a simple depolarization arising from the action of acetylcholine on the receptor, the ganglion potential consists of at least three components (Figure 6.3a). The first is an early negative wave (N wave) or excitatory postsynaptic potential (EPSP), which is of brief duration and represents depolarization resulting from activation of nicotinic receptors on the ganglion cells. This phase is probably responsible for initiating activity in the postganglionic fibres and it shows typical 'nicotinic' properties. The second phase consists of a positive (P wave) or inhibitory postsynaptic potential (IPSP), which follows the N wave immediately; it is greatly increased by repetitive activation of preganglionic fibres and represents postganglionic hyperpolarization. Finally, there is a late negative wave (LN wave, or late EPSP) which is again due to depolarization.

In contrast to the N wave, which is readily blocked by D-tubocurarine, neither the P nor the LN waves are blocked. On the other hand, the LN wave can be blocked by atropine, an antagonist of the muscarinic actions of acetylcholine (see Chapter 7). Catecholamines have been found to be involved with the P wave and small intensely fluorescent interneurones (SIF cells) have been identified in

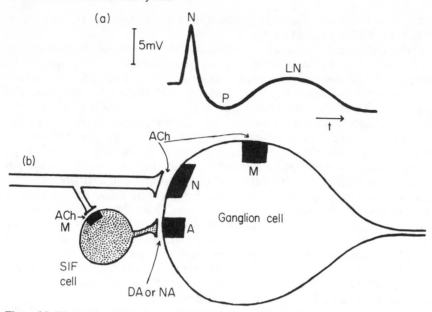

Figure 6.3 Diagrammatic representation of the transmission process at an autonomic ganglion and the electrical events associated with stimulation of the preganglionic nerve. (a) The sequence of postsynaptic potentials: N, early negative wave of depolarization; P, positive wave of hyperpolarization; LN, late negative wave of depolarization. (b) Hypothetical arrangement of synapses on the ganglion cell which could account for the potentials recorded: N, nicotinic ACh receptor; M, muscarinic ACh receptor; A, adrenergic receptor for dopamine (DA) or noradrenaline (NA); SIF, small intensely fluorescent interneurone (modified from Eccles and Libet, 1961)

autonomic ganglia (Figure 6.3b). It is therefore believed that acetylcholine, released from the terminals of the preganglionic fibres, activates not only nicotinic receptors on the ganglion neurones, to produce the N wave, but also muscarinic receptors on the same neurone, which are responsible for the LN wave. In addition, the release of acetylcholine activates muscarinic receptors on the SIF cells which themselves release noradrenaline or dopamine, and this in turn influences the activity of the ganglion cell and results in the P wave (see Figure 6.3a). Thus, while transmission at the autonomic junction is primarily nicotinic, both muscarinic and catecholaminergic mechanisms have a role, although their functional significance is not fully understood. The situation is further complicated by the fact that both 5-hydroxy-tryptamine and histamine can affect ganglionic transmission in experimental animals, although whether these actions have any physiological relevance is not known. Most of the knowledge about the function of autonomic ganglia has been obtained from studies of isolated preparations of sympathetic ganglia, as para-sympathetic ganglia are less accessible and much more difficult to study experimentally. It is worth noting that ganglionic transmission *in vivo* is blocked by nicotinic antagonists such as hexamethonium (see below) and not by atropine.

Drugs affecting transmission in autonomic ganglia

Since transmission in autonomic ganglia is essentially nicotinic, most of the drugs discussed in Chapter 5 influence ganglionic, as well as neuromuscular transmission.

There are, however, some important differences and larger doses may be needed, e.g. with tubocurarine, to produce effects on ganglia. In addition, anticholinesterase drugs are less effective at autonomic ganglia due to the removal of the transmitter by diffusion, rather than to hydrolysis by cholinesterase. Nevertheless, drugs such as physostigmine can cause a rise in blood pressure due to their ganglionic actions, but this can be blocked by atropine.

Autonomic ganglion stimulants

Nicotine

This is an alkaloid (see Figure 5.1b) which is present in the tobacco plant (*Nicotiana tabacum*) and is the most important active ingredient in tobacco. Nicotine stimulates the postsynaptic neurones in both sympathetic and parasympathetic ganglia, as well as the chromaffin cells of the adrenal medulla and the neuromuscular junction (see Figure 4.1). This action causes the release of acetylcholine, adrenaline and noradrenaline at various sites in the body and the end result is therefore complex. However, there is usually a rise in blood pressure although the heart rate may be slowed and the force of contraction of the heart reduced. These effects appear at lower doses than those which affect neuromuscular transmission. Large doses of nicotine will first cause stimulation, followed by a depolarization block. However, nicotine is not used as a ganglion blocker but its actions may be important in the development of cardiovascular disease associated with smoking.

Lobeline (Figure 6.4a)

This is also naturally occurring, being found in the lobelia plant (*Lobelia inflata*). Its action is similar to that of nicotine and it was once used as a respiratory stimulant. In addition, because it can induce nausea and vomiting, it has been used in attempts to produce conditioned aversion to tobacco.

Trimethylammonium (TMA) (Figure 6.4b)

This is a synthetic nicotinic agonist, which stimulates ganglion cells over a wider range of doses than does nicotine. It therefore only produces a block when very large doses are used and is preferred as a ganglion stimulant.

DMPP (1,1-dimethyl-4-phenylpiperazinium)

This is also a potent synthetic nicotinic agonist which, like TMA, has greater agonist than antagonist actions.

(a)

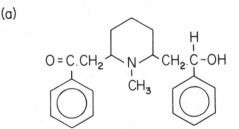

(b)

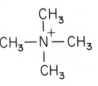

Figure 6.4 The chemical structures of (a) lobeline and (b) tetramethylammonium (TMA)

None of these stimulant drugs has any clinical or therapeutic application and they are used solely in experimental studies on autonomic ganglia.

Ganglion-blocking drugs

Drugs such as nicotine, TMA and DMPP, if used in sufficiently large doses, will block ganglionic transmission by producing a depolarizing block. Similarly, drugs such as D-tubocurarine will block transmission across autonomic ganglia as well as at the neuromuscular junction. However, there is a group of drugs which are competitive antagonists of acetylcholine and which have a more selective action at ganglia. These drugs were developed mainly for the treatment of hypertension. By blocking transmission at sympathetic ganglia, they reduce sympathetic tone and this results in a fall in arterial blood pressure (see Chapter 8). Unfortunately, reflex vasoconstriction is also abolished so that the circulation is unable to adjust to changes in the position of the body. This results in postural hypotension which can cause dizziness or even fainting when changing from a reclining to an upright posture. For, this reason, the use of ganglion blockers has been abandoned, and clinically, they are of historical interest only. In addition, more effective remedies for this condition are now available which do not have this side-effect. The structures of some typical ganglion-blocking drugs are shown in Figure 6.5.

Tetraethylammonium (TEA) (Figure 6.5a)

This is similar in structure to TMA (see Figure 6.5a). It is a specific antagonist at nicotinic receptors in autonomic ganglia and in the adrenal medulla, with little effect on the neuromuscular junction. However, it is poorly absorbed when taken orally and has a very short duration of action, making it unsuitable for clinical use.

It is interesting that substitution of the methyl groups on the TMA molecule (Figure 6.4b) with ethyl (Figure 6.5a) changes the pharmacological activity from stimulation (depolarization) to competitive antagonism.

Hexamethonium (Figure 6.5b)

This was the first ganglion blocker to be used successfully in the treatment of hypertension. In structure it resembles decamethonium (see Chapter 5) but has a 6-carbon chain separating the two quaternary nitrogen atoms instead of 10 (compare Figures 5.4a and 6.5b). This length of the methylene chain (i.e. six carbon atoms) is optimal for maximum ganglion-blocking activity, whereas decamethonium has the optimal chain length (ten carbon atoms) for maximum activity at the neuromuscular junction. However, decamethonium produces a depolarizing block whereas hexamethonium produces no initial stimulation, i.e. it is a competitive antagonist. The differences in the activity of these two drugs point to important differences in the nature of the receptors for acetylcholine at the two sites, i.e. ganglia and the neuromuscular junction (see above).

Hexamethonium is more potent than TEA and has a longer duration of action but, like TEA, it is poorly absorbed from the GI tract. These drugs will also cause a blockade of transmission at parasympathetic ganglia and this can lead to the appearance of unwanted effects, similar to those produced by the muscarinic antagonist, atropine (see Chapter 7), such as a reduction in intestinal motility, urinary retention, reduction in secretions and blurring of vision.

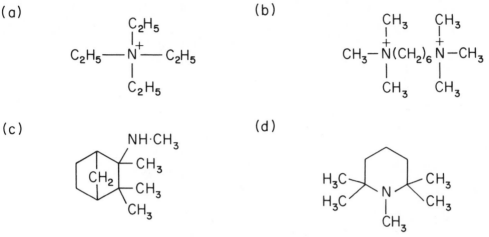

Figure 6.5 The chemical structures of (a) tetraethylammonium (TEA), (b) hexamethonium, (c) mecamyl-amine and (d) pempidine

Mecamylamine (Figure 6.5c)

This was developed as an orally active hypotensive agent which does not contain a quaternary nitrogen atom. It is well absorbed when given by mouth and has a relatively long duration of action (up to 12 h). In addition to the usual spectrum of side-effects, because of the absence of the quaternary nitrogen, this drug will penetrate into the CNS and can cause unpleasant central effects, e.g. tremor and even psychotic symptoms.

Pempidine (Figure 6.5d)

This is very similar to mecamylamine in its properties but has a shorter duration of action and this is thought to account for a reduced incidence of effects on the CNS.

Both mecamylamine and pempidine are non-competitive ganglion blockers.

Chapter 7

Drugs affecting the parasympathetic system

Transmission at parasympathetic ganglia has been discussed in Chapter 6. It is mediated by acetylcholine and is nicotinic in nature. Acetylcholine is the transmitter released by all postganglionic parasympathetic nerves (see Figures 4.1 and 7.1a). It is also the transmitter released by a few postganglionic sympathetic nerves (i.e. those that innervate sweat glands and the smooth muscle walls of blood vessels in skeletal muscle). All other postganglionic sympathetic nerves release noradrenaline (see Chapter 8).

The actions of acetylcholine released from postganglionic nerve endings are mimicked by the alkaloid muscarine (Figure 7.1b) and are antagonized by atropine, a competitive antagonist of acetylcholine at 'muscarinic' junctions. Acetylcholine produces effects at muscarinic receptors in much smaller concentrations than are needed for nicotinic stimulation, and it does so by combining with a 'muscarinic receptor which has different properties to those of the nicotinic receptor. Thus, whereas a two-point interaction appears to be satisfactory for the binding of nicotinic agonists (see Figure 4.6), which in general lack stereospecificity for the nicotinic receptor, in the case of the muscarinic receptor a third point of interaction is needed to account for the high degree of stereoselectivity of muscarinic agonists. This third binding site is thought to be the methyl group, corresponding to the acetyl methyl in acetylcholine, and which is present in potent muscarinic agonists. The reason why acetylcholine can act at both nicotinic and muscarinic receptors is probably the fact that the acetylcholine molecule is relatively flexible and can assume different conformations. Nicotine and muscarine, and related agonists, contain ring systems and therefore have more rigid structures, thus limiting the range of receptor conformations with which they can interact, and hence the range of pharmacological activity.

The arrangement of postganglionic parasympathetic nerve endings on the effector organs that they innervate (mainly smooth muscle and glands) is anatomi-

(a)

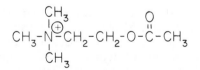

(b)

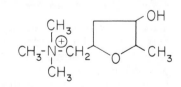

Figure 7.1 The chemical structures of (a) acetylcholine and (b) muscarine

69

cally quite different from the arrangement in ganglia or at the neuromuscular junction. Furthermore, although acetylcholine released from the presynaptic nerve terminals is excitatory at some sites, causing smooth muscle to contract (e.g. intestine, bladder detrusor muscle, bronchioles, etc), at others it is inhibitory (sphincters, heart muscle, blood vessels, etc). In addition, the response may be graded rather than being 'all-or-none', and the events may take seconds, compared with a duration of milliseconds for comparable events at the neuromuscular junction. In some organs the ratio of pre- to postganglionic parasympathetic fibres may be 1:1, but for others (e.g. Auerbach's plexus), it can be as high as 1:8000.

There is evidence for the existence of more than one type of muscarinic receptor and so far two subtypes, designated as M_1 and M_2, have been identified. If, as has been suggested, the relative distribution of these receptor subtypes varies in different tissues, then it should be possible to develop drugs with selective actions at these sites. This appears, in fact, to be the case although most of the evidence for the selective agonists and antagonists at subtypes of muscarinic receptors has come from binding studies *in vitro*. However, one drug, pirenzepine, with such a selective action is now in use.

Drugs mimicking parasympathetic stimulation

These are often called 'parasympathomimetic' drugs, which strictly should also include ganglion stimulants, but the term is usually confined to muscarinic agonists acting at the junctions formed by postganglionic parasympathetic nerve terminals. Acetylcholine itself, of course, will stimulate muscarinic receptors, but it is rarely used as a drug, partly because the effects will be widespread but mainly because any effects produced will be extremely transient due to the rapid hydrolysis of acetylcholine by cholinesterases. However, acetylcholine can be used to produce miosis when applied directly to the eye (see below). Substitution on the acetylcholine molecule results in drugs which are resistant to the action of cholinesterases and also which are, in the main, muscarinic agonists.

Methacholine (acetyl β-methylcholine) (Figure 7.2a)

This differs from acetylcholine in having a methyl group on the β-carbon atom. The potency at muscarinic receptors is relatively unchanged but nicotinic actions are almost absent. In addition, methacholine is only slowly hydrolysed by acetylcholinesterase and is virtually unaffected by other, less specific, cholinesterases in plasma and other tissues. Thus, methacholine has more prolonged actions than acetylcholine and is fairly specific for muscarinic receptors.

Carbachol (carbamoylcholine) (Figure 7.2b)

This is derived from acetylcholine by the substitution of an amide group on the acyl carbon atom. This renders carbachol immune to hydrolysis by cholinesterases and reduces the nicotinic but not the muscarinic potency. Carbachol is therefore a potent muscarinic stimulant, with a long duration of action, and it is active when taken orally. Its nicotinic effects, although less than those of acetylcholine, are more pronounced than those of other parasympathomimetic stimulants.

(a) 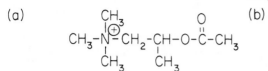 (b)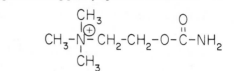

(c)

$CH_3-N^{\oplus}(CH_3)-CH_2-CH(CH_3)-O-C(=O)-NH_2$

Figure 7.2 Parasympathetic stimulants: (a) methacholine, (b) carbachol and (c) bethanechol

Bethanechol (carbamoylmethylcholine) (Figure 7.2c)

This drug combines the amide group of carbachol and the β-methyl substitution of methacholine. Both substitutions combine to reduce the nicotinic potency and render bethanechol immune to hydrolysis by cholinesterases. It is therefore a long-acting muscarinic stimulant, almost devoid of nicotinic activity.

Pilocarpine (Figure 7.3a)

This naturally occurring alkaloid is present in the leaflets of S. American shrubs of the genus *Pilocarpus*. Pilocarpine is a potent muscarinic stimulant with relatively weak nicotinic activity. It is a particularly potent stimulant of glandular tissue such as sweat and salivary glands. Hence the leaves of *Pilocarpus* shrubs were chewed to produce salivation.

Muscarine (Figure 7.1b)

Also an alkaloid, muscarine is present in the poisonous fungus *Amanita muscaria*. It is the prototype parasympathomimetic drug and has no nicotinic activity. Apart from peripheral effects due to stimulation of muscarinic receptors, it also has stimulant effects on the CNS.

(a)

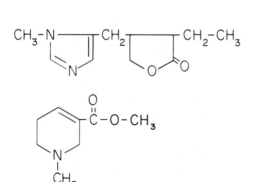

Figure 7.3 Muscarinic agonists: (a) pilocarpine; (b) arecoline

Arecoline **(Figure 7.3b)**

This alkaloid is present in betel nuts, which are the seeds of the plant *Arecha catechu*. Betel is chewed habitually in parts of Asia to promote salivary secretion and to aid digestion. However, there may also be some central stimulation.

The pharmacological actions of muscarinic agonists

In general the actions of muscarinic agonist drugs mimic the effects of stimulation of parasympathetic postganglionic nerves, although there are some minor differences between the actions of the different drugs. The effects are widespread throughout the body due to the large number of organs which receive an innervation through postganglionic parasympathetic nerves (see Figure 6.2). These are the actions of acetylcholine which predominate when it is administered to an animal. They are summarized in Table 7.1 and can be considered under the following headings: (1) effects on smooth muscle (other than blood vessels); (2) effects on the eye; (3) effects on glands, and (4) cardiovascular effects.

Table 7.1 Responses to stimulation of parasympathetic nerves

Effector organ	*Response*
Eye	
Sphincter muscle of iris	Contraction (miosis)
Ciliary muscle	Accommodation for near vision
Heart	
S-A node	Decrease in rate
Atria	Decrease in contractility
A-V node	Decrease in conduction velocity
Blood vessels	
Arterioles*	Dilatation
Lungs	
Bronchial muscle	Contraction (bronchoconstriction)
Bronchial glands	Stimulation (secretion)
GI tract	
Motility and tone	Increased
Sphincters	Relaxation
Secretion	Stimulation
Urinary bladder	
Detrusor muscle	Contraction
Trigone and sphincter	Relaxation
Uterus	Contraction in some species
Glands	
Salivary, lachrymal	Increased secretion
Sweat**	Increased secretion

* Mostly not innervated
** Part of the sympathetic system, not innervated

Effects on smooth muscle

Smooth muscles, other than those of blood vessels, which receive a parasympathetic innervation (see Figure 6.2), are those of the GI tract, urinogenital tract, respiratory tract and muscles of the eye, all of which contract in response to acetylcholine released from the postganglionic nerve endings. The actions of acetylcholine in causing the contraction of smooth muscle appear to be similar to those which cause contraction of skeletal muscle, i.e. at the neuromuscular junction. However, much less is known about the actions of acetylcholine at junctions on smooth muscle and no organized endplate appears to be present at such junctions, the nerves ramifying widely over the smooth muscle fibres. Nevertheless, acetylcholine produces changes in the permeability of the postjunctional muscle membrane, associated with increased permeability to Na^+ and K^+ ions, and this results in depolarization, the production of action potentials in the muscle fibre and activation of the contractile mechanism.

Stimulation of the smooth muscle of the GI tract leads to contraction of the walls of the gut and relaxation of the sphincters. In general the effects are increased tone and motility (increased peristaltic movements), together with increased secretion (see 'Effects on glands' below). Stimulation of the smooth muscle of the bladder results in contraction of the detrusor muscle and relaxation of the trigone and sphincter muscles. Overstimulation by muscarinic agonists or by parasympathetic stimulation will result in defaecation and voiding of the bladder.

An increase in the frequency of contraction of the uterus may occur in many species in response to administration of muscarinic agonists, although the sensitivity of the uterus to acetylcholine decreases during pregnancy. However, the human uterus is relatively insensitive to acetylcholine.

Stimulation of the smooth muscle of the respiratory tract (bronchi and bronchioles) can cause bronchoconstriction, which, with increased secretion of mucus from the bronchial glands (see 'Effects on glands' below), can be undesirable, particularly where there may be a history of respiratory problems or a susceptibility to asthma.

Effects on the eye

Parasympathetic postganglionic fibres innervate the sphincter muscle of the iris as well as the ciliary muscle which regulates the shape of the lens for accommodation (Figure 7.4). When these nerves are stimulated, or a muscarinic agonist or acetylcholine is administered, the sphincter muscle contracts and the pupil becomes smaller (miosis). In addition, the ciliary muscle contracts and this in turn leads to relaxation of the suspensory ligaments of the lens which becomes more convex or adjusted for near vision. An important secondary effect of these actions is that when the sphincter muscle of the iris contracts, the canal of Schlemm is less obstructed mechanically and this allows for better drainage of the intraocular fluid from the anterior chamber (see Figure 7.4). This action is utilized in the treatment of glaucoma in which a raised intra-ocular pressure occurs (see below).

Effects on glands

Muscarinic agonists and acetylcholine stimulate increased secretion from exocrine glands of the digestive and respiratory systems. Thus, there is increased lachrymation and salivation, as well as increased secretion of mucus from bronchial

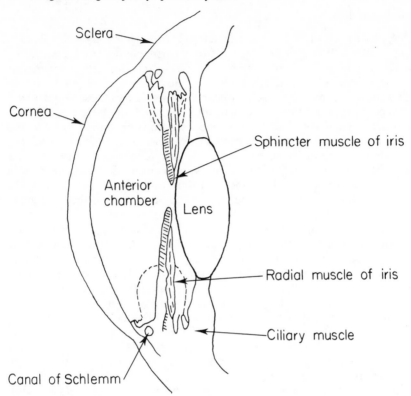

Figure 7.4 The structures in the eye referred to in the text. The ciliary muscle and the sphincter muscle of the iris are innervated by parasympathetic fibres from the oculomotor (IIIrd cranial) nerve and the radial muscle of the iris by sympathetic fibres from the superior cervical ganglion (see Figures 6.1 and 6.2)

glands and increased activity of parietal glands in the stomach and of enzyme-secreting glands in the intestine. Profuse salivation is a sign of overstimulation of the parasympathetic system.

The sweat glands in the skin also respond to muscarinic stimulation although these are innervated by the sympathetic system (see Figure 4.1 and Chapter 8).

Cardiovascular effects

Acetylcholine has three main effects on the cardiovascular system, all of which appear to be mediated by muscarinic receptors: they are vasodilatation, a decrease in cardiac rate (negative chronotropic effect) and a decrease in the force of cardiac contraction (negative inotropic effect). Muscarinic agonists cause dilatation of most vascular beds although few of these are innervated by postganglionic parasympathetic nerves. The action appears to be related to muscarinic receptors in the endothelial cells of vascular smooth muscle which are not innervated by the autonomic nervous system.

The vagus nerve, which is a parasympathetic nerve, innervates the S-A (sinu-atrial) and A-V (atrioventricular) nodes of the atrial muscle, whereas parasympathetic innervation of the ventricular muscle is sparse. When the vagus is stimulated, acetylcholine is released to act on muscarinic receptors in the heart and there is a selective increase in the permeability of the S-A pacemaker cells and the A-V nodal tissue to K^+. This increased permeability leads to hyperpolarization and a decrease in the rate of discharge of the S-A node, together with a decrease in the rate of conduction of impulses through the A-V node. Thus, there is a slowing of the heart rate and sufficiently intense vagal stimulation can result in heart block. Muscarinic agonists produce similar effects. The decreased force of contraction is due to the action of acetylcholine, or a muscarinic agonist, on the atrial muscle. This overall decrease in myocardial activity, i.e. decreased rate and decreased force of contraction, is associated with reduced oxygen demand by the heart and, together with the peripheral vasodilatation, leads to a fall in blood pressure accompanied by bradycardia. However, the effects may be partially obscured by the release of catecholamines and compensatory effects through baroreceptor and other reflexes.

The clinical uses of muscarinic agonists

Acetylcholine is rarely used as a drug for the reasons already given, except as an intra-ocular solution (1% solution with 3% mannitol) where rapid short-lasting miosis is required, e.g. in corneal grafting operations. Carbachol and bethanechol are the only muscarinic agonist drugs to be used systemically for their actions on the GI tract and urinary bladder. They may be used to relieve postoperative urinary retention and gastric atony after vagotomy. Side-effects may occur due to parasympathetic stimulation and these may include nausea, vomiting, sweating, blurred vision, bradycardia and intestinal colic. Due to the bronchoconstriction produced, these drugs are contra-indicated in patients with asthmatic conditions or other respiratory problems. Methacholine has been used in the treatment of atropine poisoning or belladonna intoxication but is no longer used clinically and physostigmine is preferred to counteract the parasympathetic effects associated with atropine poisoning or overdose with tricyclic antidepressant drugs (see Chapter 18).

As all muscarinic agonists produce miosis, they are useful for relieving the raised intra-ocular pressure which occurs in glaucoma. However, of the drugs available, pilocarpine or carbachol are mainly used, sometimes in combination with the anticholinesterase, physostigmine.

Muscarinic antagonists

These are drugs which block the actions of acetylcholine at muscarinic sites and also the effects of muscarinic agonists, by competitive antagonism. They also tend to block responses evoked by stimulation of parasympathetic nerves and are therefore sometimes called 'parasympatholytic' drugs. However, this term is incorrect as the drugs have no direct action on the nerves. Furthermore, because they block the muscarinic actions of acetylcholine at sites other than postganglionic parasympathetic nerve terminals, more appropriate terms are 'antimuscarinic' or 'muscarinic cholinergic blocking' drugs. As atropine is the prototype, they are sometimes called 'atropine-like' drugs.

In general, these drugs have little effect on the actions of acetylcholine at nicotinic receptors. Thus, large doses of atropine are needed to cause any blocking of ganglionic transmission and the effect may be due, at least in part, to the presence of muscarinic receptors on autonomic ganglia (see Chapter 6). The doses needed to produce any blockade of the effects of stimulation of parasympathetic nerves are usually larger than those needed to antagonize the effects of acetylcholine or of muscarinic agonists (see below).

Atropine (Figure 7.5a)

This is the prototype antimuscarinic drug and is a naturally occurring alkaloid which is present in Solanaceae plants, the best-known of which is the deadly nightshade, *Atropa belladonna*. However, atropine is also found in a number of other plants. Its actions have been known for many centuries and, in the Middle Ages, it was popular as a poison. Chemically, atropine consists of a racemic mixture of (+)- and (−)-hyoscyamine, of which the (−)-isomer is the more potent. However, the racemic form (atropine) is used because the (−)-isomer racemizes in solution. Atropine has also been synthesized.

Atropine is a tertiary amine and readily crosses the blood–brain barrier; it therefore produces effects in the CNS (see below). However, its quaternary ammonium analogue, *N*-methylatropine or atropine methyl-nitrate, does not penetrate into the CNS and can be used where central effects need to be avoided. The quaternary ammonium derivatives of atropine and of related atropine-like drugs lose some of their selectivity for muscarinic receptors and may interfere with ganglionic or neuromuscular transmission in doses which produce the muscarinic blockade.

Hyoscine (Figure 7.5b)

This is also known as scopolamine, which is (−)-hyoscine, and is a naturally occurring alkaloid found in the shrub, black henbane (*Hyocyamus niger*), and is similar in structure to atropine (see Figure 7.5a). The peripheral antimuscarinic actions of hyoscine are similar to those of atropine although it is more potent in some respects (see below). However, the two drugs differ markedly in their actions on the CNS.

Homatropine (Figure 7.5c)

This is one of the large number of synthetic or semisynthetic atropine-like drugs that has been made in an attempt to produce selectivity for those functions under parasympathetic control which might profitably be blocked in various diseases, e.g. actions on the GI tract and the eye. Like atropine, it is a tertiary amine and can therefore produce central effects. It resembles atropine in its pharmacological properties but is less potent and has a shorter duration of action.

Propantheline (Figure 7.5d)

This is an example of a synthetic quaternary ammonium muscarinic-blocking drug. It has potent peripheral antimuscarinic actions but, as it does not penetrate the blood–brain barrier, it lacks central actions.

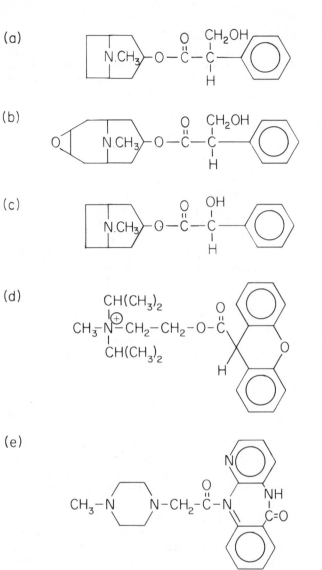

Figure 7.5 Muscarinic antagonists: (a) atropine, (b) hyoscine, (c) homatropine, (d) propantheline and (e) pirenzepine

Pirenzepine (Figure 7.5e)

This is a tricyclic compound that does not cross the blood–brain barrier and therefore has no central actions. Whereas most antimuscarinic drugs are equally effective at all muscarinic receptors, pirenzepine is an example of an antagonist with selective actions at the M_1 subtype of muscarinic receptor. Thus, pirenzepine has been shown to reduce gastric secretion in doses which do not have appreciable effects on the receptors in other organs, e.g. the eye and heart (see below).

The pharmacological actions of antimuscarinic drugs

In general, the effects produced by muscarinic antagonists are the opposite of those of the muscarinic agonists discussed above, i.e. dilatation of the pupil and loss of the ability to focus for near vision, reduced secretions, reduced tone and motility of the gut and tachycardia. However, in view of the importance of these actions and the fact that some of them are utilized clinically, they are discussed here in detail.

The gastrointestinal tract

Gastrointestinal movements and the tone of intestinal smooth muscle, which are increased by acetylcholine and muscarinic agonists, are correspondingly reduced by atropine and other muscarinic-blocking drugs. However, although responses to acetylcholine and muscarinic agonists are completely blocked, atropine does not abolish responses mediated by the vagus nerve. The reason for this discrepancy in the action of atropine is not known, although one possible explanation is that, as the motility of the gut is controlled by a complex system of intramural nerve plexuses, influences from the CNS (i.e. via the vagus) may perhaps only modify or modulate the effects of the intrinsic reflexes and cannot block them completely. Other explanations, e.g. that a transmitter other than acetylcholine or other mediator substances are involved, are also possible. Nevertheless, both in normal subjects and in patients with gastrointestinal disease, adequate doses of muscarinic-blocking drugs produce marked inhibitory effects on the motor activity of the stomach and intestine, characterized by a decrease in tone and a decrease in the amplitude and frequency of peristaltic contractions.

Secretions

All glands that are stimulated by cholinergic nerves are affected by muscarinic antagonists. Thus, the flow of saliva is considerably reduced, the mouth becomes dry, and swallowing and talking may become difficult. The secretion of mucus from glands lining the respiratory tract is reduced and drying of the mucous membranes of the mouth, nose, pharynx and bronchi occurs. Lachrymation is also reduced and, in addition, sweating which is under the control of cholinergic nerve fibres of the sympathetic system (see Chapter 8), is suppressed and the skin becomes hot and dry. Muscarinic-blocking drugs do not affect gastric secretion, unless given in large doses, in spite of the fact that the activity of the acid-secreting cells of the gastric mucosa is increased by vagal stimulation. Nevertheless, these drugs have been used to reduce gastric secretion (see below).

The eye

Atropine and related drugs block the responses of the sphincter muscle of the iris and the ciliary muscle of the lens (see Figure 7.4). Thus, the pupil is dilated (mydriasis) and accommodation is paralysed (cycloplegia) with the lens focused for distant vision. The normal reflex constriction of the pupil in response to light is abolished and this distinguishes the mydriasis produced by atropine from that caused by sympathomimetic amines (Chapter 8). The intra-ocular pressure is little affected when it is normal initially. However, when the intra-ocular pressure is already raised, for example in older people, the contraction of the iris back into the anterior chamber of the eye blocks the drainage of the intra-ocular fluid and may precipitate an attack of glaucoma in patients in whom it has not previously been detected. Conventional doses of atropine (i.e. less than 1.0 mg) have little effect on the eye although hyoscine, in equivalent doses, will produce mydriasis and loss of accommodation. However, local application of atropine or hyoscine to the eye produces ocular effects of long duration, and accommodation and pupillary reflexes may not recover in full for a week or more.

Cardiovascular effects

The main effect of atropine on the heart is to alter rate. With small doses (0.5–1.0 mg) there is initially a transient decrease in heart rate. This is attributed to a central action of the drug, stimulating vagal centres in the medulla. However, the effect is usually only slight and the main effect of atropine, especially when larger doses (2 mg or more) are used, is to produce tachycardia, by blocking the inhibitory influence of the vagus nerve on the heart. There is considerable individual variation in the degree of tachycardia produced by atropine, depending upon the resting level of parasympathetic activity ('vagal tone'). The tachycardia is more pronounced in healthy young adults, where vagal tone is high, and less in young children and old people in whom vagal tone is low. With hyoscine the initial bradycardia persists and, even with large doses, hyoscine does not cause tachycardia. The reason for this is not known.

The changes in heart rate produced by antimuscarinic drugs do not have any appreciable effect on arterial blood pressure due to the operation of cardiovascular reflexes which maintain cardiac output at a constant level. Similarly, these drugs have negligible effects on peripheral blood vessels, due to the absence of parasympathetic innervation, while the cholinergic innervation of blood vessels in skeletal muscle via sympathetic fibres does not appear to be involved to any great extent in the regulation of tone and the vasodilatation in exercised muscles is caused by the release of metabolites as a result of muscular activity.

Other smooth muscle

The smooth muscle of the bronchi and bronchioles is relaxed by atropine and related drugs and this results in a widening of the airway. The detrusor muscle of the bladder is relaxed but contractions of the bladder due to parasympathetic nerve stimulation are only partially blocked. Effects on the human uterus are negligible and, although the bile duct and gallbladder are slightly relaxed, this effect is not sufficient to justify the use of atropine as a biliary antispasmodic.

Central effects

Both atropine and hyoscine penetrate the blood–brain barrier and therefore produce effects in the CNS. However, whereas the central effects of atropine are stimulant, those of hyoscine are depressant. In the dose range usually used in man (0.5–1.0 mg), the signs of central stimulation with atropine are slight, although slight stimulation of respiration may occur. The relative contribution to this effect of central vagal stimulation and bronchiolar dilatation which, by increasing the 'dead space' will stimulate respiration, is not known. Large doses of atropine cause restlessness, irritability, disorientation, hallucinations and delirium (see atropine poisoning below). In contrast, hyoscine in normal therapeutic doses causes drowsiness and sedation. The sedative action of hyoscine is often accompanied by amnesia and euphoria, effects which are sometimes utilized clinically (see below) and have led to its use as a so-called 'truth drug'. In overdose, the actions of hyoscine on the CNS are stimulant and resemble those of atropine overdose.

Certain antimuscarinic drugs with central actions are used in the treatment of Parkinson's disease and others, including hyoscine, for their anti-emetic effects. These actions are discussed in Chapters 19 and 20.

The clinical uses of muscarinic antagonists

Antimuscarinic drugs have been used for a wide variety of clinical conditions, predominantly to depress the control of effectors by the activity of the parasympathetic branch of the autonomic nervous system. However, the absence of drugs with selective actions on the muscarinic receptors of different organs, or organ systems, results in the therapeutic responses often being accompanied by side-effects. This limits the usefulness of these drugs, at least when they are administered systemically. The discovery of the existence of subtypes of muscarinic receptors, already referred to, and the development of selective agonists and antagonists for these receptor subtypes, should lead eventually to the development of more selective, and therefore more effective, drugs in this area.

The gastrointestinal tract

The principal uses for antimuscarinic drugs have been in the treatment of peptic ulcer and for reducing hypermotility of the gut. All muscarinic antagonists reduce gastric secretion and gastric motility, but the doses required to produce these effects are usually associated with pronounced side-effects. The synthetic or semisynthetic quaternary compounds, such as propantheline, are preferred in order to avoid effects on the CNS. Unfortunately, these drugs are poorly absorbed when given orally and large doses are required to reduce gastric secretion effectively. Peripheral side-effects, such as dry mouth, blurred vision (due to loss of accommodation) and urinary retention, occur frequently. The advent of alternative forms of treatment for gastric ulcer, i.e. histamine H_2 antagonists, has resulted in muscarinic antagonists being less frequently used for the treatment of peptic ulcer. The exception to this is the drug pirenzepine (Figure 7.5e) which is a relatively selective antagonist at M_1 muscarinic receptors. This, drug, apart from being a useful tool in the classification of subtypes of muscarinic receptors, can be used to depress gastric secretion without producing a significant level of side-effects and, as it does not cross the blood–brain barrier, it produces no effects on the CNS.

Antimuscarinic drugs are used as antispasmodics to prevent the spasm of intestinal smooth muscle which occurs in colic. However, these drugs are effective only when the cause of the spasm is, in fact, due to excessive contraction of the smooth muscle of the gut.

Ophthalmology

When muscarinic antagonist drugs are administered locally, either in the form of eye drops or as an ointment, their effects will be mainly localized to the eye. Side-effects are less likely to occur and these drugs are therefore useful in ophthalmology: for example, examination of the retina is facilitated by mydriasis. The drugs are also used to produce cycloplegia (loss of accommodation) and they are used in the treatment of iritis and uveitis to prevent the development of adhesions between the iris and the lens. Full recovery from the effects of atropine, infused into the eye, may take up to 7 days or more and there is a risk of side-effects developing. Shorter-acting antimuscarinics, such as homatropine which has a duration of action of up to 24 hours, are therefore preferred, unless prolonged mydriasis and cycloplegia are required. However, mydriasis of short duration, i.e. of a few hours, can be conveniently produced with a sympathomimetic drug (see Chapter 8).

Prolonged mydriasis may precipitate an attack of acute narrow-angle glaucoma in patients who are predisposed to this condition, but who may not have shown any signs previously. Therefore, again, shorter-acting drugs are to be preferred.

Anaesthesia

Because of the reduction in secretions produced by antimuscarinic drugs, especially of salivary and bronchial secretions, they have been used in the premedication given before the administration of surgical anaesthesia. This use of the drugs was particularly important when inhalation anaesthetics such as ether were used, as the latter are irritant and cause a marked increase in bronchial secretion. With the replacement of ether by non-irritant gaseous anaesthetics such as halothane, premedication with antimuscarinics has become less important, although the prevention of bradycardia and hypotension produced by halothane is also important. Atropine is the most commonly used antimuscarinic drug for premedication, although hyoscine is sometime used because, as well as drying up secretions, it produces amnesia due to its central sedative action.

As mentioned in Chapter 5, atropine is given at the same time as neostigmine when the latter is used to terminate or reverse the paralysis produced by tubocurarine. The atropine is needed to prevent the stimulation of muscarinic receptors, e.g. in the heart, by neostigmine.

Central actions

Certain antimuscarinic drugs are used in the treatment of Parkinson's disease. They are also effective in the relief of motion sickness. Both of these actions relate to antimuscarinic actions in the brain and are dealt with in Chapters 19 and 20.

The use of hyoscine as a 'truth' drug has already been referred to.

Other uses

Because of the bronchial dilatation which they produce, antimuscarinic drugs were at one time used in the treatment of bronchial asthma. However, they have now largely been replaced by selective sympathomimetic drugs (see Chapter 8) which are more effective and possess fewer side-effects. However, one antimuscarinic drug, ipratropium, which is administered by aerosol, is effective, particularly in bronchoconstriction where there is obstruction of the airway, e.g. in chronic bronchitis. Ipratropium has been claimed to produce few side-effects.

The cardiovascular actions of the antimuscarinic drugs have few clinical applications, except for the occasional use of atropine to relieve bradycardia after myocardial infarction in selected cases and to reduce bradycardia in rare cases of hyperactive carotid sinus reflexes.

Large doses of atropine are used in cases of cholinergic poisoning, e.g. by anticholinesterase organophosphorous insecticides or nerve gases. A drug which crosses the blood–brain barrier is preferred for this purpose because it is necessary to counteract the central, as well as the peripheral effects of the anticholinesterase. An enzyme-reactivating agent, such as pralidoxime (see Chapter 5) is usually given concurrently. Atropine is a useful antidote for mushroom poisoning of the so-called 'rapid type', caused by the ingestion of muscarine found in *Amanita muscaria* and some other fungi.

Atropine poisoning

Because of the presence of atropine and related atropine-like alkaloids in many plants, poisoning by belladonna alkaloids, either by deliberate or accidental ingestion), is not uncommon. The symptoms are those to be expected from the blocking of parasympathetic influences, i.e. extreme dryness of the mouth and thirst, dilatation of the pupils and photophobia, blurring of vision, increased heart rate, difficulty in micturition and constipation. There is also a marked hyper-pyrexia, or rise in body temperature, which is accentuated by the absence of sweating. With large doses there may be difficulty in speech, palpitations, rapid breathing, restlessness, confusion, excitement, hallucinations and delirium. Convulsions, followed by coma, may occur in extreme cases. Treatment, apart from the removal of any remaining drug from the stomach, consists of intravenous administration of physostigmine, which, because it penetrates the blood–brain barrier will reverse both the central and peripheral effects of atropine.

A striking feature of poisoning or overdose with atropine is flushing of the skin ('atropine flush'). The skin becomes hot and dry because of decreased secretion of sweat – an antimuscarinic action – but the flush is mainly due to vasodilatation of the superficial blood vessels of the skin of the neck and face. This effect is apparently not related to the muscarinic antagonist action of atropine and is at present unexplained.

Chapter 8

Drugs affecting the sympathetic system

In the parasympathetic branch of the autonomic nervous system, acetylcholine is the transmitter released from both pre- and postganglionic nerve terminals, although the actions of acetylcholine are different at the postsynaptic and post-junctional receptors. However, in the sympathetic branch, although acetylcholine is the transmitter in the ganglia, the catecholamine noradrenaline is released from the majority of postganglionic nerve terminals. In addition, there is the adrenal medulla, which is homologous with sympathetic ganglia, and which releases a mixture of adrenaline and noradrenaline into the bloodstream.

Noradrenaline, like adrenaline, is a catecholamine (Figure 8.1). At one time it was thought that the transmitter at postganglionic sympathetic nerve endings was

(a)

(b)

HO —⟨⟩— CH.CH$_2$.NH$_2$
HO   OH

(c)

HO —⟨⟩— CH.CH$_2$.NH.CH$_3$
HO   OH

(d)

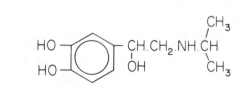

Figure 8.1 The chemical structure of (a) catechol, (b) noradrenaline, (c) adrenaline and (d) isoprenaline

adrenaline, and not noradrenaline, or even that both substances were transmitters at different sites. This concept was supported by the fact that stimulation of sympathetic nerves was found to cause stimulation at some sites and inhibition at others, and that the responses showed some differential sensitivity to adrenaline and noradrenaline. However, this hypothesis was abandoned after it was found that noradrenaline was the predominant catecholamine in peripheral tissues and sympathetic nerves, and that the differences in the responses at different sites could be attributed to different properties of the receptors (see 'Receptors for catecholamines', below). Nevertheless, the term 'adrenergic' is often still applied in a global way to include the 'noradrenergic' system.

Noradrenergic transmission

The synthesis of noradrenaline

Noradrenaline is synthesized from the amino acid precursor, L-tyrosine, which is a constituent of diet. The synthetic pathway is common to all catecholamines and occurs in the chromaffin cells of the adrenal medulla, in sympathetic nerves and ganglia and in the brain. In mammals, tyrosine can be derived from phenylalanine, which is also present in the diet, by the action of an enzyme, phenylalanine hydroxylase, which is found in the liver. As this reaction takes place outside the nervous system, the starting point for the synthesis of catecholamines is usually taken to be L-tyrosine. This substance is present in the bloodstream and is taken up into sympathetic postganglionic nerves by an active transport process. The first step in the synthesis is hydroxylation of the L-tyrosine to 3,4-dihydroxyphenylalanine (L-dopa) (Figure 8.2) by the enzyme tyrosine hydroxylase. This enzyme is a unique constituent of catecholamine-containing neurones of both the peripheral and central nervous system, and is also found in the chromaffin cells of the adrenal medulla. Tyrosine hydroxylase, together with L-aromatic amino acid decarboxylase (or dopa decarboxylase), which regulates the next stage in the synthesis, is present in the cytoplasm of noradrenergic nerve terminals. Tyrosine hydroxylase is stereospecific and converts only the naturally occurring substrate, L-tyrosine and not D-tyrosine; it is also to a large extent substrate specific and does not convert tyramine or L-tryptophan. The enzyme requires a cofactor, tetrahydropteridine, together with molecular oxygen and ferrous ions (Fe^{2+}) for its activity. The action of tyrosine hydroxylase is the rate-limiting step in the synthesis of noradrenaline, the activity of the enzyme being regulated by the concentration of the end product. Thus, large concentrations of noradrenaline in the nerve terminals inhibit the enzyme, so reducing the amount of noradrenaline formed. For this reason, interference with the synthesis at this stage can influence the activity of noradrenergic nerves, and drugs which act on the presynaptic receptors on these terminals have this type of action (see below).

The next two steps in the synthesis consist of decarboxylation of L-dopa to dopamine by the enzyme, dopa-decarboxylase, and the conversion of dopamine to noradrenaline by the hydroxylating enzyme, dopamine-β-hydroxylase (Figure 8.2). Dopa-decarboxylase is present in tissues other than the nervous system (e.g. liver, stomach and kidney) and requires pyridoxal phosphate (the active form of vitamin B_6) as a cofactor. It is not specific for L-dopa and will decarboxylate other substrates, particularly naturally occurring aromatic amino acids. In fact, it is probable that the role of this enzyme is not confined to the synthesis of

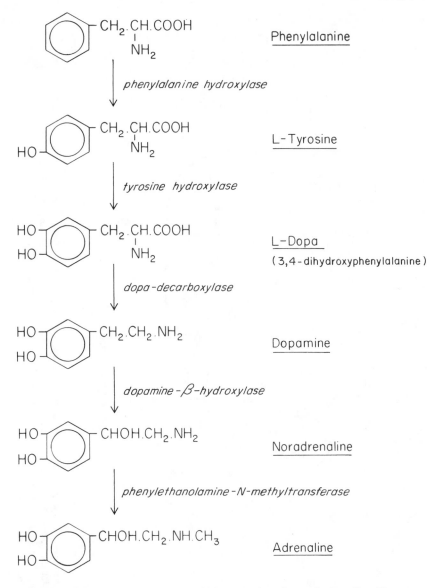

Figure 8.2 Steps in the synthesis of dopamine, noradrenaline and adrenaline. The enzymes involved at each stage are shown in italics

catecholamines. The product of the decarboxylation of L-dopa is dopamine which is itself a neurotransmitter in the brain (see Chapter 10), but peripherally, its principal role is as a precursor to noradrenaline.

Whereas both tyrosine hydroxylase and dopa-decarboxylase are mainly present in the cytoplasm of noradrenergic nerves, dopamine-β-hydroxylase is localized to the membranes of the synaptic vesicles in which the transmitter is stored (Figure 8.3). This enzyme requires ascorbic acid as a cofactor, together with molecular oxygen,

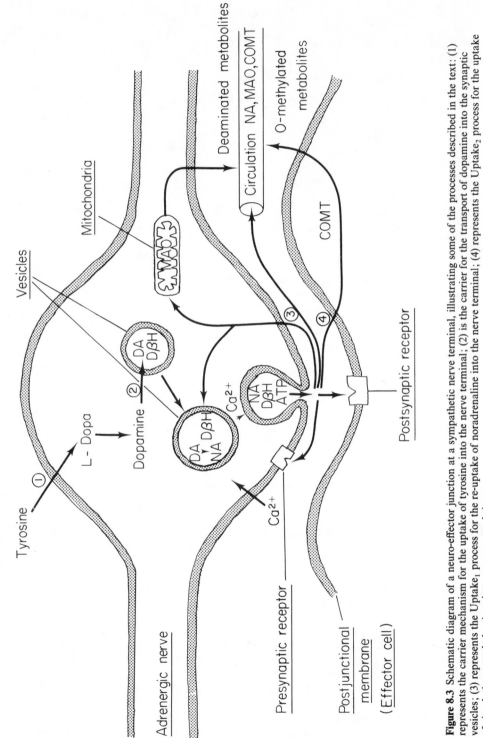

Figure 8.3 Schematic diagram of a neuro-effector junction at a sympathetic nerve terminal, illustrating some of the processes described in the text: (1) represents the carrier mechanism for the uptake of tyrosine into the nerve terminal; (2) is the carrier for the transport of dopamine into the synaptic vesicles; (3) represents the Uptake$_1$ process for the re-uptake of noradrenaline into the nerve terminal; (4) represents the Uptake$_2$ process for the uptake of circulating catecholamines into non-neuronal tissues

for its activity. It does not show a high degree of substrate specificity and will act on most phenylethylamines, converting them to the corresponding phenylethanol-amine. This can result in structurally analogous metabolites being formed, which can replace noradrenaline in the nerve endings and can be released by the same mechanisms, to function as 'false transmitters' (see page 97).

The end-product regulation of the activity of tyrosine hydroxylase, referred to above, is only one feedback process which controls the amount of neurotransmitter in noradrenergic nerve terminals in relation to the level of neuronal activity. Thus, increased activity will lead to depletion of the transmitter in the terminals and this will stimulate synthesis, whereas reduced levels of neuronal activity will cause accumulation of transmitter and this will depress synthesis. However, there are also longer-term effects which involve changes in the amount of tyrosine hydroxylase available. Prolonged neuronal activity over a period of time results in induction of the synthesis of tyrosine hydroxylase in the cell body. The enzyme then passes to the terminal region by axoplasmic flow.

The lack of specificity of the enzymes involved in the synthesis of catecholamines results in the existence of other possible pathways (see Figure 8.4), in which a number of related substances are formed: examples of these are tyramine, octopamine and synephrine, which are present in small amounts in many tissues containing adrenaline or noradrenaline. However, the amounts may be consider-ably increased when the catabolizing enzyme for the catecholamines, monoamine

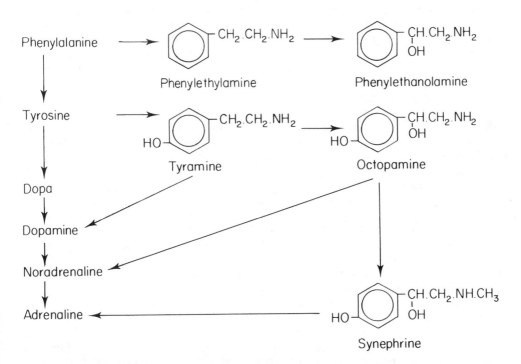

Figure 8.4 Some of the minor pathways involved in the synthesis of dopamine, noradrenaline and adrenaline. The main pathway, as in Figure 8.2, is on the left. Some of the minor products, e.g. octopamine and synephrine, are produced by the same enzymes that are involved in the main synthetic pathway

oxidase (see page 93), has been inhibited, or when large amounts of the immediate precursor have been administered. Octopamine, which is an important neurotransmitter in invertebrates, can be taken up by noradrenergic nerve terminals and acts as a false transmitter (see page 97).

The synthesis of adrenaline

In those chromaffin cells of the adrenal medulla which produce adrenaline rather than noradrenaline, there is an additional enzyme present which converts noradrenaline to adrenaline (Figure 8.2). This enzyme is phenylethanolamine-N-methyltransferase (PNMT); it is found in the cytoplasm and requires the presence of the methyl donor, S-adenosyl methionine.

The synthesis of adrenaline in the chromaffin cells is also controlled by the secretion of glucocorticoids from the adrenal cortex.

Storage and release

The noradrenaline which is synthesized in postganglionic sympathetic nerve terminals is stored in vesicles which are similar in size to those present in cholinergic nerve terminals, but which can be distinguished by their different staining characteristics when they are examined histochemically, and by their density in the electron miscroscope. Thus, the vesicles which store noradrenaline and adrenaline are dense cored whereas those which store acetylcholine are clear. In sympathetic nerve terminals the vesicles are small (0.05–0.2 μm in diameter) and also contain the nucleotide, adenosine triphosphate (ATP). Larger dense-core vesicles are present in the cell body of noradrenergic nerves and in chromaffin granules in the adrenal medulla.

As the enzyme dopamine-β-hydroxylase is localized to the vesicular membrane, it seems likely that dopamine, which is formed in the cytoplasm, then passes into the vesicles where it is converted by dopamine-β-hydroxylase to noradrenaline. The uptake of dopamine into the storage vesicles is an active transport process which requires ATP as a source of energy and magnesium ions (Mg^{2+}) to activate the enzyme ATPase. One function of the catecholamine storage vesicles, apart from providing a depot of transmitter ready to be released by the appropriate physiological stimulus, may be to protect the noradrenaline from being destroyed by the enzyme monoamine oxidase (MAO), which is present intraneuronally.

In the adrenal medulla both noradrenaline and adrenaline are stored in dense-core chromaffin granules. However, as the enzyme phenylethanolamine-N-methyltransferase is present in the cytoplasm, it seems that the noradrenaline must diffuse out of the granules in order to be converted to adrenaline in the cytoplasm and the adrenaline then re-enters the chromaffin granules.

Noradrenaline is released from the nerve terminals as a consequence of stimulation of sympathetic nerves. Furthermore, sympathetic nerves can sustain their output of transmitter over prolonged periods of stimulation, provided that the mechanisms for the synthesis and re-uptake of the transmitters are not impaired. Some of the reasons for this sustained release have been discussed above. The release process is believed to involve exocytosis, similar to that which occurs at cholinergic nerve terminals and is dependent on the presence of calcium ions (Ca^{2+}) extracellularly. There is some evidence which suggests that the more recently synthesized transmitter is released preferentially, thus leading to the concept of there being more than one pool of transmitter within the sympathetic neurone.

More is known about the release of catecholamines from the adrenal medulla. The stimulus for this is the release of acetylcholine by the preganglionic fibres and its interaction with nicotinic receptors on the chromaffin cells to produce a localized depolarization. This results in increased permeability to calcium ions which pass into the cell, mobilizing the stores of catecholamines and causing their release by exocytosis. The release of catecholamines from the chromaffin cells is accompanied by the release of ATP, chromogranins (specific proteins) and some dopamine-β-hydroxylase. In man, the catecholamines are released in the proportion 80% adrenaline and 20% noradrenaline.

Mechanisms of inactivation

Two main processes are involved in the inactivation of catecholamine neurotransmitters: (1) metabolism; (2) re-uptake.

Metabolism

The metabolism of catecholamines is a much slower process than is the hydrolysis of acetylcholine by acetylcholinesterase, the major enzymes involved being monoamine oxidase and catechol-O-methyltransferase.

Monoamine oxidase inactivates catecholamines by converting them to the corresponding inactive aldehydes which are then rapidly metabolized, usually by the enzyme aldehyde dehydrogenase, to the corresponding acid. In the case of noradrenaline and adrenaline, this is 3,4-dihydroxymandelic acid (Figure 8.5). Monoamine oxidase is widely distributed in the body, being found in almost all tissues. The largest amounts are in the liver and kidneys but it is also present in significant quantities in the intestine, brain and all parts of the sympathetic nervous system. As well as metabolizing catecholamines it also breaks down 5-hydroxytryptamine. Most of the monoamine oxidase in the nervous system is intraneuronal, where it is bound to the surface of the mitochondria (Figure 8.3). It is thought that the function of the intraneuronal monoamine oxidase is to regulate the amount of catecholamine transmitter in the cytoplasm. However, the major part of the noradrenaline which is synthesized is stored in vesicles where it is protected from the action of this enzyme. Nevertheless, the monoamine oxidase could act on catecholamines taken up by the nerve endings or released from vesicles into the cytoplasm.

Monoamine oxidase has been found to exist in two different forms that can be distinguished on the basis of differential substrate specificity and also sensitivity to inhibition by selective inhibitors. The two subtypes have been designated as MAO_A and MAO_B and appear to have a different distribution in a number of tissues. Thus, while equal amounts of both types are found in the liver and brain of most species, the human placenta contains only MAO_A and this type appears to be predominant in noradrenergic nerve terminals in the rat. On the other hand, human platelets contain only MAO_B. The physiological and pathological significance of the existence of the subtypes of monoamine oxidase is not known. Drugs which inhibit the action of monoamine oxidase are used principally for their effect on the CNS and they are discussed in Chapter 17.

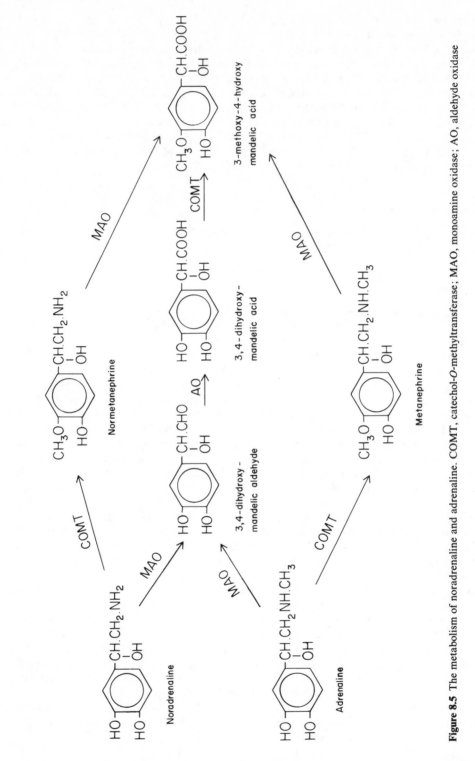

Figure 8.5 The metabolism of noradrenaline and adrenaline. COMT, catechol-*O*-methyltransferase; MAO, monoamine oxidase; AO, aldehyde oxidase

The enzyme catechol-*O*-methyltransferase (COMT) has a wide distribution in tissues and is found in the cytoplasm of many cells and also occurs extracellularly; it is not associated with membranes, however. This enzyme is not found in noradrenergic nerve terminals. The largest amounts of COMT are present in the liver and kidneys. The enzyme converts noradrenaline to normetanephrine and adrenaline to metanephrine (Figure 8.5)

It seems unlikely that COMT has any significant action on the noradrenaline released from nerve terminals. However, both the adrenaline and noradrenaline which are released into the circulation from the adrenal medulla are mainly metabolized by COMT. Monoamine oxidase and COMT seem to be able to act sequentially, the 3-methoxy compounds formed from catecholamines by the action of COMT being substrates for monoamine oxidase. Similarly, the metabolites formed by the action of monoamine oxidase can act as substrates for COMT. Thus, the breakdown of catecholamines can follow a number of different pathways and a variety of end products can be produced (Figure 8.5). Nevertheless, the metabolite of noradrenaline that is mainly excreted in the urine is 3-methoxy-4-hydroxymandelic acid.

Re-uptake mechanisms

Although metabolism by enzyme action is important for regulating the levels of catecholamines circulating in the bloodstream and of noradrenaline in the cytoplasm of sympathetic nerve terminals, it is generally accepted that the inactivation of noradrenaline, after it has been released into the synaptic cleft and produced its postsynaptic effect, is by a non-metabolic process. This process actively removes the transmitter and is known as 're-uptake'. It involves the active transport of noradrenaline against a concentration gradient and therefore requires energy. It is dependent upon the presence of sodium (Na^+) and potassium (K^+) ions and derives energy from the breakdown of ATP mediated by the enzyme Na^+-ATPase. Inhibition of this enzyme blocks the re-uptake process.

Thus, noradrenaline released into the synaptic cleft is rapidly transported back into the nerve terminal and is then taken up into the storage vesicles once again (Figure 8.3). The re-uptake process therefore serves not only to terminate the action of the released transmitter but also to conserve the supply of noradrenaline. In fact, since noradrenaline is re-used in this way, synthesis is required only in order to maintain an adequate pool of transmitter.

Uptake of noradrenaline can also take place into non-neuronal tissues, e.g. cardiac muscle and smooth muscle of the blood vessels and intestine. However, this uptake tends to occur only when there are high levels of catecholamines in the circulation, e.g. after stimulation of the adrenal medulla. These two uptake processes have been called Uptake$_1$ for uptake into neurones and Uptake$_2$ for uptake into non-neuronal tissue.

The uptake process into nerves, Uptake$_1$, is not completely specific for noradrenaline and other derivatives of phenylethylamine can be taken up. The extent to which this occurs depends upon a number of factors, one of which is the presence of substituent groups on the nitrogen atom. Thus, adrenaline is not taken up to the same extent as noradrenaline; isoprenaline (Figure 8.1d), however, is not taken up at all. On the other hand, tyramine is taken up into nerve terminals and, whereas it has little direct action of its own, it does cause the release of noradrenaline. Drugs with this type of action are known as indirectly acting sympathomimetic amines (see page 95).

Receptors for catecholamines

These are also known as 'adrenoceptors', a term used to cover both receptors for adrenaline and for noradrenaline. Not very much is known about the action of the presynaptically released noradrenaline on the postsynaptic receptor on the effector organ, which results in a physiological response. However, local application of noradrenaline mimics the effects of stimulation of sympathetic nerves and antagonists block both the effects of exogenously applied noradrenaline and of nerve stimulation. As in the case of the cholinergic system, the actions of noradrenaline released from sympathetic nerve terminals are mediated by different types of post-synaptic receptors, α- and β-receptors, which have different distributions in various tissues. The α-adrenoceptors are mainly responsible for the excitatory actions of noradrenaline and they mediate the contraction of some smooth muscles, particularly vascular smooth muscle cells, resulting in vasoconstriction, and they relax other smooth muscle (e.g. intestine). On the other hand, β-adrenoceptors mediate the actions of noradrenaline in stimulating contraction of heart muscle and relaxing smooth muscle in the bronchioles and the uterus, as well as causing vasodilatation. These two types of receptor can be readily distinguished by the potencies of the agonists. Thus, adrenaline is roughly equipotent at both types of receptor, while noradrenaline is more potent at α-receptors, and the synthetic compound isoprenaline (Figure 8.1d) is more potent at β-receptors. More important is the fact that selective antagonists with differential actions at these two receptors have been developed so that drugs are available for the control of blood pressure by regulating peripheral resistance (α-blockers) or for selective action on the heart (β-blockers). Furthermore, it is also possible to distinguish between two different types of β-receptor: β_1 is responsible for stimulation of the heart and lipolysis, and β_2 causes vasodilatation and relaxation of the smooth muscle of the respiratory tract. Again, drugs acting selectively at the two sites have important clinical applications (see 'The clinical uses of sympathomimetic drugs', below).

As well as postsynaptic α- and β-receptors, there is evidence for the existence of both receptor types on the presynaptic nerve terminal. Thus, the presynaptic α-receptor has been designated α_2 and the postsynaptic α-receptor, α_1. Drugs with selective actions at these two sites are available (see below). It is believed that the presynaptic receptors form part of a feedback circuit which controls the rate of release of noradrenaline. Thus, stimulation of the α_2-receptors by high concentrations of noradrenaline leads to a decrease in the release of noradrenaline. Conversely, presynaptic β-receptors appear to have the opposite effect as low levels of stimulation of presynaptic β_2-receptors result in the increased release of noradrenaline.

The response to stimulation of β-receptors is mediated by the formation of cyclic AMP as a second messenger (see Chapter 3), i.e. adenylate cyclase is activated by an agonist action at the receptor and catalyses the conversion of adenosine triphosphate to cyclic AMP. The contraction of smooth muscle, which is mediated by stimulation of α-adrenoceptors, appears to be correlated with an increased concentration of calcium ions. Activation of the receptor produces a change in the permeability of the cell membrane so that calcium can enter and activate the contractile mechanism. The breakdown of phosphotidylinositol in the cell membrane by the enzyme phospholipase C is thought to lead to the opening of calcium channels in the membrane (see Chapter 3). Stimulation of some α-receptors, e.g. α_2-receptors, appears to inhibit the activity of adenylate cyclase.

There are some postganglionic sympathetic fibres which, although anatomically they are part of the sympathetic branch of the autonomic nervous system, release acetylcholine (see Figure 4.1). Sweat glands, for example, are innervated by sympathetic nerves and stimulation of these nerves causes sweating, yet acetylcholine, applied locally, can also induce sweating whereas atropine blocks this effect and also the response to nerve stimulation. It is therefore thought that some post-ganglionic sympathetic fibres are cholinergic and that the receptors are muscarinic. Some cholinergic sympathetic fibres also innervate the blood vessels in skeletal muscle, mediating dilatation.

Drugs with presynaptic actions

There are a number of ways in which presynaptic mechanisms of noradrenergic transmission can be influenced by drugs. Some of these have already been referred to. The effects can be either depressant or stimulant and some are important for the clinical applications of these drugs.

Inhibitors of synthesis

Enzyme inhibitors are known which block the formation of noradrenaline, as of course does noradrenaline itself. The activity of tyrosine hydroxylase is inhibited by α-methyl-*p*-tyrosine (Figure 8.6a), which competes for the enzyme. This substance is used in the treatment of phaeochromocytoma (see below). Dopa decarboxylase can be inhibited by drugs such as carbidopa (Figure 8.6b) and benserazide (Figure 8.6c) which, as they do not penetrate into the CNS, produce depletion of catecholamines only peripherally. They are combined with L-dopa in the treatment of Parkinson's disease, to restrict the conversion of the administered L-dopa to dopamine in the CNS, thereby allowing a reduction in the dose and in the incidence of peripheral side-effects. A number of drugs inhibit the activity of dopamine-β-hydroxylase, of which disulfiram (Figure 8.6d) is probably the best known.

These enzyme inhibitors cause a decrease in the content of noradrenaline in the tissues and an increase in the amount of dopamine. Disulfiram also inhibits aldehyde dehydrogenases in the liver, including alcohol dehydrogenase and this action leads to the accumulation of acetaldehyde in the tissues when ethanol is ingested. Disulfiram (antabuse) therefore, has a role in the treatment of alcoholism (see Chapter 11) although its mechanism of action is probably more complex than simply inhibition of alcohol dehydrogenase. However, the hypotension which is also produced may well be due to the reduction in the amount of noradrenaline present in sympathetic nerve terminals.

Inhibitors of monoamine oxidase

This is a large group of drugs, most of which have other actions as well. As these drugs are mainly used for their effects on the CNS, where they have antidepressant actions, they are discussed in detail in Chapter 17. Peripherally, they cause increased levels of catecholamines, i.e. of dopamine as well as noradrenaline. The increase in intraneuronal levels of noradrenaline will, of course, lead to the inhibition of tyrosine hydroxylase. Increased amounts of other amines, such as

(a)

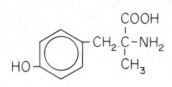

(b)

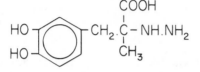

(c)

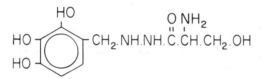

(d)

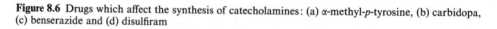

Figure 8.6 Drugs which affect the synthesis of catecholamines: (a) α-methyl-*p*-tyrosine, (b) carbidopa, (c) benserazide and (d) disulfiram

tyramine and octopamine, which are formed by the same enzymes that are concerned with the synthesis of catecholamines (Figure 8.3), may occur and these can act as 'false transmitters' (see below). The depression in peripheral noradrenergic transmission which occurs as a result of these actions may explain the hypotension which frequently occurs with the therapeutic use of monoamine oxidase inhibitors. However, monoamine oxidase inhibitors potentiate the actions of indirectly acting sympathomimetic amines, resulting in the development of hypertension, and this can be a severe adverse effect when these drugs are used clinically: it is discussed in more detail in Chapter 17. All the monoamine oxidase inhibitors have effects on other enzymes, including the microsomal enzymes in the liver. They are therefore likely to potentiate the actions of drugs which are normally metabolized by liver microsomal enzymes, e.g. barbiturates. The monoamine oxidase inhibitors are also hepatotoxic.

The activity of the enzyme COMT can be inhibited by substances such as

(a)   (b)

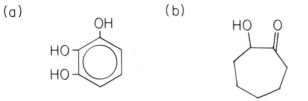

Figure 8.7 Some inhibitors of catechol-*O*-methyltransferase: (a) pyrogallol and (b) tropolone

pyrogallol and tropolone (Figure 8.7). The effect of inhibition of COMT is to prolong the actions of adrenaline and noradrenaline in the circulation. However, drugs with this action have no particular pharmacological or clinical uses.

Effects on storage

Indirectly acting sympathomimetic amines

A number of derivatives of phenylethylamine can displace naturally occurring catecholamines from the intraneuronal storage vesicles. Such drugs are known as 'indirectly acting sympathomimetic amines'. Their main action is to cause the release of noradrenaline from the presynaptic terminals of sympathetic nerves and is therefore 'stimulatory'. However, because they enter the terminals by the same transport mechanism that is responsible for the re-uptake of noradrenaline, they also prolong the actions of released noradrenaline. The indirectly acting sympathomimetic amines are not catecholamines and therefore have little action on postsynaptic receptors. Examples are tyramine (Figure 8.4), ephedrine (Figure 8.8a) and amphetamine (Figure 8.8b). Amphetamine readily penetrates the blood–brain barrier and is best known for its central stimulant effects (see Chapter 16). Ephedrine has less central stimulant action and is used for its peripheral effects (see below). Apart from tyramine, these drugs are not appreciably metabolized by monoamine oxidase and therefore have long-lasting effects. However, they produce tachyphylaxis, in which the response rapidly diminishes with repeated administration. This phenomenon is particularly marked with amphetamine and is due to the depletion of the stores of noradrenaline in the nerve terminals. The indirectly acting sympathomimetic amines do not have any appreciable effect on the storage of catecholamines in the adrenal medulla.

(a)   (b)

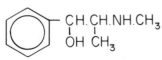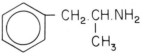

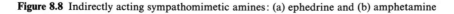

Figure 8.8 Indirectly acting sympathomimetic amines: (a) ephedrine and (b) amphetamine

Reserpine (Figure 8.9a)

This is one of the drugs which affect the storage of catecholamines by inhibiting uptake into the storage vesicles. Reserpine is a naturally occurring alkaloid, present in the shrub *Rauwolfia serpentina,* which is indigenous to India, Africa and South America. It is highly lipid soluble and therefore rapidly penetrates cell membranes. It therefore enters the nerve terminals where it binds to the membranes of the storage vesicles, preventing the uptake of catecholamines. This action is thought to be due to inhibition of the ATPase-dependent uptake mechanism in the vesicular membranes. Thus, any amine which diffuses out will not be pumped back again and will be degraded by monoamine oxidase in the cytoplasm. The ultimate effect is to cause a failure of transmission due to the gradual depletion of the stores of transmitter in the noradrenergic nerve terminals. However, reserpine causes depletion not only of catecholamines but also of 5-hydroxytryptamine, an effect which is important in the CNS (see Chapter 12).

Doses of reserpine which are just sufficient to cause a failure in transmission, produce a reversible impairment of the storage vesicles and, in this case, function

(a)

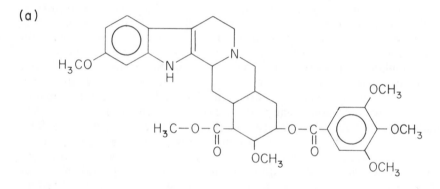

(b)

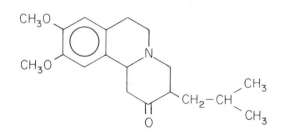

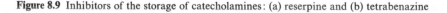

Figure 8.9 Inhibitors of the storage of catecholamines: (a) reserpine and (b) tetrabenazine

can be restored by the administration of exogenous amine, or its precursor. In addition, the depleting effect of reserpine can be largely prevented by inhibiting the action of the intraneuronal monoamine oxidase with a monoamine oxidase inhibitor, such as iproniazid. Larger doses of reserpine cause irreversible damage to the storage vesicles and the effects are then much less easily reversed. Chronic administration of reserpine can lead to increased activity of the enzymes tyrosine hydroxylase and tryptophan hydroxylase (which is concerned in the synthesis of 5-hydroxytryptamine), resulting in a compensatory increase in the synthesis of catecholamines and 5-hydroxytryptamine.

Depletion of catecholamines by reserpine also takes place in the adrenal medulla but the process is slower and less complete than in other tissues. Because it enters the brain, reserpine causes depletion of catecholamines and 5-hydroxytryptamine in the CNS, resulting in sedation. The drug was at one time used as a neuroleptic (see Chapter 12) but is no longer used for this purpose because of the severe mental depression that can occur. Reserpine still has a place in the treatment of hypertension (see Section 7 below) because of the reduction in sympathetic activity that it produces. The drug is also useful in experimental pharmacology to help to determine whether a compound with sympathomimetic actions is acting directly or indirectly. Thus, the effects of a drug with direct postsynaptic actions on adreno-ceptors will not be altered by pretreatment of the preparation with reserpine, but the effects of indirectly acting sympathomimetic amines will be lost or at least considerably reduced by reserpinization.

Tetrabenazine (Figure 8.9b)

This is similar to reserpine in its chemical structure and pharmacological properties. However, tetrabenazine has a more pronounced depleting action on the CNS than it has peripherally. The drug is largely of historical interest but it has an application in the treatment of movement disorders associated with conditions such as Huntington's chorea, senile chorea and related neurological conditions (see Chapter 19).

False transmitters

These are substances which resemble the naturally occurring transmitter and which are stored and released by the same mechanisms. However, they usually have weaker postsynaptic actions than the endogenous transmitter and consequently produce an impairment of transmission. They may also differ from the endogenous transmitter in their susceptibility to the actions of metabolizing enzymes, thereby having more prolonged effects. The ability of these substances to act as false transmitters is dependent upon the lack of specificity of the uptake mechanisms and the enzymes involved in the synthesis of noradrenaline.

Methyldopa

This is the α-methyl analogue of dopa which is converted to α-methyldopamine by dopa decarboxylase and then by dopamine-β-hydroxylase to α-methylnoradrenaline (Figure 8.10a), which is stored in vesicles and released by the same mechanism as that which releases noradrenaline. However, α-methylnoradrenaline is only slightly less potent than noradrenaline in its action on postsynaptic receptors and it is

98

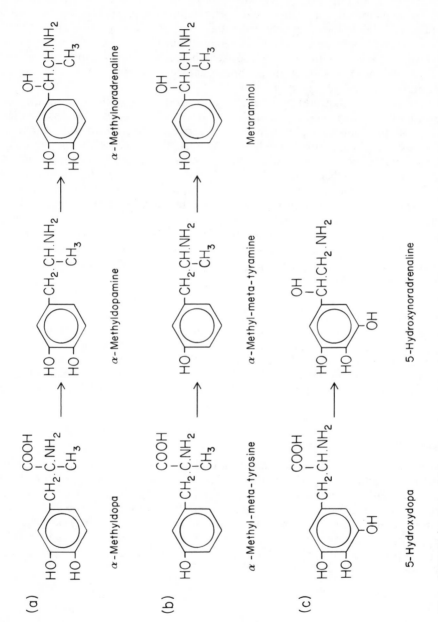

Figure 8.10 The synthesis of false transmitters: (a) α-methylnoradrenaline, (b) metaraminol and (c) 5-hydroxynoradrenaline

therefore thought that the false transmitter action is probably not involved to any great extent in the hypotensive action of this drug (see page 115).

Other substances which can act as false transmitters are α-methyl-*meta*-tyrosine, which is converted to metaraminol (Figure 8.10b), and 5-hydroxydopa, which is converted to 5-hydroxynoradrenaline (Figure 8.10c). Only methyldopa and metaraminol are used as drugs.

Effects on release

While the indirectly acting sympathomimetic amines stimulate the release of noradrenaline from nerve terminals by displacing the transmitter from the intraneuronal storage vesicles, there are also drugs which block the release of noradrenaline from sympathetic nerve terminals. These are usually called 'adrenergic neurone-blocking drugs'. The characteristic feature of the action of these drugs is that they block the response to stimulation of postganglionic sympathetic nerves without altering the response to noradrenaline. However, most of the drugs in this category have other actions as well. For example, xylocholine (TM 10) (Figure 8.11a), which was the first substance found to have this action, also has nicotinic actions.

Bretylium (Figure 8.11b)

This was developed in the search for drugs with fewer side-effects than xylocholine and was the first of the adrenergic neurone-blocking drugs to be used in the treatment of hypertension. Bretylium does not cause any depletion of noradrenaline but is itself concentrated in noradrenergic nerve terminals by the transport mechanism for the re-uptake of noradrenaline into the terminals. Once in the terminal, bretylium prevents the release of noradrenaline in response to nerve impulses and at one time it was thought that this effect might be attributable to a local anaesthetic action as bretylium and related substances are local anaesthetics. However, the release of noradrenaline can be prevented by doses of bretylium which are too small to block the conduction of nerve impulses in the terminals and an alternative explanation for its action is that it interferes with the calcium-dependent release mechanism. Bretylium is no longer used in the treatment of hypertension, because of erratic absorption from the GI tract and the development of tolerance to the drug; furthermore, the side-effects include postural hypotension. This drug does have a role in the treatment of cardiac arrhythmias, however.

Guanethidine (Figure 8.11c)

This has an action similar to that of bretylium, being taken up into noradrenergic nerve terminals, but in large doses it also causes depletion of noradrenaline. It therefore has a reserpine-like action, but this is confined to peripheral noradrenergic nerve terminals and no depletion occurs at the adrenal medulla or in the CNS. Guanethidine is used in the treatment of hypertension (see below), although postural hypotension can occur. Chronic administration of guanethidine can result in the development of supersensitivity of the postsynaptic receptors, similar to that produced by denervation. However, this is probably of little importance as the amount of noradrenaline released is so small.

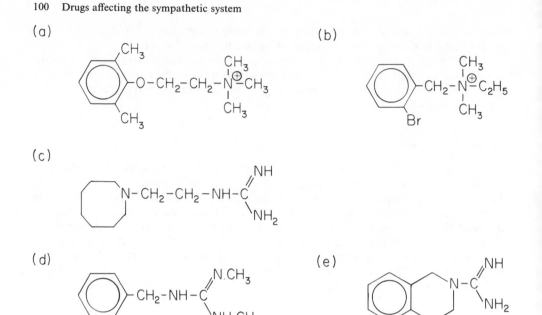

Figure 8.11 Drugs which affect release of catecholamines (a) xylocholine, (b) bretylium, (c) guanethidine, (d) bethanidine and (e) debrisoquine

Bethanidine **(Figure 8.11d)** *and debrisoquine* **(Figure 8.11e)**

These are similar to guanethidine in their effects but they have a shorter duration of action. Bethanidine also has a more rapid onset of action.

Finally, a variety of substances can influence the release of noradrenaline from the terminals of sympathetic nerves. These include acetylcholine and prostaglandins of the E series. The inhibitory effects of acetylcholine on the release of noradrenaline are due to an action on muscarinic receptors and it has been suggested that this may have a physiological role. The inhibition of the release of noradrenaline by prostaglandins occurs in many, but not all, sympathetic nerves. The mechanism for this effect is unknown although a link with the availability of calcium is a possibility, and its significance is also not known. In addition, the noradrenaline which has been released from the nerve terminals is known to inhibit further release of transmitter and this action is mediated by presynaptic or autoreceptors (Figure 8.4). There is, therefore, an inhibitory feedback mechanism which limits the amount of transmitter released. The presynaptic receptors which mediate this effect are of the α_2-type and drugs exist which have selective actions on these receptors. The actions of these drugs are considered, together with those which act on postsynaptic receptors, on page 101.

Effects on re-uptake

A wide range of substances inhibit the re-uptake of noradrenaline into the terminals, i.e. inhibition of Uptake$_1$. These include drugs such as amphetamine and tyramine, although their main action as indirectly acting sympathomimetic amines is to cause the release of noradrenaline. Certain of the adrenergic neurone-blocking drugs, such as guanethidine, can also inhibit re-uptake but, again, this is not their main action.

Cocaine (Figure 8.12a)

This is a naturally occurring substance which is present in the leaves of *Erythroxylon coca*, a plant indigenous to South America, where extracts of the leaves were taken to produce a sense of well-being or euphoria. Cocaine is, of course, a local anaesthetic (see Chapter 9), but it also inhibits the re-uptake of noradrenaline, thus prolonging and enhancing its action, as re-uptake is the principal mechanism for inactivating the transmitter. Cocaine therefore produces sympathomimetic effects although these are relatively slow to develop. The effects include mydriasis, an increase in heart rate and blood pressure, and pale skin. Large doses can cause death from cardiac failure due to a direct toxic action on the heart. Cocaine also blocks the re-uptake of noradrenaline in the central nervous system, and this action is responsible for the euphoria produced and is probably the reason why the drug is abused.

Methylphenidate (Figure 8.12b)

This is a synthetic drug, chemically related to cocaine which also resembles cocaine in its pharmacological properties. It is used as a central stimulant and is discussed in Chapter 16.

Imipramine and related drugs

These are the tricyclic drugs which are used as antidepressants. They all inhibit the re-uptake of noradrenaline (and in some instances 5-hydroxytryptamine as well). However, their peripheral actions, especially in overdose, are due to other properties (see Chapter 17).

Neurotoxic effects

The analogue of dopamine, 6-hydroxydopamine (Figure 8.12c), when administered intravenously, is taken up into noradrenergic nerves where it produces a selective destruction of the terminals and a long-lasting depletion of the stores of noradrenaline. This has been described as 'chemical sympathectomy' because the effects resemble those of surgical denervation. However, the cell bodies remain viable after treatment with 6-hydroxydopamine and eventually re-innervate the effector tissues. The adrenal medulla is less affected and 6-hydroxydopamine does not enter the CNS. However, when injected intracerebrally the drug causes degeneration of dopamine- and noradrenaline-containing neurones and it has proved to be a useful tool for studies of the functions of catecholamines in the CNS.

Drugs with agonist actions at adrenoceptors

These are the directly acting sympathomimetic amines as opposed to the indirectly acting sympathomimetic amines described above on page 95 although their effects

(a)

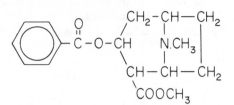

(b)

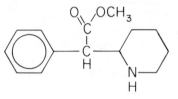

(c)

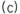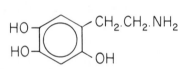

Figure 8.12 Drugs which affect re-uptake of catecholamines: (a) cocaine, (b) methylphenidate and the neurotoxic drug (c) 6-hydroxydopamine

are, of course, very similar. The two endogenous sympathomimetic amines that are released by stimulation of sympathetic nerves are adrenaline, which is released from the adrenal medulla into the circulation, and noradrenaline, released from sympathetic nerve endings. Although noradrenaline has been shown to be more potent at α-adrenoceptors than at β-receptors, it is the physiological transmitter released at both sites. Because adrenaline is roughly equipotent at both α- and β-receptors, its effects will tend to predominate at β-receptors whereas those of noradrenaline will be more apparent on α-receptors.

The distribution of α- and β-receptors

With the development of agonist and antagonist drugs with selective actions at a particular subtype of receptor, the pharmacological effects produced, together with the functional response, will depend upon the location of the receptors on which a particular drug is acting. These are summarized in Table 8.1 to which reference will be made in discussing the actions of the different drugs.

Table 8.1 Responses to stimulation of sympathetic nerves

Effector organ	Receptor type	Response
Eye		
Radial muscle of iris	α	Contraction (mydriasis)
Ciliary muscle	β	Relaxation (slight)
Heart		
S-A node	β_1	Increased rate (chronotropic)
Atria	β_1	Increased contractility (inotropic)
A-V node	β_1	Increased contractility
Blood vessels		
Vascular smooth muscle	α	Constriction
Arterioles in skeletal m.	α, β_2	Constriction
Lungs		
Bronchial smooth muscle	β_2	Relaxation
GI tract		
Motility and tone	α, β	Relaxation
Sphincters	α	Contraction
Urinary bladder		
Detrusor muscle	β	Relaxation
Trigone and sphincter	α	Contraction
Uterus	α, β	Contraction (pregnant, α)
		Relaxation (non-pregnant, β)
Skin		
Pilomotor muscles	α	Contraction
Sweat glands	M*	Increased secretion
Metabolic effects		
Liver	α, β_2	Glycogenolysis
Fat cells	α, β_1	Lipolysis

* M, muscarinic, i.e. acetylcholine receptors but part of the sympathetic system

Noradrenaline (Figure 8.1b)

When used as a drug, the main effects of noradrenaline are on the cardiovascular system and, in general, they mimic the effects of stimulation of sympathetic nerves. The contraction of vascular smooth muscle due to activation of α-receptors results in an increase in peripheral resistance and therefore a rise in blood pressure. Although the heart is stimulated due to the activation of β_1-receptors causing an initial tachycardia, the rise in blood pressure activates baroreceptor reflexes and this, in turn, causes increased activity in the vagus nerve which reduces the heart rate. Thus, the net effect of an infusion of noradrenaline is a rise in blood pressure and bradycardia. Blood flow to the kidney and liver is reduced, and usually to the skeletal muscles as well, but coronary blood flow is increased. The clinical uses of noradrenaline are few but are discussed on page 108.

Adrenaline (Figure 8.1c)

Again, the cardiovascular effects predominate. The systolic pressure is increased whereas the diastolic pressure is reduced, and thus the pulse pressure is increased although the mean pressure may be little changed. Because of stimulation of β-receptors, the heart rate will be increased. However, peripheral resistance is decreased. Thus, although vasoconstriction occurs in the splanchnic vessels and the skin, which contain mainly α-receptors, the blood vessels of skeletal muscle, which contain mainly β-receptors, will be dilated. The cutaneous vasoconstriction results in pallor of the skin. Like noradrenaline, adrenaline is inactive when given orally and is usually administered intravenously, but the tachycardia produced can be unpleasant and there is a risk of precipitating cardiac arrhythmias. Adrenaline also increases coronary blood flow but the increased myocardial oxygen consumption may result in an overall reduction in myocardial efficiency, compared with the effects of noradrenaline. Adrenaline stimulates glycogenesis and lipolysis in the liver, causing blood glucose levels to rise and also an increase in the level of free fatty acids in the plasma.

Dopamine (Figure 8.2)

Apart from being the immediate precursor to noradrenaline in the biosynthetic pathway (see 'The synthesis of noradrenaline' on page 84) and a neurotransmitter in the CNS, dopamine has some weak direct actions on adrenoceptors and also indirect sympathomimetic actions. Dopamine has an agonist action on $β_1$-receptors in the heart and exerts a positive inotropic effect on the myocardium. It increases cardiac output but does so without causing a significant increase in heart rate or peripheral resistance. It therefore has an application in the treatment of congestive heart failure. The only peripheral dopamine receptors which are known are present on renal and mesenteric vascular smooth muscle, stimulation of which causes vasodilatation. Infusion of small doses of dopamine causes an increase in glomerular filtration, renal blood flow and sodium excretion. Dopamine is used in the treatment of cardiogenic shock.

Ephedrine (Figure 8.8a)

This is a naturally occurring drug that is found in various species of the plant *Ephedra,* which is indigenous to China. In fact, ephedrine has been in use for more than 2000 years. It is not a catecholamine and part of its action is indirect, due to the release of noradrenaline, but it also has substantial postsynaptic actions which resemble those of adrenaline, on both α- and β-receptors. Ephedrine is a phenyl-ethanolamine (see Figure 8.4); it is metabolized slowly and its effects are therefore more prolonged than those of adrenaline. It is also effective when given orally. Unlike adrenaline, however, it enters the CNS and produces central stimulation although this effect is not as marked as that of amphetamine. The cardiovascular effects resemble those of adrenaline but are more persistent. A pressor response is produced due to peripheral vasoconstriction (although the coronary vessels are dilated) and cardiac stimulation. Ephedrine is an orally effective pressor agent which is used in the treatment of heart block (Stokes–Adams syndrome) in which there is a drastic fall in blood pressure, and fainting.

Although less potent than either adrenaline or isoprenaline, ephedrine causes bronchodilatation by an agonist action at $β_2$-receptors (see Table 8.1), and its more prolonged action, together with the fact that ephedrine is effective when given orally, has led to the use of this drug in the prophylactic treatment of milder forms of bronchial asthma. Ephedrine is less effective in relieving bronchospasm once this has occurred, when more efficacious drugs are required. Because of the central stimulation, insomnia, restlessness and anxiety can occur. Ephedrine is a common constituent of nasal inhalants as it reduces congestion by virtue of its vasoconstrictor action. It is also used locally in ophthalmology to produce mydriasis (see Table 8.1). Ephedrine has also been used to treat nocturnal enuresis (bedwetting) in cases where there is impaired nervous control of the bladder, by increasing the tone of the sphincters (Table 8.1).

Phenylephrine (Figure 8.13a)

This drug has actions similar to those of noradrenaline but it is less potent. As it is not a derivative of catechol, it is not metabolized by catechol-O-methyltransferase (COMT) and it therefore has a longer duration of action than noradrenaline. It is used as a decongestant because of its peripheral vasoconstrictor action and as an alternative to noradrenaline in the treatment of acute hypotension.

Agonists with selective α-adrenoceptor activity

Methoxamine (Figure 8.13b)

This has an action which is almost exclusively on α-receptors, which it stimulates directly. Its main effect therefore is to increase blood pressure due to peripheral vasoconstriction and there is little effect on the heart or bronchi. Furthermore, methoxamine has no central effects as it does not cross the blood–brain barrier. It is not taken up by adrenergic neurones and has no indirect sympathomimetic activity. It is used solely as a pressor agent in acute hypotensive states.

Imidazolines

These are drugs, many of which have agonist actions at α-receptors. They have no action at β-receptors and are not taken up into adrenergic nerves. They are used as decongestants but have central effects which include sedation. A typical example of this group is oxymetazoline (Figure 8.13c).

Clonidine (Figure 8.13d)

This is an α-agonist which is selective for the α_2-receptors that are located on the presynaptic nerve terminals. Its agonist action is therefore to reduce the release of noradrenaline from the terminals and the overall effect is therefore similar to that of an antagonist drug. Clonidine has a hypotensive action and is used in the treatment of hypertension. It is thought that the main action of clonidine is central and that it acts on α_2-receptors in the brain stem to reduce sympathetic outflow.

Agonists with selective β-adrenoceptor activity

Isoprenaline (Figure 8.1d)

This is a synthetic catecholamine which is derived from noradrenaline; it is, in fact, isopropylnoradrenaline. It is a potent agonist at β-receptors with virtually no action at α-receptors. Because of the stimulation of β-receptors on the bronchi, isopren-

106

(a)

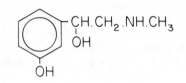

(b)

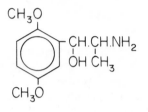

(c)

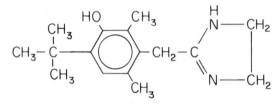

(d)

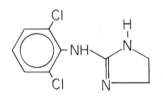

(e)

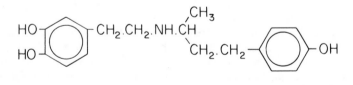

(f)

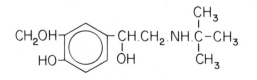

Figure 8.13 Sympathomimetic agonists (a) phenylephrine, (b) methoxamine, (c) oxymetazoline, (d) clonidine, (e) dobutamine and (f) salbutamol

aline can be used to relieve bronchoconstriction, e.g. in asthma. However, it also stimulates the β-receptors on the heart, causing tachycardia, and it produces vasodilatation of some peripheral blood vessels, especially those of skeletal muscles, causing a fall in blood pressure. In addition, isoprenaline has metabolic effects (see Table 8.1). Isoprenaline is not metabolized by monoamine oxidase, nor is it taken up into adrenergic nerves, but it is metabolized by COMT. Absorption of the drug can be erratic when it is administered orally, due to the metabolism by COMT, but it is well absorbed after sublingual administration. It is also used in the form of an aerosol for the relief of acute asthmatic attacks. However, this route can easily lead to overdose and the stimulant action on the heart can cause cardiac arrhythmias which may be fatal. The use of isoprenaline for the relief of asthma has now been superseded by safer drugs (see below). The cardiac-stimulant properties of isoprenaline are utilized in the treatment of heart block and severe bradycardia.

Dobutamine (Figure 8.13e)

This drug resembles dopamine in structure. It increases cardiac output by selectively stimulating β_1-receptors. It has little effect on the mean arterial blood pressure but increases the force of cardiac contraction without any appreciable effect on rate. It therefore has a role as a cardiac stimulant in cardiovascular failure in myocardial infarction and in cardiac surgery.

Salbutamol (Figure 8.13f)

This is one of the many non-catecholamine drugs that have been synthesized and which have a selective stimulant action on β_2-adrenoceptors. As these substances are not catecholamines, they are not metabolized by COMT and therefore have a long duration of action. More important, the absence of an action on β_1-receptors means that the drugs are relatively safe for use as bronchodilators as they do not have any undesirable cardiac effects. Salbutamol is well absorbed and can be given by all routes of administration, i.e. intravenously, orally and by inhalation.

The clinical uses of sympathomimetic drugs

Some of these have already been briefly referred to. For example, the peripheral vasoconstrictor action of adrenaline is utilized to control superficial haemorrhage when the drug is applied topically or as a spray. However, it is effective for controlling bleeding only from arterioles and capillaries and not from larger vessels. Solutions of adrenaline are used in ophthalmology for instillation into the eye to control haemorrhage and to reduce conjunctival congestion. The mydriasis produced by local application of ephedrine or phenylephrine to the conjunctiva is short lasting, i.e. a few hours, and it does not involve cycloplegia or an increase in intra-ocular pressure. Sympathomimetics are therefore often preferred to muscarinic antagonists, such as atropine, for producing mydriasis in ophthalmology. Adrenaline and phenylephrine have been found to be effective in the treatment of wide-angle glaucoma, reducing the intra-ocular pressure by their local vasoconstrictor action, which causes a decrease in the production of aqueous humour. The vasoconstrictor action of adrenaline is also used to retard the absorption of local anaesthetics and adrenaline is usually included in preparations of these drugs.

The use of sympathomimetic amines with actions on α-receptors as nasal decongestants has already been mentioned. Some, e.g. ephedrine, phenylephrine and oxymetazoline, are effective when applied topically either in the form of nose drops or in inhalers. However, phenylephrine and other sympathomimetic drugs, such as phenylpropanolamine and pseudoephedrine, also produce shrinking of the nasal mucosa when they are administered locally. These drugs, usually mixed with other agents such as antipyretic analgesics, antitussives, antihistamines and anti-muscarinics, are the basis of preparations which are promoted for the relief of colds and other conditions of the upper respiratory tract.

Some sympathomimetic amines, e.g. dopamine, have a role in relieving severe hypotension in emergency situations such as cardiogenic shock or overdose with antihypertensive drugs or CNS depressants. Noradrenaline, administered intravenously, will also relieve acute hypotension although the effect will be transient unless a continuous infusion is maintained. However, the bitartrate salt is strongly acidic and leakage from the infusion site can cause necrosis of the surrounding tissues. Infusion of noradrenaline is also used to relieve the dramatic fall in blood pressure which occurs in operations for phaeochromocytoma (see below) when the tumour has been removed. Adrenaline, given intramuscularly, can be beneficial in anaphylactic shock where the first-line treatment includes the restoration of blood pressure, although replacement of lost fluids may be more effective and also more important.

Sympathomimetic drugs with agonist actions at β-receptors are used for their bronchodilator action in the treatment of reversible airway obstruction, e.g. in bronchial asthma. However, a selective β_2-agonist, such as salbutamol, is usually preferred in order to avoid cardiac effects. Nevertheless, adrenaline may be used in emergency situations, i.e. status asthmaticus, and ephedrine can be used prophylactically.

Drugs with antagonist actions on adrenoceptors

Antagonists acting predominantly on α-receptors

A number of drugs, with varying chemical structures, block α-receptors, some of them also having other pharmacological actions. Because of the large number, only the most important are discussed here.

Phenoxybenzamine (Figure 8.14a)

This drug, together with dibenamine, is a haloalkylamine and produces an irreversible blockade of α-receptors, due to covalent bonding to the receptor site. In normal doses there is no action on β-receptors. The onset of action is slow, i.e. up to 1 h in man, and it may persist for several days. The blockade of peripheral α-receptors prevents the vasoconstriction produced by catecholamines. In normotensive subjects the effects of phenoxybenzamine on the mean arterial blood pressure are slight. However, the drug interferes with the reflex mechanisms which adjust the blood pressure and this can result in postural hypotension. In hypertensive patients, phenoxybenzamine reduces the blood pressure but, again, postural hypotension can occur. Phenoxybenzamine antagonizes the arrhythmias provoked by catecholamines and it has been used to prevent the occurrence of arrhythmias associated with the use of halogenated anaesthetics. It is useful for providing long-term blockade of α-receptors before removal of tumours of the adrenal medulla (e.g. phaeochromocytoma). Phenoxybenzamine has other pharmacological actions,

(a)

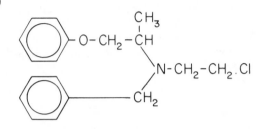

(b)

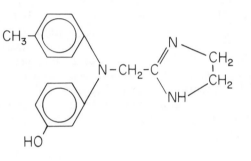

(c)

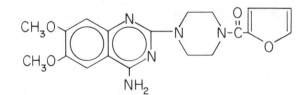

(d)

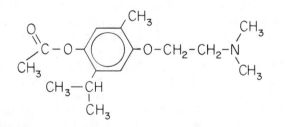

Figure 8.14 Drugs with α-antagonist actions: (a) phenoxybenzamine, (b) phentolamine, (c) prazosin, (d) thymoxamine

including antagonism at receptors for acetylcholine, histamine and 5-hydroxy-tryptamine.

Phentolamine (Figure 8.14b)

This is an imidazoline and closely resembles those imidazolines that are α-receptor agonists (see page 105). It is a competitive antagonist at α-receptors with no action on β-receptors. It has a direct vasodilator action and, when administered intravenously, can cause a fall in blood pressure, together with tachycardia which, in part, is reflexly induced. Phentolamine is mainly used to treat hypertensive crises caused by circulating catecholamines, e.g. in phaeochromocytoma. Phentolamine is also an agonist at receptors for 5-hydroxytryptamine.

Prazosin (Figure 8.14c)

This is a selective α-receptor antagonist with an action mainly on α_1-receptors, which are postsynaptic, and little effect on presynaptic α_2-receptors; thus it does not enhance the release of noradrenaline. Prazosin causes peripheral vasodilatation by antagonizing the vasoconstrictor action of endogenous catecholamines and this results in a fall in blood pressure. However, the action of prazosin in lowering the blood pressure differs from the effects of other α-adrenoceptor antagonists, such as phenoxybenzamine, as postural hypotension is less likely to occur and there is no significant increase in heart rate. The absence of reflex tachycardia with prazosin is thought to be due to the absence of an α_2-blocking action with this drug. Prazosin is used as a peripheral vasodilator in the treatment of hypertension (see below).

Thymoxamine (Figure 8.14d)

This is a phenoxyalkylamine which has antagonistic actions at α-receptors. It is used in the treatment of peripheral vascular disease, including Raynaud's disease. It also has some weak antihistaminic activity.

Ergot alkaloids

These were the first adrenergic antagonists to be discovered. The members of this group vary in their properties, some being α-receptor antagonists and also antagonists at receptors for 5-hydroxytryptamine and dopamine and some being partial agonists. Many of the drugs occur naturally and ergot is a fungus which can infect rye. Outbreaks of poisoning by ergot (ergotism) due to the consumption of bread made from infected grain were associated with a characteristic spectrum of symptoms. These include initial tingling, leading to an intense sensation of burning and pain in the extremities. This is due to intense and prolonged vasoconstriction. Later the ischaemic extremities become gangrenous, the limbs blacken and might even fall off. These symptoms probably gave rise to the old name for the disease – St Anthony's fire. Central effects were also associated with the poisoning, including vomiting, dizziness, headache, confusion, drowsiness, uncosciousness and convulsions. As ergot can produce powerful contractions of the uterus, it also caused abortion. The ergot alkaloids are derivatives of lysergic acid and are best known for their actions on the cerebral circulation, or on the brain itself. For example, dihydroergotoxine, which is a mixture of the three alkaloids dihydroergocornine, dihydroergocristine and dihydroergocryptine (Figure 8.15), has little vasoconstrictor activity and does not contract the uterus, but it does have α-adrenergic antagonist properties and is used as a vasodilator for the treatment of peripheral vascular disease. Although it has little effect on normal levels of blood pressure, dihydroergo-toxine lowers blood pressure in hypertension. The drug is effective in the treatment of migraine although the mechanism for this action is not clear because attacks of migraine are associated with vasodilatation of the cerebral blood vessels. On the basis that improved cerebral blood flow might have a beneficial effect on depressed mental function, e.g. in senile dementia, dihydroergotoxine has been given to geriatric patients. Although some improvement in psychological tests has been claimed, it is doubtful if the drug has any appreciable therapeutic action in this condition.

Other α-antagonists include yohimbine, which is an indolealkylamine and is chemically related to reserpine. Apart from blocking α-receptors, it also blocks receptors for 5-hydroxytryptamine. Yohimbine readily penetrates into the CNS where it blocks α_2-receptors. Its effects are therefore the opposite to those of clonidine and in the CNS yohimbine is stimulatory. It is also reputed to be an

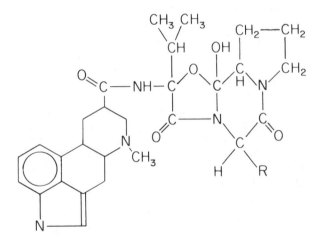

Dihydroergocornine   R = $-CH.(CH_3)_2$

Dihydroergocristine   R = $-CH_2-\bigcirc$

Dihydroergocryptine   R = $-CH_2-CH(CH_3)_2$

Figure 8.15 Ergot alkaloids. The general structure of the amino acid alkaloids and of the three derivatives present in dihydroergotoxine

aphrodisiac. The dibenzazepine, azatepine, and benzodioxanes, such as piperoxane, are α-antagonists. Some of the phenothiazine neuroleptic drugs, such as chlorpromazine, have an α-blocking action among their other pharmacological properties. These drugs are discussed in Chapter 12. Some antidepressant drugs also block α_2-receptors (see Chapter 17).

Antagonists with predominant actions on β-receptors

These drugs, commonly called β-blockers, were developed as selective agents in the search for compounds which might prove useful in the treatment of hypertension, angina pectoris and cardiac arrhythmias. They are mostly analogues of isoprenaline (Figure 8.1d) and the first drug of this type was dichloroisoprenaline. It has a selective action at β-receptors but is a partial agonist. Because of the stimulant action, which appears before the antagonist effect, this drug has not been used clinically but its discovery stimulated the search for antagonist drugs with less agonist activity. A large number of these compounds is now known, many of them having very similar actions and only the major ones are reviewed here.

Propranolol (Figure 8.16a)

This is a potent competitive antagonist at β-receptors and produces a dose-dependent reduction of the responses to stimulation of sympathetic nerves at all sites where β-receptors occur. It has no agonist activity and it is equally effective at β_1- and β_2-receptors. Propranolol exists in two isomeric forms, the β-blocking activity being mainly in the (−)isomer. Thus, the (−)isomer is 50–100 times more potent than the (+)isomer in blocking β-receptors but both isomers have local anaesthetic actions and are roughly equipotent in this respect.

The blocking of β-receptors on the heart causes a reduction in the sympathetic influence on the heart and this leads to bradycardia and reduced force of cardiac contraction. The net result is a fall in cardiac output. In normotensive subjects, there may be no change or only a slight fall in blood pressure. However, in hypertensive individuals, propranolol produces a marked fall in systolic and diastolic blood pressure, which is slow to develop. It is thought that during the early stages in the chronic administration of propranolol, there may be an increase in peripheral resistance, due to the blocking of β_2-receptors which mediate vasodilatation of blood vessels in skeletal muscle (see Table 8.1). Propranolol is therefore a useful drug in the treatment of hypertension and can be combined effectively with a peripheral vasodilator (see below). However, its mechanism of action in producing a lowering of blood pressure is probably more complex than simply a reduction in cardiac output. For example, the release of renin from the juxtaglomerular cells of the kidney is stimulated by β-agonists and this effect can be blocked by β-blockers. Thus, it has been proposed that propranolol may exert at least part of its antihypertensive action by inhibiting the secretion of renin by the kidney. In support of this theory, it has been found that propranolol in relatively modest doses had a greater hypotensive effect in individuals with elevated plasma renin activity than in patients with low renin levels. Nevertheless, patients with low levels of renin activity still respond to propranolol. It is possible, therefore, that different mechanisms may operate to reduce a raised blood pressure in different groups of hypertensive patients.

(a)

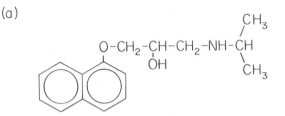

(b)

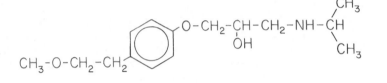

(c)

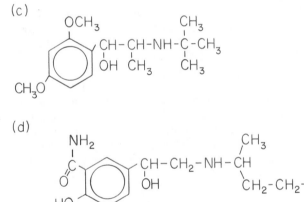

(d)

Figure 8.16 Drugs with β-antagonist actions: (a) propranolol, (b) metoprolol, (c) butoxamine, the non-selective antagonist and (d) labetolol

Propranolol is a useful drug in the prophylactic treatment of angina pectoris, reducing both the number and the severity of attacks. This is particularly true for attacks of angina related to exertion and stress. Blockade of β-receptors in these circumstances will obviously reduce the response of the heart to sympathetic stimulation. However, propranolol produces a reduction in the myocardial oxygen consumption at rest as well as during exertion and it is thought that, after blockade of the β-receptors, the myocardium is able to extract a larger proportion of oxygen from the blood perfusing it.

Propranolol is also effective in the treatment of cardiac arrhythmias, especially supraventricular tachycardias. The drug increases the refractoriness of the A-V node by blocking β-adrenergic influences. β-Blockers have also been found to reduce the recurrence of myocardial infarction.

Propranolol has central effects but it is not known whether these can be attributed to β-blockade in the CNS. The membrane-stabilizing action is apparent only with large doses and it is thought that this is unlikely to be responsible for the central effects. Propranolol can have adverse effects in patients whose hearts are severely compromised by disease or by other drugs, and it may precipitate heart failure, either suddenly or slowly. Supersensitivity of β-adrenergic receptors may develop with chronic administration of the drug and abrupt withdrawal can lead to severe anginal attacks or fatal cardiac arrhythmias. Thus, if administration of the drug is to be stopped, it must be done gradually.

An important adverse effect of propranolol is due to blockade of the β-receptors on the bronchi (Table 8.1), which leads to bronchoconstriction, and this must be avoided in patients suffering from asthma or with a history of bronchospasm. Because of the blocking of the β_2-receptors subserving vasodilatation of peripheral blood vessels, propranolol can cause symptoms of ischaemia, such as cold extremities, and can exacerbate these symptoms in patients suffering from Raynaud's disease and other peripheral vascular disorders.

Examples of other β-adrenoceptor antagonists which affect both β_1- and β_2-receptors, i.e. are 'non-selective', are alprenolol, sotalol, oxprenolol, pindolol and timolol, but there are many more. Their actions are similar to those of propranolol but they vary in potency. However, some, e.g. alprenolol, oxprenolol and pindolol, have some intrinsic activity, i.e. agonist activity. This activity is greatest in pindolol. It is thought that the intrinsic sympathomimetic activity is likely to reduce the development of supersensitivity of the β-receptors with chronic administration and that abrupt withdrawal of the drug will be less likely to produce untoward effects. Drugs with intrinsic activity are also less likely to cause cold extremities. Sotalol does not possess the membrane-stabilizing property of propranolol but is equally effective in the treatment of cardiac arrhythmias. Thus the theory that this action of propranolol is due to its local anaesthetic action can be largely discounted.

Metoprolol (Figure 8.16b)

The tendency of propranolol and related 'non-selective' drugs to produce undesirable effects such as bronchoconstriction due to blockade of β_2-receptors, led to the development of 'cardioselective' β-blockers with a greater potency for β_1-receptors than for β_2-. The selectivity, however, is relative and bronchospasm can occur with large doses. The first drug of this type to be used was practolol but it was withdrawn because of its toxic effects which are not associated with the β-blocking action. Metoprolol is a typical cardioselective β-blocker which is used for the treatment of hypertension, angina and cardiac arrhythmias.

Other drugs of this type are acebutolol and atenolol. They are all similar in their actions.

Drugs also exist with selective antagonist actions at β_2-adrenoceptors, an example being butoxamine (Figure 8.16c) which is related to isoprenaline, but such substances do not have any therapeutic applications and their only use is in the analysis of mechanisms and in the characterization of receptors.

Labetolol (**Figure 8.16d**)

This is an antagonist drug which is not selective for either α- or β-receptors and is also equally effective at both β_1- and β_2-sites. It is an effective antihypertensive agent when given orally. The reduction in blood pressure results from reduction in peripheral resistance due to the blockade of α-receptors on vascular smooth muscle, combined with the β-blocking action on the heart which reduces both systolic and diastolic blood pressure. However, postural hypotension can occur with labetol.

Clinical uses of antagonist drugs

Some of these have been mentioned already. However, perhaps the most important application for drugs which reduce sympathetic activity is in the treatment of essential hypertension, a condition in which many different kinds of pharmacological manipulation have been tried and discarded. For example, the ganglion-blocking drugs which were described in Chapter 6 are no longer used, and the adrenergic neurone-blocking drugs (see page 99) are used only where other forms of treatment have failed. Similarly, drugs with presynaptic actions, e.g. depletion (reserpine), false transmitter actions (methyldopa) or on presynaptic receptors (clonidine), are used only infrequently. These three drugs are thought to produce their hypotensive effects by acting on the CNS, but reserpine can induce mental depression, and both methyldopa and clonidine cause sedation; in addition, the sudden withdrawal of clonidine can produce a hypertensive crisis.

Although they vary in their other properties, e.g. membrane-stabilizing actions, partial agonist activity and penetration of the CNS, all the known β-blockers produce a lowering of blood pressure in doses that are equipotent for β-blockade. These drugs, together with the diuretics, represent the drugs of choice for the treatment of essential hypertension, mainly because of their ability to lower a raised blood pressure without producing undesirable side-effects. However, the use of combinations of drugs with actions on different mechanisms, each of which contributes to a reduction in blood pressure, appears to have advantages. Thus, the combination of a β-blocker, which will reduce cardiac output, with a thiazide diuretic, which will reduce blood volume, and a peripheral vasodilator (such as hydralazine) to reduce peripheral resistance, can be effective in the management of hypertension. Such a combination has the advantage that, as the effects of the drugs on blood pressure are additive, smaller doses are required than would be needed if each drug was used on its own, thus reducing the incidence of side-effects. There may, furthermore, be other advantages: for example, the reflex tachycardia associated with the vasodilator action of hydralazine will be prevented by the β-blocker.

The use of β-blockers in the treatment of angina has been discussed above.

The α-adrenergic antagonists are effective in relieving secondary hypertension, such as that caused by high levels of circulating catecholamines in phaeochromocytoma. In this condition, a tumour of the adrenal medulla causes the excretion of excessive amounts of adrenaline and noradrenaline. There is usually a fairly constant level of hypertension, together with intermittent paroxysmal attacks in which the blood pressure rises still further. Drugs such as phenoxybenzamine and α-methyl-p-tyrosine are effective in reducing the hypertension, while phentolamine, given intravenously, can be used for diagnosis. Phenoxybenzamine can also be used to provide prolonged α-blockade before removal of the tumour and the infusion of a pressor agent, such as noradrenaline, may be needed after the tumour has been removed.

The α-adrenergic blocking drugs are also used in the management of hypertensive emergencies associated with overdose of sympathomimetic drugs, withdrawal of clonidine and use of monoamine oxidase inhibitors (see Chapter 17). They are also effective in the treatment of peripheral vascular disease, such as Raynaud's syndrome, and reverse the ischaemia caused by local vasoconstriction due to inadvertent infiltration of α-agonists into subcutaneous tissue during intravenous administration. A paradoxical use of α-adrenoceptor antagonists is in the treatment of shock associated with hypotension, in which the intense peripheral vasoconstriction which occurs can lead to an inadequate blood supply to vital tissues. The use of a vasodilator drug, together with intravenous administration of blood or fluids, will restore perfusion of the tissues and aid recovery.

Chapter 9

Drugs with non-synaptic actions

Although most drugs with actions on the nervous system produce their effects at synapses, by interfering with or mimicking the actions of the endogenous transmitters, there are some drugs which act in a different manner and affect the generation or conduction of nerve impulses. Many of these drugs are important because they are used clinically as local anaesthetics; others are used experimentally. In fact, a wide variety of substances are able to stabilize cell membranes and some of these have been referred to in earlier chapters, e.g. propranolol (see Chapter 8). They include alcohol, inhalation anaesthetics, barbiturates, antiepileptic drugs and neuroleptics, and they are all highly lipid soluble. It seems that, because of their lipid solubility, these substances can enter the cell membrane and produce a stabilizing effect if their concentration is high enough.

Local anaesthetics

These are substances which prevent both the generation and conduction of action potentials in nerve cells by a reversible, membrane-stabilizing action. They also stabilize the membranes of other excitable tissues, such as muscle. Their principal use is to produce a reversible block of conduction in nerve fibres, particularly fibres mediating the conduction of pain, thus producing a localized 'anaesthesia' or 'analgesia'. However, some derivatives of local anaesthetics are used as antiarrhythmic drugs, to depress the activity of cardiac muscle. Local anaesthetics block impulse conduction in all types of nerve fibres but smaller fibres are more susceptible to their action than larger fibres. As pain fibres are usually of small diameter, and are also unmyelinated, they will be affected preferentially by smaller concentrations of local anaesthetics than will fibres conducting other sensations or motor fibres.

All local anaesthetics are composed of two components, a hydrophilic centre and a lipophilic centre, which are separated by an intermediate alkyl chain. The hydrophilic group is usually a tertiary amine but may be a secondary amine. The lipophilic group is an aromatic residue which is linked to the alkyl chain by an ester or an amide link (see Figure 9.1). Many of these drugs are derivatives of *para*-aminobenzoic acid, e.g. procaine (Figure 9.2b). Changes in any part of the molecule can alter the anaesthetic potency and toxicity and it is necessary for the hydrophilic and lipophilic centres to be in balance. Thus, if the hydrophilic centre dominates, the local anaesthetic action will be weak because the drug cannot penetrate the

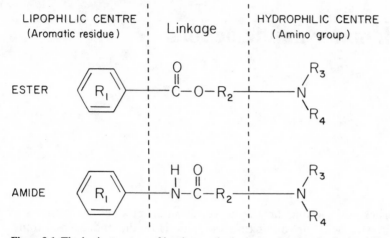

Figure 9.1 The basic structure of local anaesthetic drugs, showing the hydrophilic centre (amino group) and the lipophilic centre (aromatic residue) linked by either an ester or an amide chain. Slight variations in the moieties R_1 to R_4 do not affect the local anaesthetic action

nerve membrane. On the other hand, dominance of the lipophilic centre will result in low solubility in water. Apart from these factors, which affect the pharmacokinetic properties of the drugs, it appears that all three parts of the local anaesthetic molecule participate in the binding of the drug to the nerve membrane. The physicochemical properties of these drugs and their structure–activity relationships have received considerable attention.

In the concentrations needed to produce local anaesthesia, the drugs do not affect the resting potential of the nerve membrane but they prevent the development of action potentials by a stabilizing action on the membrane. Thus, they do not block the sodium pump but prevent the transient increase in the permeability of the nerve membrane to sodium ions, which is the necessary preliminary to the influx of sodium ions constituting the first phase of the action potential. There is also a reduction in the secondary increase in permeability to potassium ions, but this is of less importance to the blocking of sodium permeability and requires larger concentrations of the drug. The membrane-stabilizing action is also dependent on the extracellular concentration of calcium ions and a high concentration of calcium ions can itself produce a stabilizing effect, as well as either increasing or reducing the effect of a local anaesthetic.

As most local anaesthetics are secondary or tertiary amines, they can exist in charged or uncharged forms, depending upon the pH (see Chapter 2). They are more effective in alkaline solutions because increasing the pH increases the proportion of uncharged molecules present and these penetrate the tissues more readily. However, once the drug has penetrated the nerve membrane, it appears that it is the cationic form which is active, and that the action is on the inner surface of the nerve membrane. This concept is supported by the experimental finding that quaternary analogues of local anaesthetics are effective when applied internally to the giant axon of the squid, but not when applied externally. The precise mechanism through which local anaesthetic drugs affect sodium permeability is not known, but it is thought that the receptor on which they act is within the sodium channel itself. One possibility is that the drugs increase the surface pressure of the lipid layer which constitutes the nerve membrane, thereby closing the pores through which the sodium ions pass. Some local anaesthetics, e.g. benzocaine, are only slightly water soluble and probably act from inside the membrane, rather than passing through to its inner surface.

Cocaine (Figure 9.2a)

This drug has already been discussed in Chapter 8 (page 101) because of its action of blocking the re-uptake of noradrenaline, but it is also the prototype local anaesthetic, as well as being a naturally occurring drug. It is a potent drug but its use as a local anaesthetic is restricted because of its toxicity, due to potentiation of the action of noradrenaline and the central effects of cocaine, together with the fact that it is addictive. As cocaine readily penetrates mucous membranes, it is an effective surface anaesthetic when applied to the cornea or laryngeal mucous membrane.

Procaine (Figure 9.2b)

This is one of the first synthetic local anaesthetics, which is less toxic than cocaine, but also weaker in its anaesthetic action; however, it is not addictive. It does not penetrate mucous membranes well and is therefore of little use for surface anaesthesia. Like cocaine, procaine has some stimulant action on the CNS and can interact with sympathomimetic amines. However, because it is also rapidly metabolized, solutions of procaine for local injection usually contain a vasoconstrictor substance such as adrenaline. This prevents the absorption of the drug into the systemic circulation and also retards its metabolism. Procaine is metabolized in the blood and liver to p-aminobenzoic acid and diethylaminoethanol, by a plasma esterase. The p-aminobenzoic acid inhibits the action of sulphonamide antibiotics. Therefore, where sulphonamide therapy is being employed, local anaesthetics which are not derivatives of p-aminobenzoic acid should be used.

Procaine has an anti-arrhythmic action on the heart but is not very effective for this purpose because it is metabolized very quickly and large doses, given intravenously, can cause convulsions. A related substance, procainamide, has a similar anti-arrhythmic action and is a therapeutically useful drug. It is less rapidly metabolized in the blood and does not have excitatory actions on the CNS because it does not penetrate the blood–brain barrier.

Lignocaine (Figure 9.2c)

This is the most widely used local anaesthetic drug. It is more stable than most other local anaesthetics as it is not hydrolysed by plasma esterases and it has a rapid onset of action. It is effectively absorbed from mucous membranes and can be used as a surface anaesthetic. When lignocaine is used for infiltration anaesthesia, solutions containing adrenaline are usually employed. Lignocaine has depressant effects on the CNS and can cause sedation. It has an anticonvulsant action and, when given intravenously, has been found effective in relieving status epilepticus (see Chapter 13), although other drugs, such as benzodiazepines, are now preferred.

A number of other synthetic local anaesthetic drugs are in current use. Examples of these are bupivacaine (Figure 9.2d), which has a long duration of action, mepivacaine (Figure 9.2e) and prilocaine (Figure 9.2f), the latter two being similar to lignocaine in action, but having a longer duration of action.

(a)

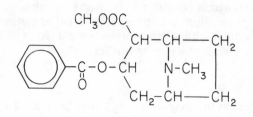
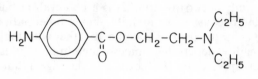

(b)

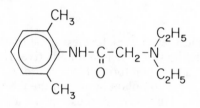

(c)

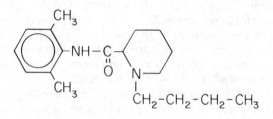

(d)

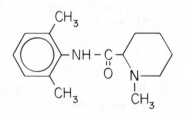

(e)

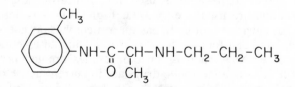

(f)

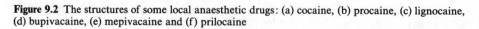

Figure 9.2 The structures of some local anaesthetic drugs: (a) cocaine, (b) procaine, (c) lignocaine, (d) bupivacaine, (e) mepivacaine and (f) prilocaine

The clinical uses of local anaesthetic drugs

Local anaesthetics are used to abolish the sensation of pain in relatively restricted areas of the body. They enable operative procedures, e.g. dental extractions, to be carried out without the necessity for a general anaesthetic. All local anaesthetics have a similar mechanism of action and block the conduction of nerve impulses. However, because they vary in their other properties, some are more useful for certain applications than others.

The sites of application of local anaesthetics

The various locations to which local anaesthetics are applied are illustrated in Figure 9.3.

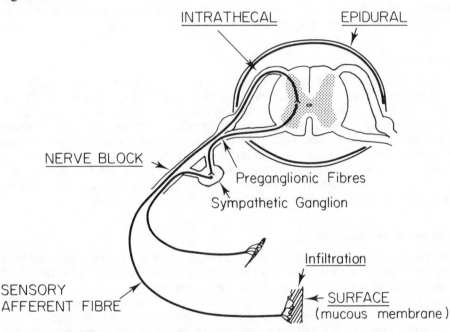

Figure 9.3 Diagrammatic transverse section of the spinal cord showing the sites at which local anaesthetics are applied (modified from Crossland, 1980)

Surface anaesthesia

This involves topical application of the drug in the form of a solution or ointment to the site at which anaesthesia is required. It usually is restricted to mucous membranes, e.g. the conjunctiva and upper respiratory tract. The drugs used are those which are well absorbed from mucous membranes, e.g. lignocaine, cocaine and benzocaine.

Infiltration anaesthesia

A solution of the local anaesthetic is injected into the site which is to be incised surgically (Figure 9.3). The object is to ensure that the finer nerve endings which supply the region are anaesthetized. The infiltration may be superficial, i.e. limited to the skin, or it may include subcutaneous structures. It is mainly used for minor surgical procedures, e.g. extraction of teeth, draining of abscesses) etc. The drugs used are lignocaine, bupivacaine (for a longer duration) and prilocaine.

Nerve block

In this case, the local anaesthetic is injected as close as possible to the main nerve trunk supplying the region in which anaesthesia is required (Figure 9.3). Conduction in both motor and sensory fibres will be blocked, thus enabling surgery to be carried out on a limb, for example. Because the fibres in nerve trunks are considerably larger than the fine fibres encountered in the skin, larger concentrations of local anaesthetic are needed for nerve block than those used for infiltration anaesthesia. The method can also be used for the relief of postoperative pain. Again, lignocaine, bupivacaine and prilocaine are suitable drugs.

Epidural anaesthesia

This is also known as extradural anaesthesia and is a special form of regional nerve block. If the local anaesthetic is injected into the extradural space (Figure 9.3), the drug will reach the roots of the spinal nerves and anaesthetize them. Some of the drug may penetrate the dura, entering the subarachnoid space and anaesthetizing the nerve roots. In the thoracic region there is a significant interdural space formed between the layers of the dura and epidural anaesthesia is produced by injecting the drug into this space. This method is used for operations on the thorax and abdomen, as well as in obstetrics, and for the relief of postoperative pain. A longer-acting drug, such as bupivacaine, tends to be used.

Spinal or intrathecal anaesthesia

In this case the local anaesthetic is injected into the subarachnoid space so that it reaches the roots of the spinal nerves (Figure 9.3). To avoid damage to the spinal cord, the injection is usually made in the lumbar region, below the termination of the cord. The level at which anaesthesia is produced will depend upon the specific gravity of the solution injected, compared with CSF. Thus, isobaric solutions (the same specific gravity as CSF) will produce an effect at the same level as the intrathecal injection, hypobaric solutions at a higher level and hyperbaric solutions at a lower level. Hyperbaric solutions can be readily obtained by the addition of glucose to the solution of local anaesthetic and the level at which anaesthesia is produced can be varied by tilting the patient. The local anaesthetic within the subarachnoid space penetrates the superficial layers of the spinal cord to reach the spinal nerve roots and so produce nerve block. Lignocaine, bupivacaine and prilocaine can all be used.

Solutions of local anaesthetics containing catecholamine vasoconstrictor substances, e.g. adrenaline or noradrenaline, should not be used in patients who are taking antidepressant drugs such as tricyclics or monoamine oxidase inhibitors (see Chapter 17) because of the risk of cardiac arrhythmias and hypertension. In such cases felypressin, a derivative of vasopressin, can be used as it does not interact with antidepressants. Local anaesthetics for use in digits or appendages should not contain a vasoconstrictor because of the risk of ischaemia.

Veratrum alkaloids

These are substances present in plants belonging to the genus *Veratrum*. They have an effect on nerve membranes opposite to that of the local anaesthetics, delaying closure of sodium channels after an action potential has been produced. However, the end result is the same, as a block of conduction will occur as the result of prolonged depolarization.

Toxins

A number of toxins act directly on nerve fibres, unlike those which act at the neuromuscular junction (see Chapter 5). Thus, tetrodotoxin (which is present in the puffer fish and Californian newt), saxitonin (which is found in dinoflagellates that are ingested by certain clams and mussels) and maculotoxin (present in the salivary glands of the Australian blue-ringed octopus), all block the conduction of action potentials in nerves without altering the membrane potential. The effects they produce are, therefore, similar to those of the local anaesthetics and it has been shown that these toxins block sodium channels in the nerve membrane. Both tetrodotoxin and saxitoxin contain a guanidine group which is ionized at body pH. Guanidine ions have been shown to substitute for sodium ions under certain circumstances; it is possible that the guanidine group of tetrodotoxin and saxitoxin could enter the sodium channels of the nerve membrane but that the channels become blocked by the bulk of the rest of the molecule. Maculotoxin does not contain a guanidine group and a different mechanism of action must be postulated if this hypothesis is true.

Another group of toxins includes batrachotoxin, obtained from the skin of a S. American frog (*Phyllobates aurotaenia*) and used as an arrow poison, ciguatoxin, present in certain moray eels, and grayotoxins, which are found in the leaves of rhododendrons. These all produce an irreversible depolarization of nerve membranes by keeping the sodium channels open. Initially the membrane is excited but the persistent depolarization eventually leads to a block of conduction.

None of these toxins has any therapeutic application but their highly specific actions have helped in the analysis of the mechanism of nerve conduction.

Part 3

The central nervous system

Chapter 10

Synaptic transmission in the central nervous system

The central nervous system (CNS), which comprises the brain and spinal cord, is considerably more complex in its organization than the peripheral nervous system and, in the CNS, more substances are involved in the process of synaptic transmission. Thus, while peripheral nerves are mainly concerned with conveying signals to the effector organs and with relaying information from the sense organs to the brain, the CNS is involved with the control and co-ordination of movement (behaviour), together with higher functions such as consciousness, emotion, language, memory and learning, and in man, with attributes like imagination, abstract reasoning and creative thought.

It has been estimated that the human brain contains about 10^{10} neurones and, while some of these form well-defined pathways, many are linked together in the form of diffuse networks, e.g. in the cerebral cortex. The numbers of synapses on individual neurones in the CNS can be measured in hundreds or thousands, the largest recorded number being around 80 000. Various types of synapses, i.e. axo–somatic, axo–dendritic and axo–axonal (see Chapter 3, Figure 3.2), as well as dendro–dendritic, exist in the brain and can be either excitatory or inhibitory in nature, although excitatory synapses tend to be of the axo–dendritic type and inhibitory synapses, axo–somatic. The influences on an individual neurone in the CNS, particularly in the brain, can therefore be extremely complex, and the integration of spatial and temporal patterns of excitation and inhibition over the surface and in different parts of the neurone, will determine the level of activity, together with the probability of its firing. Another aspect of the structure of the CNS which is important for synaptic transmission is the presence of non-neuronal cells, or neuroglia. Although the function of glial cells is mainly to provide the neurones with mechanical support and with insulation through the production of myelin, they are also involved in metabolic processes, including the uptake and removal of some neurotransmitters. Compared with the peripheral nervous system, where single synapses can be isolated relatively easily, the complexity of the CNS makes it extremely difficult to study the events taking place at a single synapse and our knowledge in this area has been dependent on advances in the techniques which can be used.

The criteria which must be satisfied before a substance can be considered to be a neurotransmitter have been outlined in Chapter 3. These same criteria also apply to the CNS and, in fact, there is a degree of similarity between many of the characteristics of peripheral and central synapses, especially where the same transmitter is involved.

NEUROTRANSMITTERS IN THE CNS

Acetylcholine

The mechanisms through which acetylcholine functions as a synaptic transmitter in the CNS resemble very closely the peripheral mechanisms, for example those at the neuromuscular junction (Chapter 4). Thus, the synthesis of acetylcholine from acetate and choline is mediated by the enzyme choline acetyltransferase within the nerve terminals, where the transmitter is stored in vesicles and released by the process of exocytosis, which is calcium-dependent. The released transmitter diffuses across the synaptic gap to act upon the postsynaptic receptor and is then inactivated by being hydrolysed by the enzyme, acetylcholinesterase. Apart from postsynaptic receptors, it is known that presynaptic receptors for acetylcholine exist on many nerve terminals in the CNS. They may be present on cholinergic nerve terminals (autoreceptors) but the best evidence for the existence of presynaptic receptors for acetylcholine is on the terminals of other neurotransmitter systems. The function of these presynaptic receptors is to modulate the release of the transmitter.

Cholinergic pathways in the CNS

The first cholinergic pathway in the CNS to be identified was that between the terminals of recurrent collateral axons of lower motor neurones in the spinal cord and inhibitory neurones known as Renshaw cells (Figure 10.1). Acetylcholine is, of course, the transmitter released from the terminals of the motor neurones (at the neuromuscular junction), and its release from the collateral terminals excites the Renshaw cells, but the influence of these cells on the motor neurones is inhibitory. This pathway therefore forms a negative feedback loop.

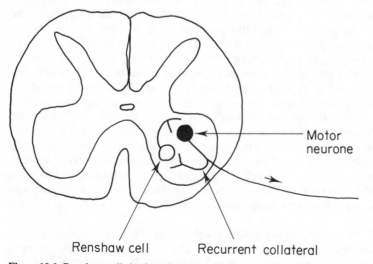

Figure 10.1 Renshaw cells in the spinal cord. Recurrent collaterals of the axons of motor neurones in the ventral horn activate the Renshaw cells which then inhibit the motor neurones. The synapse between the recurrent collateral and the Renshaw cell is cholinergic

In the brain, the identification of cholinergic pathways has been hampered by the lack of suitable techniques. Acetylcholine, together with the enzymes responsible for its synthesis and destruction, is widely distributed throughout the brain and the regional differences which have been detected are small and appear to have no functional significance. Early attempts to map cholinergic pathways using histochemical staining methods, based on the localization of acetylcholinesterase, produced somewhat misleading results as this enzyme is not localized exclusively to cholinergic neurones. More reliable information about the distribution of cholinergic neurones in the CNS and of the existence of pathways in the brain has been obtained more recently by the use of immunohistochemical staining techniques coupled with microiontophoresis.

The principal cholinergic pathways in the brain of the rat are illustrated schematically in Figure 10.2. There is a widespread distribution of cholinergic fibres in the cerebral cortex, the majority of which originate in the nucleus basalis

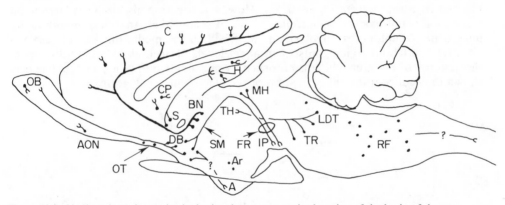

Figure 10.2 Cholinergic pathways in the brain, shown on a sagittal section of the brain of the rat. A, amygdala; AON, anterior olfactory nucleus; Ar, arcuate nucleus; BN, nucleus basalis; C, cerebral cortex; CP, caudate putamen; DB, nucleus of diagonal band; FR, fasciculus retroflexus; H, hippocampus; IP, nucleus interpeduncularis; LDT, lateral dorsal tegmental nucleus; MH, medial habenula; OB, olfactory cortex; RF, hindbrain reticular formation; S, septum; SM, stria medullaris; TH, thalamus; TR, tegmental reticular system; OT, olfactory tract (modified from Cuello and Sofroniew, 1985)

(which is thought to be homologous with the nucleus of Maynert in primates). Another pathway which has been known for some time is from the septum to the hippocampus. The striatum is known to contain the highest concentration in the brain of acetylcholine and its associated enzymes. In this region, as well as in the nucleus accumbens, there are cholinergic interneurones. Intrinsic cholinergic neurones are also present in the cerebral cortex and in the brain stem, including the respiratory centre in the medulla. Although Figure 10.2 illustrates cholinergic pathways in the brain of the rat, the presence of these pathways has been confirmed in many other species, including primates.

Cholinergic mechanisms in the CNS and function: effects of drugs

Most of the information concerning the involvement of cholinergic mechanisms in the brain with function has come from studies of the central effects of drugs which modify cholinergic transmission. Many drugs, for example anaesthetics, hypnotics and sedatives, increase the level of acetylcholine in the brain, but this is probably an indirect effect which comes about through the depression of the activity of cholinergic neurones and is probably unrelated to the mechanism of action of these drugs (see Chapter 11). Both nicotinic and muscarinic receptors are present in the brain and their properties are similar to those of the peripheral receptors. However, muscarinic receptors predominate by a factor of between 10 and 100 to 1 and are also present presynaptically, in which case their function is to modulate the release of the transmitter. Many of the drugs which have actions at peripheral cholinergic receptors are without central effects as they do not cross the blood–brain barrier.

Agonists

Oxotremorine and arecoline (Figure 10.3a,b), both of which are muscarinic agonists, cause tremor when given in sufficiently large doses and the effect is blocked by atropine (see Figure 7.5a). However, nicotine also induces tremor but this action is not blocked by atropine. Thus, it seems likely that both nicotinic and muscarinic receptors are involved in the mechanisms mediating tremor (see also Chapter 19). Cholinergic agonists can affect levels of arousal and wakefulness and the quantity of nicotine which is absorbed from a single puff of a cigarette has been shown to produce transient activation of the electroencephalogram.

(a)

(b)

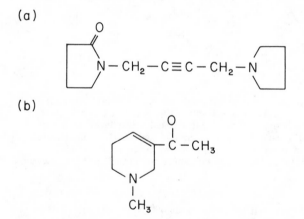

Figure 10.3 The chemical structures of (a) oxotremorine and (b) arecoline

Physostigmine, which produces agonist-like effects by inhibiting the breakdown of acetylcholine (see Chapter 5), and which readily penetrates the blood–brain barrier, has been found to enhance memory and learning in experimental animals and has also been tested in Alzheimer's disease (see Chapter 20).

Antagonists

Apart from antagonizing the tremor induced by muscarinic agonists, muscarinic antagonists are effective in relieving the symptoms of Parkinson's disease. They also have useful anti-emetic properties and some, e.g. hyoscine (Figure 7.5b), form the basis of remedies for motion sickness (see Chapter 20). Some muscarinic antagonists have been found to have effects on short-term memory. For example, hyoscine, which is also sedative, produces amnesia and has been used as a so-called 'truth' drug. Large doses of atropine, on the other hand, are stimulant in the CNS and certain esters of glycolic acid (glycolates), such as Ditran which is a mixture of two glycolate esters, are psychotomimetics (Chapter 18). The uses of anticholinergic drugs in the treatment of Parkinson's disease and as anti-emetics are discussed in Chapters 19 and 20. Cholinergic mechanisms in the respiratory centre in the medulla are important for the actions of anticholinesterases (see Chapter 5) and paralysis of the respiratory centre is an important factor in the toxicity of these compounds.

Noradrenaline

As with acetylcholine, the processes involved in the synthesis, storage, release and actions of noradrenaline in the CNS appear to be very similar, if not identical, to those at the periphery, i.e. at sympathetic noradrenergic nerve terminals (Chapter 8). An important factor is that the amino acid precursor of the catecholamines, L-tyrosine, readily crosses the blood–brain barrier and is therefore transported into the brain from the bloodstream. Another is that, whereas acetylcholine is widely distributed throughout the CNS, the catecholamines have an uneven distribution, which is similar in most mammalian species. Thus, noradrenaline is present in the highest concentrations in the hypothalamus and brain stem.

Noradrenergic pathways in the CNS

The mapping of catecholamine pathways in the CNS has been facilitated by the development of histochemical techniques that utilize a reaction between catechol-amines (and also 5-hydroxytryptamine) and formaldehyde, which produces a derivative that is fluorescent under suitable conditions. This technique has been used in conjunction with lesioning.

Noradrenergic pathways in the CNS arise from cell bodies in two main regions: (1) the locus coeruleus,which is within the caudal central grey matter of the brain stem and is composed only of noradrenaline-containing neurones and (2) groups of cells scattered through the ventral and lateral tegmental regions of the medulla (Figure 10.4).

A major ascending pathway arises from the cell bodies in the locus coeruleus, the fibres projecting rostrally to form a dorsal bundle (Figure 10.4) and giving off branches to many other regions of the brain, e.g. the cerebellum, thalamus, hypothalamus, hippocampus, olfactory area, etc. Eventually, these ascending fibres terminate diffusely in the neocortex. A second ascending pathway arises from the noradrenergic neurones, which are more diffusely distributed throughout the brain stem, and these fibres form a ventral bundle and terminate in the hypothalamus and amygdala. Where the two ascending bundles of noradrenergic fibres run together, they form a structure known as the median forebrain bundle.

Many of the neurones in the lateral ventral tegmentum of the brain stem give rise to short axons and are probably interneurones. There is also a descending noradrenergic tract arising in this region which projects caudally into the spinal cord.

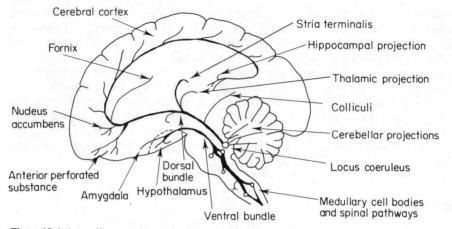

Figure 10.4 Ascending noradrenergic pathways in the brain shown, in this case, on a diagrammatic sagittal section of the primate brain (modified from Kruk and Pycock, 1983)

Noradrenergic mechanisms and function

The dorsal nucleus of the vagus and the nucleus of the tractus solitarius receive a noradrenergic innervation from the neurones in the lateral tegmentum and it is believed that these neurones are concerned with the central control of sympathetic tone and hence, with blood pressure. In the spinal cord, the descending noradrenergic pathway has three components, one in each of the dorsal and ventral horns and the other in the lateral sympathetic column. The latter is associated with vasomotor control, while the noradrenergic neurones in the ventral horn participate in the control of flexor muscles, an effect which is mediated by α-adrenoceptors. The ascending noradrenergic systems appear to be involved in a variety of functions although the evidence, in some cases, is inconclusive. For example, the locus coeruleus has been associated with the maintenance of behavioural attention and vigilance, and noradrenergic mechanisms in the brain have been shown to be involved in the process of reinforcement, a process which facilitates learning.

Noradrenergic mechanisms are important in the control of sleep and wakefulness and it is likely that the ascending noradrenergic pathways mediate 'phasic' arousal, because this response is lost when these pathways are interrupted. Furthermore, drugs which release noradrenaline from nerve terminals, e.g. amphetamine (Chapters 8 and 16), produce their alerting effects by an action in the brain stem where there are many noradrenaline-containing neurones. However, the arousal associated with the response to stress is probably mediated reflexly, as the increased levels of adrenaline and noradrenaline circulating in the blood do not penetrate the blood–brain barrier, at least in appreciable quantities. Noradrenergic mechanisms in the hypothalamus are associated with thermoregulation.

Noradrenergic mechanisms in the brain are also concerned with the control of mood and emotional behaviour and many drugs used to treat psychiatric conditions have effects on noradrenergic mechanisms (see Chapters 12 and 17).

Receptors for noradrenaline in the CNS

Both α- and β-adrenoceptors are present in the CNS but their distribution is not well known. Presynaptic receptors are also present. For example, presynaptic α-receptors, which appear to be mainly autoreceptors, have been designated α_2- to distinguish them from postsynaptic α_1-receptors. The drug clonidine, which is used in the treatment of hypertension (Chapter 8), is a selective agonist at α_2-receptors and it is possible that this action may contribute to its antihypertensive effect. However, in large doses, clonidine is not selective and stimulates both α_1- and α_2-receptors. There is also some evidence that presynaptic β-receptors are present in the CNS, although their precise function is not known. Most postsynaptic β-receptors in the CNS are linked to adenylate cyclase as the second messenger (see Chapter 3). How responses to α-receptors in the CNS are mediated is not known, although cyclic AMP, calcium ions and potassium have all been proposed as second messengers.

Dopamine

The principal role for dopamine in the peripheral nervous system is that of a precursor in the synthesis of noradrenaline, although the possibility exists that dopamine may have a neurotransmitter role in autonomic ganglia (Chapter 6). However, in the CNS, dopamine is a neurotransmitter in its own right, in addition to being the precursor to noradrenaline. Nevertheless, dopaminergic neurones are very similar in many ways to noradrenergic neurones and the mechanisms concerned with synthesis, storage and release, as well as inactivation, are similar in the two types of neurone. The most important difference is that the terminals of dopamine-containing neurones lack the enzyme dopamine-β-hydroxylase, which converts dopamine to noradrenaline (see Chapter 8, Figures 8.2 and 8.3); thus the synthesis stops with dopamine which is stored in dense-cored vesicles and is released by a calcium-dependent mechanism.

Dopamine pathways in the CNS

The largest concentrations of dopamine in the brain are in the basal ganglia and the limbic system. There are three main neuronal systems in the brain which utilize dopamine as the neurotransmitter, and these are described below.

Nigrostriatal pathway

This arises from dopamine-containing cell bodies in the substantia nigra (A9 in Figure 10.5), which send axons to terminate in the caudate nucleus–putamen complex (the neostriatum). This pathway forms part of the extrapyramidal system of the brain (see also Chapter 19).

Mesolimbic forebrain system

The cell bodies of the neurones forming this pathway are in the ventral tegmentum of the midbrain, close to and some within the substantia nigra (A8 and A10 in Figure 10.5) and the axons project forward to the neostriatum (caudate and putamen), the limbic system, including the limbic cortex, amygdala, nucleus accumbens, septum and olfactory tubercle, and also to the frontal cortex.

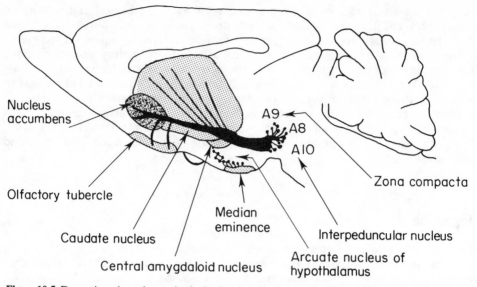

Figure 10.5 Dopaminergic pathways in the brain, shown on a representative sagittal section of the brain of the rat. A8, A9 and A10 refer to identified groups of dopamine-containing neurones. A8 and A9 are in the substantia nigra and A10 is in the ventral tegmentum (modified from Ungerstedt, 1971)

Tubero-infundibular system

The cell bodies of the neurones forming this pathway lie within the region of the arcuate nucleus of the hypothalamus (Figure 10.5) and possess relatively short axons which terminate in the median eminence.

In addition to the three dopaminergic pathways described above, there are dopamine-containing neurones with ultra-short axons in the retina and also interneurones within the hypothalamus and olfactory bulb.

Although Figure 10.5 illustrates the principal dopamine-containing pathways in the brain of the rat, similar pathways have been found in the brains of most mammalian species. The olfactory tubercle in the rat and some other species is probably homologous with the anterior perforated substance of the human brain.

Dopamine in the CNS and function

Of the neurotransmitter pathways identified in the brain to date, those in which dopamine is the transmitter are probably the best known, at least in so far as their functional role is concerned. The basal ganglia have long been known to be involved in the fine control of movement, and diseases which affect these structures have profound effects on motor activity. Drugs acting at dopamine receptors, particularly those of the nigrostriatal pathway, are used in the treatment of neurological disorders, such as Parkinson's disease (Chapter 19). Dopamine in the CNS has also been linked to disturbances of behaviour, especially emotional behaviour, and drugs which are antagonists at dopamine receptors are used in the treatment of certain psychiatric disorders, such as schizophrenia (Chapter 12). Finally, the tubero-infundibular dopaminergic pathway is concerned with the functions of the hypothalamic–pituitary endocrine system and drugs which act on dopamine receptors can influence functions controlled by this system, e.g. emesis (Chapter 20).

Dopamine receptors

The existence of more than one type of dopamine receptor in the CNS has been suggested from the results of various studies, both biochemical and behavioural. Unfortunately, there has been a tendency to use different criteria in the different types of study and, as a result, several schemes of nomenclature exist. However, as far as the mechanism of action of drugs acting on dopamine receptors in the CNS is concerned, two subtypes of dopamine receptor, D_1 and D_2, must be considered.

The D_1 subtype of dopamine receptor is linked to stimulation of the enzyme adenylate cyclase as second messenger and hence to increased levels of cyclic AMP. It is present in the nigrostriatal and mesolimbic dopamine pathways in the brain, as well as in the superior cervical ganglion peripherally. The D_2 receptor, on the other hand, is characterized by either no effect on levels of cyclic AMP, or a reduction, i.e. inhibition of the synthesis of cyclic AMP. This subtype of dopamine receptor is found in the anterior lobe of the pituitary gland and in the nigrostriatal and mesolimbic pathways. The two subtypes of dopamine receptors show different sensitivities to agonist and antagonist drugs, effects which are considered in more detail in Chapter 12. Other subtypes of dopamine receptors, i.e. D_3 and D_4, have been postulated on the basis of ligand-binding studies, but as yet have had no precise functions ascribed to them. In fact the D_1 receptor, which is linked to adenylate cyclase, shows a poor correlation with function and its precise functional role in the brain is not clear.

There is good evidence for the existence of presynaptic receptors on nerve terminals which release dopamine in the CNS. For example, autoreceptors are present on terminals of the nigrostriatal pathway and stimulation of these causes a reduction in the release of dopamine. These receptors may well be important for the mechanisms of action of drugs which control the function of dopamine in the CNS (see Chapter 12). As well as autoreceptors, presynaptic receptors for transmitters other than dopamine, e.g. acetylcholine and 5-hydroxytryptamine, are present on dopamine-containing nerve terminals in the striatum. This type of synaptic mechanism can allow for subtle interactions between different neurotransmitter systems in the brain to take place.

5-Hydroxytryptamine

5-Hydroxytryptamine (serotonin, 5-HT) is an indole (Figure 10.6), which is present in many neurones in the CNS. It is also found in many other tissues, e.g. blood platelets, mast cells and the enterochromaffin cells of the gut. It is also found widely in nature, for example in many plants and their fruit (e.g. bananas) and in insect stings. Peripherally, 5-HT acts as a local hormone or autacoid. That released from platelets, for example, has a powerful vasoconstrictor action on many blood vessels (although some are dilated) and in the gut it causes contraction of smooth muscle resulting in increased tone and motility. It has been generally assumed that only the 5-HT present in the CNS is associated with neurones, i.e. acts as a neurotransmitter. However, there is some evidence, albeit tentative, that 5-HT-containing nerve fibres may be present in the gut.

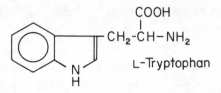

L-Tryptophan

tryptophan hydroxylase

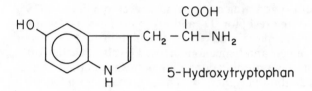

5-Hydroxytryptophan

L-aromatic acid decarboxylase

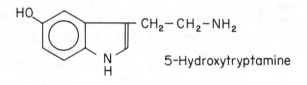

5-Hydroxytryptamine

monoamine oxidase

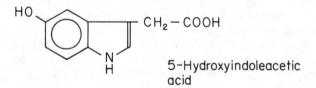

5-Hydroxyindoleacetic
acid

Figure 10.6 The synthesis and metabolism of 5-hydroxytryptamine (5-HT). The enzymes involved are shown in italics

The 5-HT in the CNS represents only about 1–2% of the total amount in the body and as the indole does not cross the blood–brain barrier, the 5-HT-containing neurones in the CNS must synthesize their own transmitter. However, the processes involved both for synthesis and metabolism are similar in the CNS and peripherally.

The synthesis of 5-HT in neurones

The primary substrate for 5-HT is the aromatic amino acid, L-tryptophan, which is present in plasma and arises mainly from diet. L-Tryptophan readily crosses the blood–brain barrier and is taken up into serotonergic nerve terminals by a neutral amino acid carrier which also transports other amino acids, such as tyrosine and phenylalanine, across the nerve membrane. Competition for this carrier mechanism can influence the intraneuronal levels of these amino acids. In the cytoplasm of the 5-HT-containing nerve terminals there is an enzyme, tryptophan hydroxylase, which converts the L-tryptophan to 5-hydroxytryptophan (5-HTP) (Figure 10.6). This enzyme requires molecular oxygen and reduced pteridine cofactor for its activity. The reaction is the rate-limiting step in the synthesis of 5-HT but the enzyme tryptophan hydroxylase is not saturated under normal conditions (compared with tyrosine hydroxylase, see Chapter 8). Therefore, increasing the amount of substrate available, by increasing the level of L-tryptophan in the diet, can result in increased synthesis of 5-HT in the CNS. This has, in fact, been done by feeding large quantities of tryptophan to psychiatric patients (Chapter 17) but with equivocal results. However, the relationship between the rate of synthesis of 5-HT in the CNS and plasma levels of L-tryptophan is not simple. For example, a fraction of the L-tryptophan in plasma is bound to plasma proteins and feedback mechanisms can alter the activity of tyrosine hydroxylase.

The next stage in the synthesis of 5-HT is the decarboxylation of 5-hydroxytryptophan to 5-hydroxytryptamine by the enzyme, 5-hydroxytryptophan decarboxylase (Figure 10.6). This reaction also takes place in the cytoplasm and requires pyridoxal phosphate (vitamin B_6) as cofactor. The decarboxylase enzyme is relatively non-specific and it was at one time thought to be identical to dopa-decarboxylase (see Chapter 8). However, it is now known that these are two distinct enzymes.

The 5-HT which is formed in the cytoplasm is actively taken up into dense-core vesicles, where it is bound in a complex with proteins, ions and adenosine triphosphate. These vesicles appear to be very similar to those which store the catecholamine neurotransmitters. The release process is also very similar, 5-HT being released into the synaptic cleft by a calcium-dependent process in response to action potentials arriving at the nerve terminals.

The removal of the neurotransmitter from the synaptic gap and from the vicinity of the postsynaptic receptor is by a high-affinity transport system, which causes the re-uptake of the transmitter into the presynaptic terminals where the 5-HT is taken up into synaptic vesicles. However, 5-HT is also metabolized to 5-hydroxindole-acetic acid (5-HIAA) (Figure 10.6) by monoamine oxidase which is located intracellularly on mitochondria, as well as extracellularly. The plasma level of 5-HIAA has been used as an indicator of the turnover of 5-HT in the CNS.

Pathways for 5-HT in the brain

The histochemical method, utilizing formaldehyde-induced fluorescence, which is used for detecting catecholamines, can also be used for 5-HT, but in this case it is less sensitive. Thus, the localization of cell bodies containing 5-HT is relatively easy, but 5-HT-containing terminals are more difficult to detect. Cell bodies containing 5-HT are clustered in the midline region of the pons and upper brain stem, in the raphe nuclei (Figure 10.7). From these cell groups ascending fibres innervate the basal ganglia, hypothalamus, thalamus, hippocampus, limbic fore-brain and neocortex. There are also projections to the cerebellum. In addition, 5-HT-containing cell bodies in the brain stem give rise to descending axons which terminate in the medulla and spinal cord. Similar pathways have been found in the primate brain (including man).

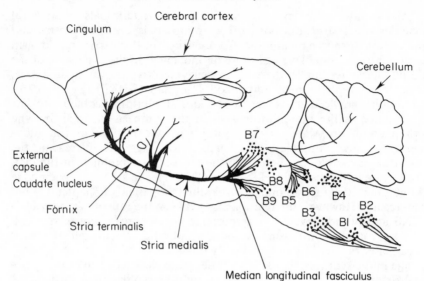

Figure 10.7 Diagrammatic sagittal section of the brain of the rat, showing ascending and descending pathways for 5-hydroxytryptamine. The raphe nuclei are represented by cell groups B4 to B9, inclusive (modified from Cooper, Bloom and Roth, 1986)

The functional role of 5-HT in the CNS

Most of our knowledge of the functional role of 5-HT as a neurotransmitter in the CNS has come from experimental studies with drugs which are known to modify the actions of 5-HT. These studies have shown that 5-HT is involved in the control of sleep and wakefulness, mood and emotion, feeding, thermoregulation, sexual behaviour and also some drug-induced hallucinatory states. However, in most cases, other neurotransmitter systems are also involved.

Drugs affecting 5-HT mechanisms in the CNS

Effects on synthesis

The levels of 5-HT in the CNS can be lowered by administering drugs which inhibit synthesis. For example, p-chlorophenylalanine (Figure 10.8a) inhibits the activity of tyrosine hydroxylase and consequently depletes the brain of 5-HT. The result, in experimental animals, is increased wakefulness and alertness (as indicated by the EEG), increased motor activity and insomnia. The effect of p-chlorophenylalanine can be reversed by the administration of the precursor of 5-HT, 5-hydroxytryptophan (5-HTP), to restore the levels of 5-HT in the brain. The administration of large amounts of 5-HTP has been found to increase the amount of slow-wave sleep and rapid-eye-movement sleep, characteristic of deep sleep, in the EEG (see Chapter 11); this is presumably due to higher levels of 5-HT than normal. The involvement of 5-HT in the brain with the control of wakefulness and sleep has been studied extensively and it is likely that the ascending 5-HT pathway (Figure 10.7) is concerned with slow 'tonic' changes in the sleep/wakefulness continuum, whereas the ascending noradrenergic pathway (Figure 10.4) is more likely to be involved in fast responses, i.e. 'phasic' arousal. Lesions of the raphe nuclei have

(a)

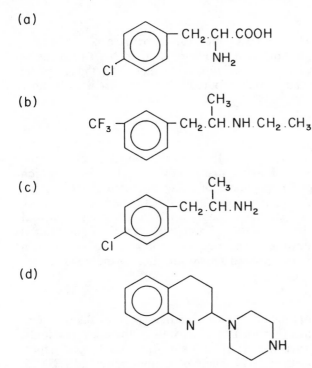

(b)

(c)

(d)

Figure 10.8 The chemical structures of (a) *p*-chlorophenylalanine, (b) fenfluramine, (c) *p*-chloro-amphetamine and (d) quipazine

been found to cause increased wakefulness. However, some of the experimental data should be treated with caution as, for example, 5-HTP is known to be taken up by non-5-HT-containing neurones and lesions of the raphe nuclei are bound to affect other neurotransmitter systems.

Storage and release

Drugs which disrupt the storage of catecholamines in synaptic vesicles, e.g. reserpine and tetrabenazine (Chapter 8, Figure 8.9), also deplete intracellular stores of 5-HT, both in the CNS and peripherally. It has been suggested that the mental depression and sedation which accompany the administration of reserpine (as an anti-hypertensive drug) might be due to depletion of 5-HT, but it is difficult to correlate this with the observation that depletion of 5-HT by inhibition of synthesis (in experimental animals) causes increased alertness and motor activity. Certainly, the release of 5-HT from peripheral stores can account for the increased motility of the gut, abdominal cramps and diarrhoea produced by reserpine, and drugs which block 5-HT receptors can be used to treat these symptoms.

Drugs which stimulate the release of 5-HT from nerve terminals, e.g. fenfluramine and *p*-chloroamphetamine (Figure 10.8b,c), cause suppression of food intake and fenfluramine is used as an anorectic agent (Chapter 20). However, these drugs also block the re-uptake of 5-HT and fenfluramine can cause disturbances of mood, including depression, when the administration of the drug is discontinued.

Re-uptake and metabolism

Drugs which inhibit the activity of the enzyme monoamine oxidase cause accumulation of 5-HT, as well as of catecholamines, and are used in the treatment of depression. Similarly, some of the tricyclic antidepressant drugs block the re-uptake of 5-HT as well as that of noradrenaline. Both groups of drugs are discussed in more detail in Chapter 17.

Agonists of 5-HT

Various substitutions can be made on the 5-HT molecule without loss of agonist activity and a number of indoles are known, structurally related to 5-HT, which have agonist actions at 5-HT receptors. Some of these are naturally occurring substances; others are synthetic. Most are psychotomimetic and are therefore discussed in Chapter 18. There are, however, some 5-HT receptor agonists that are not indoles. They include quipazine [1-(2-quinolyl)piperazine] (Figure 10.8d) which, in animals (cats and rats), produces sham-rage reactions, loss of responsiveness to external stimuli, catatonic postures and synchronization of the EEG.

Antagonists of 5-HT

Drugs which block 5-HT receptors include cyproheptadine (Figure 10.9a), cinanserin (Figure 10.9b) and ketanserin (Figure 10.9c), as well as the ergot alkaloids, methysergide, D-lysergic acid diethylamide (LSD 25) and Brom-LSD (see Chapter 18, Figure 18.2). Certain antagonists of 5-HT, such as methysergide and LSD 25, cause increased wakefulness, which is consistent with the proposed role of 5-HT in the control of wakefulness and sleep. Cyproheptadine and methysergide are used for their peripheral actions, to relieve diarrhoea and the malabsorption syndrome in patients with carcinoma of the gut.

Methysergide and cyproheptadine are effective in relieving vascular headaches and for the prophylactic treatment of migraine, a condition in which there is good evidence for an involvement of 5-HT, the action of these two drugs being on the cerebral blood vessels. Both ketanserin and cinanserin block the vasoconstrictor action of 5-HT and ketanserin lowers the blood pressure in hypertension. Most of these actions are against the peripheral autacoid actions of 5-HT. However, none of the 5-HT antagonists is completely selective, most having actions against other autacoids, such as histamine, or other neurotransmitters.

Receptors for 5-HT

The existence of more than one subtype of receptor for the peripheral actions of 5-HT was proposed by Gaddum more than 30 years ago. They were designated 'D' and 'M' and could be distinguished by the ability of different drugs to antagonize the actions of 5-HT on the gut. More recently, two sites in the brain have been identified on the basis of radioligand binding and these have been termed 5-HT$_1$ and 5-HT$_2$, and the 5-HT$_1$ site has been further subdivided into 5-HT$_{1A}$ and 5-HT$_{1B}$, again on the basis of binding studies. However, it is important, at least in considering the actions of drugs at different subtypes of receptors, that they should be distinguishable on the basis of function as well as on binding characteristics. The situation with regard to the subtypes of 5-HT receptors is not completely clear

(a)

(b)

(c)

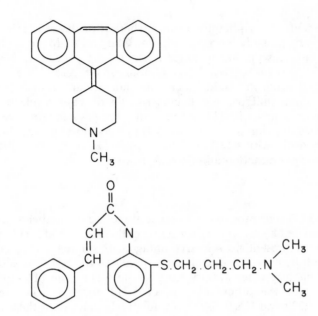

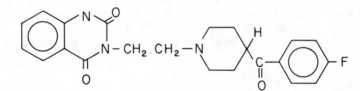

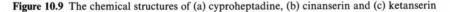

Figure 10.9 The chemical structures of (a) cyproheptadine, (b) cinanserin and (c) ketanserin

and is likely to change with the development of new drugs with more selective actions than those currently available. Nevertheless, three subtypes of 5-HT receptors can be distinguished on the basis of functional criteria, as follows.

5-HT₂ receptor

This is the principal postsynaptic 5-HT receptor in brain. It can be excitatory or inhibitory and is probably responsible for most of the central effects of 5-HT, including behavioural effects. Peripherally, the $5\text{-}HT_2$ receptor is present on various types of smooth muscle, where it mediates contraction, e.g. of blood vessels and gut, and on platelets, where it mediates aggregation. The $5\text{-}HT_2$ receptor corresponds reasonably well to Gaddum's 'D' receptor. This receptor has been characterized by the selective antagonist ketanserin, which is relatively inactive at the other subtypes of 5-HT receptor. However, ketanserin also blocks α-adrenoceptors and it is possible that this action may account, at least in part, for the antihypertensive effects of this drug.

5-HT$_3$ receptor

This receptor is present on peripheral neurones where it mediates the depolarizing actions of 5-HT and possibly corresponds to Gaddum's 'M' receptor. It is characterized by being susceptible to antagonism by drugs such as (−)cocaine, MDL 72222 (1αH,3α,5αH-tropan-3-yl-3,5-dichlorobenzoate) and ICS 205-930 [(3α-tropanyl)-1H-indole-3-carboxylic acid ester] but not to antagonists which are effective at other receptor subtypes, e.g. ketanserin. There is also a selective agonist for the 5-HT$_3$ receptor, 2-methyl-5-HT. At present there is some tentative evidence from binding studies for the presence of 5-HT$_3$ receptors in the brain. The development of new drugs with selective actions on 5-HT$_3$ receptors in brain raises the prospect of new types of action and new applications.

5-HT$_1$-like receptor

This third type of 5-HT receptor exists because there are a number of actions of 5-HT which are mediated by receptors distinct from the 5-HT$_2$ and 5-HT$_3$ subtypes. However, there are at present no selective antagonists for the 5-HT$_1$ site and it therefore cannot be fully characterized. It corresponds to the 5-HT$_1$ binding site in brain where 5-HT has a greater affinity than at the 5-HT$_2$ site. The antagonists which are selective for the other subtypes of 5-HT receptors, i.e. ketanserin, (−)cocaine, MDL 72222 and ICs 205-930, are relatively inactive at these receptors. Some 5-HT$_1$, receptors appear to be located presynaptically and probably represent the 5-HT autoreceptor (see below). Peripherally, the 5-HT$_1$ receptor mediates the inhibitory actions of 5-HT, i.e relaxation of smooth muscle, e.g vasodilatation. The 5-HT$_1$-like receptor has been further subdivided, on the basis of binding data; however, the functional characterization of these subtypes has yet to be elucidated.

Presynaptic receptors for 5-HT

There is evidence that, in the brain, 5-HT released from nerve terminals regulates the further release of neurotransmitter by a feedback mechanism. This is through the activation of autoreceptors on the nerve terminals, stimulation of these receptors inhibiting the release of more transmitter. Autoreceptors on 5-HT terminals have been found only in the CNS and at present there appear to be no drugs which act selectively on these receptors. On the other hand, drugs which act on postsynaptic 5-HT receptors have been shown, by the use of appropriate *in vitro* techniques, to affect autoreceptors. The autoreceptors for 5-HT appear to be of the 5-HT$_1$ type.

Presynaptic 5-HT receptors are present on nerve terminals which release other neurotransmitters, e.g. dopamine in the brain and acetylcholine peripherally (enteric cholinergic neurones).

Neurotoxins for 5-HT

Two derivatives of 5-HT, 5,6-dihydroxytryptamine and 5,7-dihydroxytryptamine, are selective toxins for 5-HT-containing neurones. Both are rapidly oxidized *in vivo*, a reaction which is probably the basis of the toxicity. They are taken up selectively by 5-HT neurones through the active transport process and cause degeneration of the nerve terminals. They are only used experimentally.

Amino acids

Amino acids are ubiquitous substances, all those present in the body being also found in the brain where a number function as neurotransmitters. They can be divided into two groups: those which have excitatory effects on neuronal activity and those which are inhibitory. In the first group, glutamic and aspartic acids need serious consideration, although cysteic and homocysteic acids may also be important. The main inhibitory transmitters are γ-aminobutyric acid and glycine although other substances, such as taurine and β-alanine, probably have a role.

Excitatory amino acids

Both L-glutamate and L-aspartate are important constituents of diet and are involved in a number of metabolic processes, including the tricarboxylic acid (or Krebs) cycle (Figure 10.10), which is concerned with carbohydrate metabolism. They are both dicarboxylic acids (Figure 10.11a,b) and are formed from the corresponding ketoacids (2-oxoglutarate and oxaloacetate). The synthesis of glutamate is mediated by the enzyme glutamate dehydrogenase and that of aspartate by aspartate aminotransferase. Glutamic acid is the most abundant amino acid in the brain, where it is present in larger amounts than in any other organ of the body. The enzymes responsible for the synthesis of these two amino acids are present on mitochondria and they are therefore formed in the cytoplasm of the nerve terminals. Although both glutamate and aspartate have been found to be present in nerve endings extracted from brain tissue, there is no evidence for their storage in

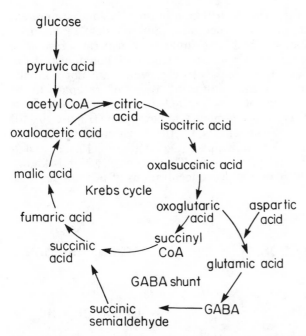

Figure 10.10 The tricarboxylic or Krebs cycle showing the relationship between the formation of γ-aminobutyric acid (the GABA shunt) and the metabolism of glucose

synaptic vesicles. However, they are released under conditions similar to those which govern the release of other neurotransmitters and the release process is calcium dependent. Inactivation of the amino acid neurotransmitters is by re-uptake into the tissues, by two processes. One process is a low-affinity system which also transports other amino acids and the second is a high-affinity sodium-dependent transport system into the nerve terminals which release the transmitter, and also into surrounding glial cells where it enters the Krebs' cycle. While both high- and low-affinity transport systems exist for amino acid neurotransmitters, only the low-affinity system exists for other amino acids.

Glutamate, taken up into glial cells, is oxidized through the Krebs' cycle or is converted to glutamine by the enzyme glutamine synthetase, which is located exclusively in glial cells. The glutamine so formed is released from the glia and can enter the nerve terminals where it can be converted back to glutamate.

Both glutamate and aspartate have powerful excitatory actions when applied to neurones by microiontophoresis and an extremely wide range of neurones through-out the CNS is affected. The excitation results from depolarization of the nerve membrane due to an increase in the conductance of the membrane to sodium ions. The ubiquitous occurrence of these amino acids in high levels throughout the CNS and their widespread actions on neurones militates against the identification of specific types of neurones using glutamate or aspartate as neurotransmitters, and also against the mapping of systems or pathways. Nevertheless, in the spinal cord there is an unequal distribution of glutamate, which is present in larger amounts in dorsal than in ventral regions.

Receptors for excitatory amino acids

Receptors for glutamate have a very wide distribution in the CNS and are present on neurones which receive inputs from other neurotransmitter systems. Glutamate receptors appear to be a population which is distinct from aspartate receptors. Evidence for this has come from the use of substances which are potent agonists at receptors for excitatory amino acids. These substances, which are not normally present in the CNS, have enabled three different types of receptor to be characterized. The first type of receptor is excited by N-methyl-D-aspartate (NMDA) (Figure 10.11c), as well as by L-glutamate, L-homocysteate (Figure 10.11d) and other analogues of aspartate. The effects of these agonists are blocked selectively by antagonists such as D-α-aminoadipate (DαAA)(Figure 10.12a) and 2-amino-5-phosphonovalerate (APV) (Figure 10.12b). This receptor, which is known as the NMDA receptor, is also blocked by low concentrations of magnesium ions.

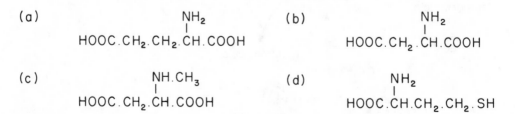

Figure 10.11 The chemical structures of (a) glutamic acid, (b) aspartic acid, (c) N-methyl-D-aspartic acid (NMDA) and (d) homocysteic acid

The two other types of amino acid receptor are excited preferentially by either quisqualate (Figure 10.12c) or kainic acid (Figure 10.12d), both of which are analogues of glutamate but with a ring structure which imparts rigidity to the molecule. Neither of these agonists is blocked by APV but the actions of quisqualate and glutamate are blocked by glutamate diethylester (GDEE) (Figure 10.13a), whereas the actions of kainic acid are resistant to GDEE and also to DαAA. However, the excitations produced by NMDA, aspartate and kainic acid in the spinal cord are blocked by γ-D-glutamylglycine (γDGG)(Figure 10.13b), which is less effective against glutamate and quisqualate.

(a)

$$NH_2$$
$$HOOC.CH_2.CH_2.CH_2.CH.COOH$$

(b)

$$NH_2$$
$$HO_3P.CH_2.CH_2.CH_2\ CH.COOH$$

(c)

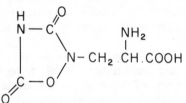

(d)

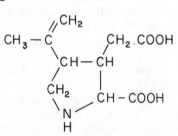

Figure 10.12 The chemical structures of (a) D-α-aminoadipic acid (DαAA), (b) 2-amino-5-phosphono-valeric acid (APV), (c) quisqualic acid and (d) kainic acid

(a)

$$O \qquad NH_2$$
$$C_2H_5.C.CH_2.CH_2.CH.COOH$$

(b)

$$O \qquad NH_2$$
$$HOOC.CH_2.NH.C.CH_2.CH.COOH$$

Figure 10.13 The chemical structures of (a) glutamate diethylester and (b) γ-D-glutamylglycine

Thus, there is evidence for the existence of three subpopulations of receptors for excitatory amino acids: (1) NMDA receptors, which could be aspartate receptors; (2) quisqualate receptors, which could be glutamate receptors, and (3) kainic acid receptors for which no endogenous neurotransmitter is as yet known.

Excitatory amino acids and function

In the spinal cord, where glutamate is most highly concentrated in the dorsal roots, it is thought that this transmitter may be involved in the transmission of sensory information in the primary afferent fibres and in the regulation of motor activity and spinal reflexes at this site. Aspartate, on the other hand, has been proposed as an excitatory transmitter on spinal interneurones, again functioning in the regulation of motor and spinal reflexes.

The excitatory amino acids are thought to be important in epilepsy (see Chapter 14). Glutamate receptors are widely distributed throughout the brain and the administration of glutamate or aspartate into the brain can cause convulsions. Glutamate has also been found to be released from experimentally induced epileptic foci. Finally, drugs which block the actions of glutamate and aspartate, as well as those of other agonists at excitatory amino acid receptors, also block experimental convulsions in animals. Although there is no direct link between the actions of the excitatory amino acids and human epilepsy, the possibility exists that new types of anti-epileptic drugs, related to the antagonists of excitatory amino acids, might be developed in the future.

Kainic acid, which is isolated from seaweed, has a toxic action on neurones in the CNS. It is about 50 times more potent than glutamate in depolarizing neurones and, when injected directly into discrete regions of the brain, it causes degeneration of the cell bodies of the neurones in the vicinity of the injection site, the axons and nerve terminals being more resistant. One theory is that the neurotoxic action is due to excessive excitation of the neuronal soma, but it is probable that the mechanism is more complex and involves receptors for kainic acid and the presence of a presynaptic glutamate input.

No therapeutically useful drugs are known which interact with receptors for excitatory amino acids, nor are these substances, at least as neurotransmitters, known to be directly involved in any diseases. However, there is a phenomenon, known as the 'Chinese restaurant syndrome', which results from the excessive use of monosodium glutamate as a flavour-enhancing agent. The symptoms, which are unpleasant, can include tachycardia, flushing, nausea and gastrointestinal discomfort.

Inhibitory amino acids

γ-Aminobutyric acid (GABA) (Figure 10.14a)

In mammals, GABA is present almost exclusively in the CNS, only trace amounts being found peripherally (e.g. in autonomic ganglia). It is formed by the decarboxylation of L-glutamic acid by the enzyme, glutamic acid decarboxylase (GAD) (Figure 10.15). This enzyme is found only in the cytoplasm of nerve terminals containing GABA and, like other amino acid decarboxylases, requires pyridoxal

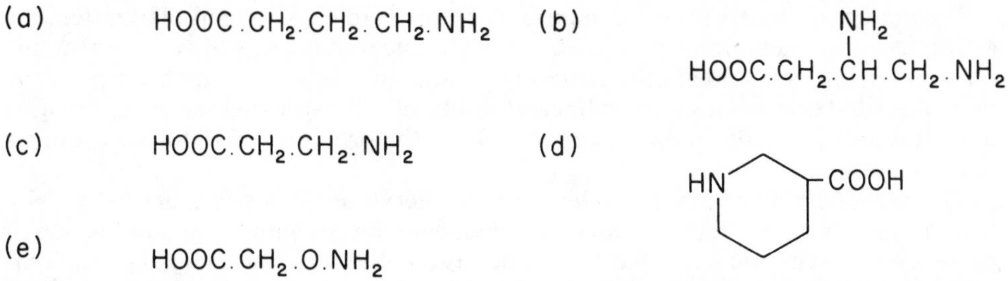

(a)   HOOC.CH$_2$.CH$_2$.CH$_2$.NH$_2$ (b)

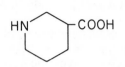

(c)   HOOC.CH$_2$.CH$_2$.NH$_2$ (d)

HN⟩—COOH

(e)   HOOC.CH$_2$.O.NH$_2$

Figure 10.14 The chemical structures of (a) γ-aminobutyric acid, (b) diaminobutyric acid, (c) β-alanine, (d) nipecotic acid and (e) amino-oxyacetic acid

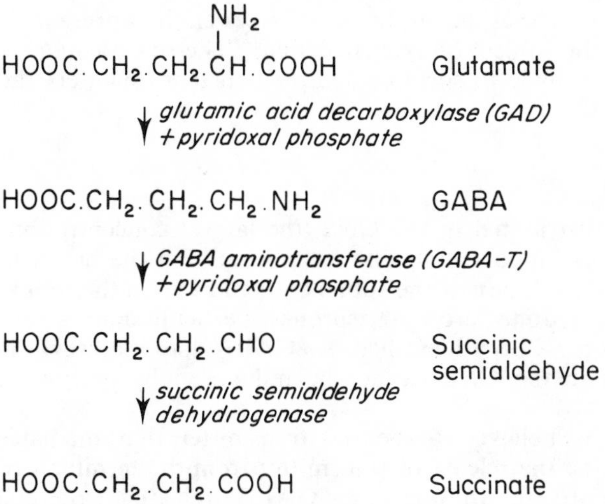

$$\overset{\text{NH}_2}{\underset{|}{}}$$

HOOC.CH$_2$.CH$_2$.CH.COOH   Glutamate

↓ glutamic acid decarboxylase (GAD)
  + pyridoxal phosphate

HOOC.CH$_2$.CH$_2$.CH$_2$.NH$_2$ GABA

↓ GABA aminotransferase (GABA-T)
  + pyridoxal phosphate

HOOC.CH$_2$.CH$_2$.CHO   Succinic
                          semialdehyde

↓ succinic semialdehyde
  dehydrogenase

HOOC.CH$_2$.CH$_2$.COOH   Succinate

Figure 10.15 The synthesis and metabolism of γ-aminobutyric acid (GABA). The enzymes involved are shown in italics

phosphate (vitamin B$_6$) as cofactor. This reaction is closely related to the oxidative metabolism of carbohydrates in the CNS, where the formation of GABA is an alternative pathway, the 'GABA shunt', to the normal route in the metabolism of glucose in the tricarboxylic acid (Krebs) cycle (Figure 10.10). The reaction is probably the rate-limiting step in the formation of GABA and it is likely that the amount of GABA formed can influence the activity of glutamic acid decarboxylase by end-product inhibition.

The enzyme, glutamic acid decarboxylase, is localized to nerve terminals in the CNS, where it is present in the cytoplasm. There is no evidence that the GABA that is synthesized in nerve terminals is stored in vesicles; nevertheless, it is released under conditions similar to those which apply to other neurotransmitters and the release is calcium dependent.

The action of GABA on postsynaptic receptors is to cause hyperpolarization, i.e. an increase in membrane potential, which reduces the possibility of an action potential being propagated and, therefore, results in inhibition. The hyperpolarization is attributable to an increased permeability of the nerve membrane to chloride ions. It is now generally accepted that GABA is the principal inhibitory transmitter in the mammalian CNS.

The GABA which has been released from nerve terminals is inactivated by a high-affinity uptake process which is dependent on sodium ions, and which is present on presynaptic nerve terminals and also on the surrounding glial cells. Some of the GABA therefore returns to the nerve terminal, where it can be metabolized or re-used, and some enters the glial cells, where it will be metabolized. The metabolism of GABA is in two stages, both of which form part of the GABA shunt of the Krebs cycle (Figure 10.10). First, the GABA is transaminated to succinic semialdehyde by the enzyme GABA-aminotransferase or GABA-transaminase (GABA-T), which requires pyridoxal phosphate as coenzyme (Figure 10.15). This enzyme has a wide distribution in tissues but in the nervous system it is present on mitochondria; it has also been the subject of extensive study. The second stage is the oxidation of succinic semialdehyde to succinic acid, which then re-enters the Krebs cycle (Figures 10.15 and 10.10).

THE DISTRIBUTION OF GABA IN THE CNS

γ-Aminobutyric acid is widely distributed in the CNS, the largest concentrations being found in the hypothalamus, hippocampus and basal ganglia in the brain, in the substantia gelatinosa of the dorsal horn of the spinal cord and also in the retina. Most of the GABA-containing neurones are interneurones, i.e. with short axons, although a few longer pathways have been identified. As GABA does not cross the blood–brain barrier, the levels in the CNS cannot be influenced by peripheral administration of GABA.

In the spinal cord, GABA is believed to be the transmitter that mediates presynaptic inhibition by reducing the release of transmitter from the terminals of primary afferent fibres (Figure 10.16). In this case, GABA, released from the terminals of neurones making axo–axonal synapses with the excitatory terminals of primary afferent neurones, causes depolarization of the afferent terminals (primary afferent depolarization) to reduce the release of transmitter and thus produce presynaptic inhibition. This indicates a major functional role for GABA in the control of spinal reflexes.

In the brain, GABA is known to be present in the Purkinje cells of the cerebellum. These cells exert an inhibitory influence on the neurones in Deiter's nucleus in the medulla; this indicates a functional role for GABA in the control of cerebellar reflexes. Large concentrations of GABA are also found in the basal ganglia, particularly the substantia nigra, globus pallidus and nucleus accumbens. In the caudate nucleus and putamen, GABA is associated with short-axon inhibitory interneurones, but there is also a long axon pathway, projecting from the globus pallidus and striatum to the substantia nigra, which releases GABA. This pathway runs in the opposite direction to the ascending dopaminergic nigrostriatal pathway (Figure 10.5 and see also Figure 19.1), and is believed to exert an inhibitory controlling influence on the activity of the dopaminergic nigrostriatal projection. Thus, GABA has an important role in the extrapyramidal system. This is discussed further in Chapter 19.

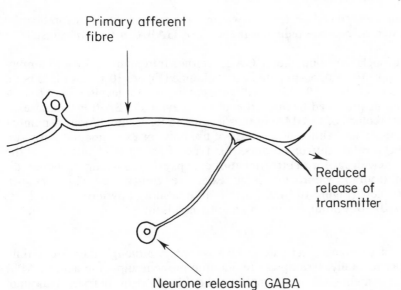

Primary afferent
fibre

Reduced
release of
transmitter

Neurone releasing GABA

Figure 10.16 Presynaptic inhibition in the spinal cord. GABA, released near the terminals of primary afferent fibres, causes depolarization (primary afferent depolarization) which reduces the amplitude of the action potentials in the primary afferent fibres and hence the amount of neurotransmitter released from the terminals

The retina contains large amounts of GABA, which is mainly localized to the horizontal cell layer where it mediates lateral inhibition.

GABA AND FUNCTION

The involvement of GABA in presynaptic inhibition in the spinal cord has been described above, as has the role of GABA in the cerebellum and basal ganglia. Together, these indicate an important role for GABA in the central mechanisms which control movement and there is evidence for the malfunction of GABA systems in certain movement disorders (Chapter 19). As with the other neurotransmitters, much of the evidence for the functional role of GABA has come from knowledge of the mechanism of action of drugs that affect GABA-mediated transmission in the CNS. Thus, GABA is certainly involved with the induction of convulsions and therefore probably with epilepsy (see Chapter 14); there is evidence that GABA may also be important in anxiety states. (Chapter 13).

DRUGS AFFECTING GABA SYSTEMS

Drugs affecting synthesis, uptake and metabolism
A number of inhibitors of glutamic acid decarboxylase are known. For example, the hydrazide, isoniazid, causes the loss of pyridoxal phosphate and thus reduces the activity of glutamic acid decarboxylase. However, as the metabolizing enzyme GABA-transaminase depends upon the same cofactor, its activity will also be affected, although this effect requires larger doses of the inhibitor. Other inhibitors

of glutamic acid decarboxylase are known but they are only of theoretical or experimental interest, because reducing the level of GABA in the brain results in convulsions.

Drugs which block the re-uptake of GABA, either into neurones, e.g. diaminobutyric acid (Figure 10.14b), or into glia, e.g. β-alanine (Figure 10.14c), or into both, e.g. nipecotic acid (Figure 10.14d) , will produce increased levels of GABA. A similar effect can be produced by inhibition of the enzyme GABA-transaminase, so reducing the metabolism of GABA and thus leading to its accumulation. A number of drugs have this action, although most are of use only for experimental purposes. However, as they are all anticonvulsants, this type of action is of interest for the development of new drugs for the treatment of epilepsy. One such drug, sodium di-n-propylacetate (sodium valproate), is in extensive clinical use (Chapter 14). Amino-oxyacetic acid (Figure 10.14e), which is an inhibitor of pyridoxal phosphate, also inhibits GABA-transaminase and is an anticonvulsant.

GABA agonists
A wide variety of substances activate GABA receptors although they are mainly only of use experimentally. Examples are 3-amino-propanesulphonic acid (3-APS) (Figure 10.17a), which does not penetrate the blood–brain barrier, muscimol (Figure 10.17b), which is found in the mushroom *Amanita muscaria* (along with muscarine) and isoguvacine (Figure 10.17c), which can enter the brain. Baclofen, which is the β-chlorophenyl derivative of GABA (Figure 10.17d), is a GABA agonist in the spinal cord but is mainly notable because it has a selective action at

(a)
$$SO_3H.CH_2.CH_2.CH_2.NH_2$$

(b)

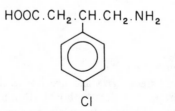

(c)

(d)
$$HOOC.CH_2.CH.CH_2.NH_2$$

Figure 10.17 The chemical structures of (a) 3-amino-propanesulphonic acid (3-APS), (b) muscimol, (c) isoguvacine and (d) baclofen

GABA$_B$ receptors (see below). Although there are no GABA agonist drugs in clinical use at the present time, there is interest in the development of new drugs with this type of action because they could well have an application in the treatment of epilepsy and in the control of movement disorders.

There are a number of drugs which modify neuronal responses to GABA, not by acting directly on GABA receptors, but by an action on receptors which are closely associated with, and have a regulatory action on, the GABA receptor. Examples are the benzodiazepines and barbiturates, the mechanisms of action of which are discussed in Chapters 11 and 13.

GABA antagonists

The principal GABA antagonists are bicuculline (Figure 10.18a) and picrotoxin (Figure 10.18b), both of which act at postsynaptic GABA receptors, bicuculline competitively and picrotoxin non-competitively. Both drugs are potent convulsants and are of experimental interest only.

Subtypes of GABA receptors

Two subtypes of receptors for GABA have been proposed, designated GABA$_A$ and GABA$_B$. The distinction between the two has been made mainly on the basis of

(a)

(b)

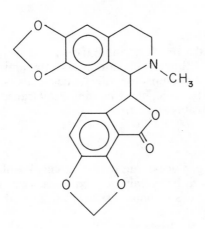

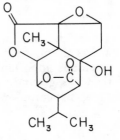

(c)

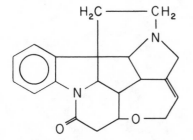

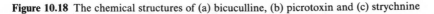

Figure 10.18 The chemical structures of (a) bicuculline, (b) picrotoxin and (c) strychnine

the potencies of the available agonists and the selective action of antagonists. Thus, GABA itself is the only agonist which is potent at both receptor sites; baclofen is as potent as GABA at the $GABA_B$ receptor but is inactive on $GABA_A$ receptors. On the other hand, 3-amino-propanesulphonic acid, muscimol and isoguvacine (Figure 10.17a,b,c) have potencies similar to or greater than GABA at $GABA_A$ receptors but are inactive or only weakly active at $GABA_B$ receptors. The effects of the $GABA_A$ agonists are blocked by bicuculline and picrotoxin which are inactive at $GABA_B$ receptors. In addition, the actions of drugs which modulate responses to GABA, e.g. benzodiazepines and barbiturates, are associated with $GABA_A$ and not $GABA_B$ receptors.

It is thought that the postsynaptic GABA receptors in the CNS which mediate the classic inhibitory actions of GABA by changes in permeability to chloride ions, are $GABA_A$ receptors. In contrast, $GABA_B$ receptors are probably located on presynaptic terminals and control the release of GABA and other neurotransmitters in the CNS, e.g. dopamine and noradrenaline. Certainly baclofen, which is only active at $GABA_B$ sites, causes a reduction in the release of neurotransmitters, whereas isoguvacine is inactive and muscimol only weakly active in this respect; this effect of baclofen is not blocked by bicuculline. The $GABA_B$ receptors are not linked to chloride channels, although they may be linked to calcium channels. In this case, the effect on the release of neurotransmitters could be mediated by an influence on the entry of calcium ions into the nerve terminals; $GABA_B$ receptors have also been found outside the CNS where GABA itself does not exist.

Glycine

This is an amino acid which is found in the free form in all tissues and body fluids, and is an important constituent of diet. Although it is not an essential amino acid, glycine is important in the metabolism of proteins, peptides, nucleic acids, etc. In the CNS, glycine also has a neurotransmitter role, being an inhibitory transmitter in the spinal cord, lower brain stem and possibly the retina.

SYNTHESIS

Glycine is formed from carbohydrates, e.g. glucose and pyruvate, via phosphoserine and serine. In the CNS, glycine appears to be mainly derived from serine (Figure 10.19), the reaction being controlled by the enzyme, serine hydroxymethyltrans-ferase, which is the rate-limiting enzyme.

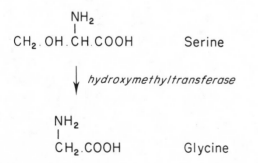

Figure 10.19 The synthesis of glycine from serine. The enzyme involved is shown in italics

STORAGE, RELEASE, UPTAKE AND METABOLISM

The mechanisms for the storage of glycine within presynaptic terminals are not known, but depolarizing stimuli, i.e. electrical stimulation or large concentrations of potassium ions, evoke the release of glycine from the spinal cord, the release being calcium dependent. As with GABA, the released glycine is removed by a high-affinity transport system and taken up into the neurones from which it was released and, also, into glial cells. It is not known whether the metabolism of glycine plays any part in its role as a transmitter.

THE DISTRIBUTION OF GLYCINE IN THE CNS

The greatest concentrations of glycine are found in the spinal cord and lower brain stem. In the spinal cord there is more glycine in the grey matter than in the white matter. When applied to neurones by microiontophoresis, glycine produces hyper-polarization which is thought to be the basis of its inhibitory action, and it has been shown to be released from inhibitory interneurones in the spinal cord and brain stem. For example, the inhibitory transmitter released by Renshaw cells on to motor neurones (see 'Cholinergic pathways in the CNS', page 128, and Figure 10.2) is glycine. The receptors for glycine, at least in the spinal cord, are exclusively postsynaptic. Therefore glycine does not mediate presynaptic inhibition as does GABA, but it does mediate recurrent inhibition. In this way, glycine is thought to have an important role in the regulation of spinal and brain stem reflexes. It is possible that glycine may play a part in spastic states involving motor neurones.

DRUGS AFFECTING GLYCINE SYSTEMS

No drugs are known to act as agonists at glycine receptors, but the convulsant drug, strychnine (Figure 10.18c), is a competitive antagonist. Small doses of strychnine, administered to man or animals, are known to enhance spinal reflexes and larger doses produce convulsions which are spinal in origin. In the medulla, strychnine stimulates the vasomotor and vagal centres. Strychnine also has effects on vision: for example, when instilled into the eye, it enhances colour vision. This action provides support for the presence of glycine receptors in the retina.

Peptides

Of all the various neurotransmitters and putative neurotransmitters, the 'neuro-active' peptides represent the group which has been expanding most rapidly in recent years. Some are substances which have been known for a long time but for which no definite function had been found, e.g. substance P; others are well-known hormones, such as the gastrointestinal hormones vasoactive intestinal peptide and cholecystokinin, which have subsequently been found to be present in the CNS where they are physiologically active. A third group of neuroactive peptides is represented by the substances which have been isolated from the CNS in the search for endogenous ligands of opiate receptors: these are the enkephalins and endorphins.

The synthesis, storage, release and inactivation of peptides

Peptides differ in many ways from other 'classic' neurotransmitters. They are very potent and are present in much smaller quantities than other transmitters. The classic neurotransmitters are synthesized in the neurone from dietary precursors by one or two enzymatic steps; they are then stored in the nerve terminals, usually in synaptic vesicles, until release, after which the transmitter, or its metabolite (e.g. choline), can be taken up into the nerve terminal and used again. In the case of the peptides (Figure 10.20), synthesis takes place in the cell body on ribosomes, directed by messenger RNA. The peptide so formed is much larger than the transmitter peptide and has no biological activity. It is known as a pre-propeptide as it contains not only the amino acid sequence from which the transmitter is derived, but also a sequence of amino acid residues which act as signals for the processing of the propeptide into its storage form. After synthesis, the pre-propeptide enters the endoplasmic reticulum from which it is transported to the Golgi apparatus where the pre- sequence is removed. The propeptide is then packaged into granules suitable for transport to the nerve terminal through the microtubule system. The propeptide is stored in the terminal but the process of final cleavage into the transmitter peptide is not well known. The peptide neurotransmitters resemble the classic transmitters in that their release from nerve terminals is calcium dependent.

No membrane transport systems for peptides that would mediate their re-uptake into nerve terminals have been identified. It is therefore assumed that inactivation of the peptide neurotransmitters is by enzymatic breakdown by peptidases. It appears, therefore, that the peptides are not recycled as, for example, are the monoamine neurotransmitters; consequently, their action depends upon adequate stores of precursor proteins. The peptidases, which are generally assumed to inactivate the peptide neurotransmitters released from nerve terminals, are not selective in their actions, however.

It is thought that neuropeptides, released from nerve terminals, act on specific receptors. However, very few such receptors have been identified, let alone characterized. In many cases neuropeptides have been found to be present in the same terminals as classic neurotransmitters and are released together with the classic transmitter. This phenomenon, which is known as 'co-transmission', is discussed below. If the action of a peptide, 'co-released' in this way, is to modulate the actions of the classic neurotransmitter, then 'neuromodulator' would be a better descriptive term for the peptide rather than neurotransmitter. Unfortunately, although the term neuromodulator is sometimes used, there has been no general agreement as to its precise definition.

The classification of neuropeptides

There is no satisfactory way of classifying neuropeptides at present and many arbitrary systems have been used.

Substance P

This is probably the first neuropeptide to be discovered. It was found in 1931, in both the brain and intestine. However, although it was found to be biologically active, substance P was not identified chemically until comparatively recently. It is a tachykinin and is known to contain 11 amino acids (Figure 10.21a); it is present

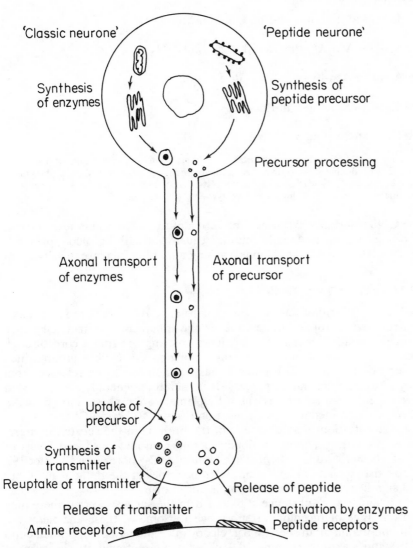

'Classic neurone'

'Peptide neurone'

Synthesis
of enzymes

Synthesis of
peptide precursor

Precursor processing

Axonal transport
of enzymes

Axonal transport
of precursor

Uptake of
precursor

Synthesis of
transmitter

Reuptake of transmitter

Release of peptide

Release of transmitter

Inactivation by enzymes

Amine receptors

Peptide receptors

Figure 10.20 Diagram comparing the processes involved in 'classic' neurotransmission and 'peptidergic' transmission, showing the processes of synthesis, packaging, transport and release (see text for further details; redrawn from Kruk and Pycock, 1983)

in many tissues in a wide range of species. In the CNS there are large concentrations of substance P in the substantia nigra, hypothalamus and dorsal horn of the spinal cord. However, it is also present, although in smaller concentrations, in many other regions of the brain. Two polypeptide precursors of substance P have been isolated from brain: they are α- and β-preprotachykinin; the latter contains not only the amino acid sequence for substance P but also that for substance K (see below). Thus, it is possible that some neurones may be able to synthesize substance P, and others both substance P and substance K. Immunohistochemical methods have been used to map neuronal pathways containing substance P.

(a)   Arg-Pro-Lys-Pro-Gln-Gln-Phe-Phe-Gly-Leu-Met-NH$_2$

(b)   Pyr-Pro-Ser-Lys-Asp-Ala-Phe-Ile-Gly-Leu-Met-NH$_2$

(c)   Pyr-Ala-Asp-Pro-Asn-Lys-Phe-Tyr-Gly-Leu-Met-NH$_2$

(d)   Asp-Val-Pro-Lys-Ser-Asp-Gln-Phe-Val-Gly-Leu-Met-NH$_2$

(e)   His-Lys-Thr-Asp-Ser-Phe-Val-Gly-Leu-Met-NH$_2$

Figure 10.21 The amino acid sequences of (a) substance P, (b) eledoisin, (c) physalaemin, (d) kassinin and (e) substance K. Ala, alanine; Arg, arginine; Asn, asparagine; Asp, aspartic acid; Gln, glutamine; Gly, glycine; His, histidine; Ile, isoleucine; Leu, leucine; Lys, lysine; Met, methionine; Phe, phenyl-alanine; Pro, proline; Ser, serine; Thr, threonine; Tyr, tyrosine; Val, valine

Outside the CNS, substance P causes contraction of the smooth muscle of the gut, but it also dilates vascular smooth muscle, causing a fall in blood pressure. Substance P stimulates the salivary glands, causing a marked increase in salivation.

SUBSTANCE P AS A NEUROTRANSMITTER

When applied to the cut end of sensory nerves, substance P causes pain and it has a depolarizing action when applied to neurones in the spinal cord. In fact, substance P is present in the small-diameter afferent fibres entering the spinal cord through the dorsal roots. These small fibres probably belong to the C-fibre group which mediate the sensation of pain. Substance P has been shown to be released from these fibres by a calcium-dependent process. It is therefore generally accepted that substance P is the neurotransmitter released by primary afferent (sensory) fibres in the dorsal horn, where it mediates pain sensation (Figure 10.22 and Chapter 15).

The largest concentration of substance P in the brain is in the substantia nigra, where it has an excitatory action on dopaminergic neurones. Reduced levels of substance P have been found in patients with Huntington's chorea (see Chapter 19). Substance P co-exists with 5-HT in the brain (in neurones of the raphe nuclei), but the functional significance of this association is not known.

Studies with analogues of substance P have led to the suggestion that there may be more than one type of receptor for substance P. Some of these analogues are endogenous in non-mammalian species, e.g. eledoisin (Figure 10.21b), physalaemin (Figure 10.21c) and kassinin (Figure 10.21d), which are found in the skin of amphibia. All tachykinins, including substance P, show approximately equal potency at one type of substance P receptor (the SP-P receptor), whereas the other receptor (SP-E) is more sensitive to eledoisin and kassinin than to other tachy-kinins. A peptide which is related to kassinin is known as 'substance K' (Figure 10.21e) and has a common precursor with substance P. The distribution of the two subtypes of substance P receptor is not known, but it seems likely that both are present in the substantia nigra.

The association of substance P with the transmission of pain has attracted interest in the possibility that antagonists of substance P might have analgesic actions. Unfortunately, specific antagonists of substance P have not been found, although a number of its analogues have weak antagonistic activity. The discovery of more specific and potent antagonists of substance P might well lead to significant developments.

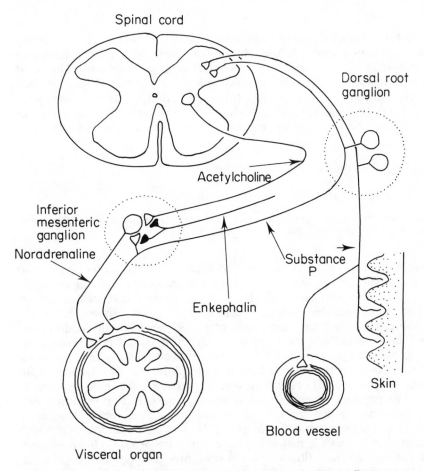

Spinal cord

Dorsal root
ganglion

Acetylcholine

Inferior
mesenteric
ganglion

Noradrenaline

Substance
P

Enkephalin

Skin

Blood vessel

Visceral organ

Figure 10.22 Schematic representation of somatic and visceral primary afferent neurones and the sympathetic nervous system. The primary visceral afferent fibres release substance P in the dorsal horn of the spinal cord (redrawn from Konishi *et al.*, 1980)

Capsaicin, a substance found in red peppers, which gives them their pungent flavour (Figure 10.23), causes the release of substance P from primary afferent terminals when it is given acutely. However, with chronic administration, capsaicin is neurotoxic and causes the degeneration of the primary afferent neurones conducting pain. This action is not restricted to neurones containing substance P; the mechanism of this effect is not known.

Figure 10.23 The chemical structure of capsaicin

Opioid peptides

An 'opioid' substance is one which has agonist activity at opiate receptors, whereas an 'opiate' is a substance derived from the opium poppy that has an analgesic action, e.g. morphine. These terms are, nevertheless, often confused. The most important opioid peptides are the enkephalins, leucine enkephalin (Figure 10.24a) and methionine enkephalin (Figure 10.24b), both pentapeptides, which were discovered in 1975. It is perhaps remarkable that the mechanism of action of morphine, which has been in use for centuries, should have been discovered so recently.

(a)   Tyr-Gly-Gly-Phe-Leu-OH

(b)   Tyr-Gly-Gly-Phe-Met-OH

Figure 10.24 The amino acid sequences of (a) leucine enkephalin and (b) methionine enkephalin. Amino acids as in Figure 10.21; Cys, cysteine; Glu, glutamic acid; Trp, tryptophan

   The discovery of the enkephalins was stimulated by the observation that morphine bound to sites in the brain which were not associated with the receptors for any of the known neurotransmitters. Thus, it was thought that an endogenous ligand for these morphine (or opiate) receptors must exist. Shortly after the discovery of the enkephalins, another group of opioid peptides, the endorphins, was found and, more recently, a third group, the dynorphins, has been discovered. Each of these groups of opioid peptides has its own precursor: pro-enkephalin for the enkephalins, pro-opiomelanocortin for the endorphins and pro-dynorphin for the dynorphins (Figure 10.25). However, the precursors contain a number of biologically active peptides, some of which are not opioids. For example, pro-opiomelanocortin contains the amino acid sequences for melanocyte-stimulating hormone (MSH) and adrenocorticotropin (ACTH), as well as β-lipotropin which itself contains the sequences for met-enkephalin and β-endorphin. However, met-enkephalin is not derived from this source but from pro-enkephalin. Leu-enkephalin, on the other hand, can be derived from both pro-enkephalin and pro-dynorphin (Figure 10.25). β-Lipotropin, which was known long before the enkephalins and endorphins were discovered, consists of 91 amino acids.

   The three precursors of the opioid peptides undergo complex proteolytic processing which can vary in different parts of the body and hence, influences the distribution of the peptides formed.

THE DISTRIBUTION OF OPIOID PEPTIDES

The peptides derived from pro-enkephalin and pro-dynorphin are widely distributed throughout the CNS and are often found together in the same area, although not in the same neurones. Those peptides derived from pro-opiomelanocortin, e.g. β-endorphin, have a more restricted distribution, being found in the anterior and intermediate lobes of the pituitary and in a group of neurones forming the arcuate nucleus of the hypothalamus. The latter project mainly to the limbic system and the brain stem. The enkephalins are present in large concentrations in the basal ganglia (striatum, caudate nucleus and globus pallidus) and an enkephalinergic pathway projects from the caudate-putamen to the globus pallidus. However, it is thought that many short-axon neurones, i.e. interneurones, contain enkephalins. In the

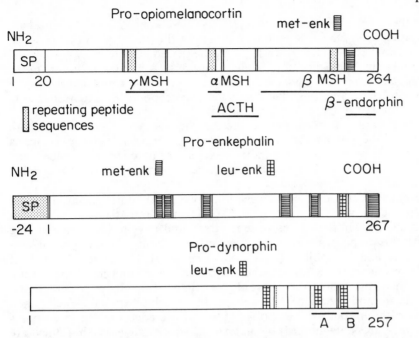

Figure 10.25 Structural relationship between the three precursors of the opioid peptides, pro-opiomelan-ocortin, pro-enkephalin and pro-dynorphin, and the peptides which are derived from them. The length, in terms of amino acid residues, is indicated by the numbers. Both pro-opiomelanocortin and pro-enkephalin have signal peptides (SP) at their N-terminals. Cleavage sites for processing are indicated by single or double vertical lines. A, dynorphin A; B, dynorphin B; MSH, melanocyte-stimulating hormone; ACTH, adrenocorticotropin; met-enk, met-enkephalin; leu-enk, leu-enkephalin (modified from Cooper, Bloom and Roth, 1986)

spinal cord, laminae I and II of the substantia gelatinosa of the dorsal horn contain the highest levels of enkephalins, together with the spinal trigeminal nucleus and the periaqueductal grey. They are also present in the hypothalamus, thalamus, raphe nuclei and nucleus locus coeruleus. In general, the enkephalins tend to be present in those regions of the brain which are rich in the monoamine neurotransmitters (noradrenaline, dopamine and 5-HT) and also substance P.

Opioid peptides are found in many tissues outside the nervous system. Endorphins, for example, are found in the adrenal medulla and enkephalins are present in the amacrine cells of the retina. There is a rich enkephalinergic innervation of the gastrointestinal tract and the presence of opiate receptors in this tissue has resulted in its use as an experimental preparation for the study of these receptors.

THE FUNCTIONS OF OPIOID PEPTIDES

As the 'endogenous ligand' for the opiate receptor, the enkephalins are thought to mimic the actions of opiate drugs such as morphine. Certainly, the actions of the enkephalins can be antagonized by the opiate antagonist naloxone. However, the enkephalins are only weak analgesics, unless injected directly into the brain, but it is thought that their rapid degradation by peptidases may be responsible for their lack of potency and analogues of the enkephalins, which are resistant to the action of peptidases, are more potent as analgesics, as is β-endorphin. There is good evidence for the involvement of the enkephalins and endorphins in pain mechanisms (see Chapter 15). Thus, the opiate receptors in the dorsal horn of the spinal cord (laminae I and II), together with those in the periaqueductal grey and medial parts of the thalamus, are believed to mediate analgesia, while the receptors in the limbic system, an area more associated with the perception and expression of emotion, are probably involved in the decreased perception of, and response to pain. This is discussed in more detail in Chapter 15.

The enkephalins have been called the 'endogenous analgesics' and both β-endorphin and the enkephalins are thought to be involved in the analgesia produced by acupuncture. It is clear that the enkephalins produce effects other than analgesia, e.g. at opiate receptors in the gut, where morphine reduces peristaltic movements.

Endorphins have been found to produce a variety of behavioural effects. They are released from the pituitary together with ACTH and from the adrenal glands together with catecholamines, in response to stress, and have a role in modulating pain during stress responses. When injected intracerebrally, β-endorphin causes muscular rigidity and immobility (a catatonia-like state). However, a variety of effects can be produced with intracerebral injection, depending upon the precise site of injection in the brain: these include locomotor stimulation, hyperactivity, seizures, catalepsy and sedation. The enkephalins produce similar effects when injected intracerebrally but are less potent. Most of the effects of the endorphins and enkephalins are antagonized by naloxone, which suggests that they are mediated by opiate receptors in the brain. Some studies have indicated that endorphins may be involved in 'reward' systems in the brain. Such an action could have important implications for the mechanisms concerned with dependence and addiction.

MECHANISMS OF ACTION OF OPIOID PEPTIDES

It is clear that there are many neurones in the brain and spinal cord that contain opioid peptides and that the precursors are also present, together with the enzyme systems for breaking down the large precursor molecules into the smaller, biologically active fragments. Furthermore, the release of enkephalins and endorphins from nerve terminals has been demonstrated and the release process is similar to that for the classical neurotransmitters. In addition, a number of pathways have been identified, including pathways in the hippocampus and the enkephalinergic pathway in the basal ganglia (already mentioned); many interneurones in the brain also contain enkephalins. There are specific receptors for these substances but how they are activated by the opioid peptides is not known, although both cyclic AMP and calcium ion permeability have been suggested as possible mechanisms. What is also lacking is evidence for specific inactivation mechanisms. The enkephalins appear to be inactivated by enzymatic breakdown due to the action of non-specific aminopeptidases which are present in neuronal tissues, rather than by a re-uptake process. It is quite possible, therefore, that the enkephalins (and endorphins) may have a neurotransmitter role in the CNS, or, alternatively, that they may function as neuromodulators, or that they may act in both roles.

RECEPTORS FOR OPIOID PEPTIDES

The possibility that there might be subtypes of opiate receptors arose from observations of the effects of morphine and morphine-like drugs with mixed agonist–antagonist actions on the spinal cord of the dog. This idea was later confirmed in bioassay studies, in which it was found that agonist drugs showed different potencies in different preparations (i.e. different tissues) and that the sensitivity of the tissues to antagonists also varied. Three main subtypes of opiate receptors have been proposed and have been designated μ, δ and κ. A fourth type, the σ-receptor, has been found, but there is doubt as to whether it is a true opiate receptor (the σ-receptor is discussed in Chapter 18). The existence of the subtypes of opiate receptors in various tissues has been confirmed in binding studies.

The μ-receptor
This receptor, at which morphine and β-endorphin are potent agonists and the enkephalins less potent, is thought to be the receptor at which analgesia is mediated in the brain, i.e. supraspinal analgesia. It is also thought to be responsible for respiratory depression, euphoria and the development of physical dependence, together with the withdrawal syndrome after dependence has occurred, as this syndrome can be blocked by morphine and other μ-agonists but not by κ-agonists. Naloxone is a more potent antagonist at μ-receptors than at δ- or κ-receptors.

The δ-receptor
Leu-enkephalin is the most potent agonist at this receptor, followed by met-enkephalin, β-endorphin and morphine. The functional role of δ-receptors is not completely clear, mainly because the same drugs act at both μ- and δ-sites. However, it seems probable that these receptors mediate the sedative actions of opiate drugs and also changes in affective behaviour. In many cases both μ- and δ-receptors appear to be present on the same neurone, although the proportion can vary in different tissues and in different species.

The κ-receptor
The endogenous ligand at this site is dynorphin and the agonist drugs are pentazocine and ethylketocyclazocine which differ in their analgesic and other properties from μ-agonists, such as morphine. Thus, κ-agonists do not cause respiratory depression to the same extent as μ-agonists. Furthermore, they cannot reverse the symptoms caused by withdrawal of morphine after chronic treatment. Their actions can be readily distinguished from those of μ-agonists. The κ-receptor is thought to mediate spinal analgesia and sedation but not respiratory depression. The drugs which act at κ-receptors, on the other hand, are liable to produce mental disturbances, such as dysphoria and hallucinations. Naloxone acts as a competitive antagonist at κ-receptors, but it is much less potent than at μ-receptors.

As there are three precursors for opioid peptides, it was thought at one time that the products of each precursor might be assigned to one of the three subtypes of receptor. However, this is not the case as all the derivatives of the three precursors are active at all three receptors, although with varying potencies. Peptides have now been synthesized which have greater selectivity for the μ- and δ-receptors. Whether these agents will lead to a clarification of the functional roles of the subtypes of opiate receptors remains to be seen, and there is a view that the three subtypes might not be distinct entities but a continuum of receptors. What is needed in order to improve our understanding of this area is the development of specific antagonists for the three receptor subtypes.

INTERACTIONS WITH OTHER NEUROTRANSMITTERS

Many of the actions of opioid peptides are mediated by presynaptic receptors which modulate the release of other neurotransmitters. In the gastrointestinal tract, for example, morphine acts presynaptically to reduce the release of acetylcholine and this action accounts, at least partly, for the reduction in intestinal motility produced by morphine. In the spinal cord, morphine and the enkephalins reduce the release of substance P in the dorsal horn. This is a presynaptic action mediated by specific opiate receptors and, since substance P mediates the conduction of pain sensation at this site, it is a possible explanation for the production of spinal analgesia (see Figure 10.22). In the brain, opiate receptors modulate the the release of noradrenaline from neurones in the locus coeruleus and the cerebral cortex. The precise mechanism by which these inhibitory effects are produced is not known, although the opening of potassium channels, leading to hyperpolarization of the terminal membrane and hence reduction in the release of transmitter, has been proposed.

The receptors for the opioid peptides and opiate drugs are therefore present not only postsynaptically but also on presynaptic terminals where they influence the release of other neurotransmitters. In this sense, the endogenous opioid peptides probably act as 'neuromodulators' rather than as neurotransmitters. A third role, which seems to be a distinct possibility, is that these substances can co-exist with the classic neurotransmitters and can be released with them from the same nerve terminals. This concept is discussed further below.

Other peptides

The list of peptides, mostly known for their role as hormones outside the nervous system, but which have now been found to be present in the CNS, grows daily. Only the main ones are reviewed here.

SOMATOSTATIN

This is a tetradecapeptide (14 amino acid residues, Figure 10.26a), which was originally found in the hypothalamus, but is also present in the cerebral cortex, hippocampus, limbic system and striatum and in dorsal root ganglia in the spinal

(a)   Ser-Ala-Asn-Ser-Asn-Pro-Ala-Met-Ala-Pro-Arg-Glu-Arg-Lys-Ala-Gly-

Cys-Lys-Asn-Phe-Phe-Trp-Lys-Thr-Phe-Thr-Ser-Cys-OH

Phe-Tyr-Cys
| |
(b)   Gln-Asn-Cys-Pro-Arg-Gly-NH$_2$

Ile-Tyr- Cys
| |
(c)   Gln-Asn-Cys-Pro-Leu-Gly-NH$_2$

(d) p-Glu-His-Pro-NH$_2$

Figure 10.26 The amino acid sequences of (a) somatostatin, (b) vasopressin, (c) oxytocin and (d) thyrotropin-releasing hormone (TRH). Amino acids as in Figures 10.21 and 10.24

cord. Apart from the CNS, it is present in the stomach, pancreas and small intestine. Somatostatin blocks the release of growth hormone and of ACTH from the pituitary and, in the gastrointestinal tract, it blocks the release of insulin, glucagon, vasoactive intestinal polypeptide (VIP), gastrin and renin.

In the CNS, somatostatin, together with its precursor prosomatostatin, has been found in nerve terminals from which it is released by a calcium-dependent process. There is, herefore, some evidence to support a neurotransmitter role for somato-statin. Is presence in dorsal root ganglia in the spinal cord suggests a possible role as a primary afferent transmitter (cf. substance P). Somatostatin has also been found to 'co-exist' with noradrenaline in neurones in sympathetic ganglia and with γ-aminobutyric acid in neurones in the thalamus.

Somatostatin has a depressant action on the brain, causing sedation and reduced motor activity. It also potentiates the sedative actions of other drugs such as barbiturates. Applied iontophoretically to single neurones it produces a reduction in firing rate. A reduction in the level of somatostatin in the cerebral cortex has been found in Alzheimer's disease (see Chapter 20), but the significance of this is not known.

A somatostatin molecule consisting of 28 amino acids has also been identified and another, with 25 amino acids. Both are biologically active and both somato-statin-25 and -28 are more potent in their effects on the pituitary gland than somatostatin-14.

VASOPRESSIN AND OXYTOCIN (Figure 10.26b,c)

These are major hormones secreted by the posterior pituitary and are nonapeptides (nine amino acids). They are present in, and also synthesized in, large neurones of the paraventricular and supra-optic nuclei of the hypothalamus, from which they are released into the bloodstream. Peripherally, vasopressin (or antidiuretic hormone) facilitates the reabsorption of water in the distal tubules of the kidney, while oxytocin stimulates contraction of uterine muscle. The neurones of the supra-optic and paraventricular nuclei of the hypothalamus give off axon collaterals which feed back to the same neurones, as well as projecting to the median eminence. Both vasopressin and oxytocin have potent inhibitory actions on these neurones and are thought to be released from the collaterals as neurotransmitters. The projections to the median eminence cause the release of vasopressin, together with ACTH.

Projections from the neurones in the supra-optic and paraventricular nuclei have been found in other parts of the brain, e.g. the hippocampus, limbic system, cortex, substantia nigra and locus coeruleus, and also in the spinal cord. However, it is not known whether vasopressin and oxytocin are released from these terminals, or whether they act as neurotransmitters. Nevertheless, it seems that these two peptides are present in nerve terminals of neuronal systems which are not related to their endocrine functions.

The behavioural effects of vasopressin are quite marked. When it is injected intracerebrally in animals, vasopressin alters blood pressure and has some analgesic activity. However, more striking is the fact that, both in animals and in man, vasopressin and oxytocin have been found to facilitate learning and memory and they are effective in extremely small quantities, so that even with systemic administration, effects on the CNS can be observed. Attempts have been made to improve cognitive function in elderly patients and in cases where memory has been affected by trauma, by administering vasopressin in a nasal spray, but with doubtful results (see Chapter 20).

(see Chapter 20)

THYROTROPIN-RELEASING HORMONE (TRH, Figure 10.26d)

This is a tripeptide which is synthesized in the hypothalamus, in neurones in the mediobasal region, and is then released into the hypothalamo–hypophyseal portal system in which it is carried to the anterior pituitary, where it causes the release of thyrotropin and prolactin into the bloodstream. However, immunohistochemical techniques have demonstrated the presence of TRH in regions of the brain other than the hypothalamus: these are the brain stem, midbrain, basal ganglia and cerebral cortex, where it is present in neurones. The TRH in these 'extrahypothalamic' sites is synthesized there, although the precise mechanisms are not known. However, TRH can be released from the neurones by a calcium-dependent process. Thyrotropin-releasing hormone has been found to interact with the catecholamine neurotransmitters in the CNS and has effects on sleep patterns and on arousal. It seems likely, therefore, that TRH may have a role outside the hypothalamus either as a neurotransmitter or as a neuromodulator.

NEUROTENSIN

This is another hypothalamic peptide which contains 13 amino acids (Figure 10.27a). As a hormone, its main action is to cause local vasodilatation and hypotension. Outside the hypothalamus, it has been found to occur in regions associated with the transmission of pain, e.g. the dorsal horn of the spinal cord, the trigeminal nerve nucleus and the periaqueductal grey matter in the brain stem. Local injection of neurotensin into these regions causes analgesia, an effect that is not blocked by opiate antagonists such as naloxone, which suggests that it is not mediated by opiate receptors. Apart from analgesia, central injections of neurotensin cause hypothermia and increased release of other hormones, such as growth hormone and prolactin. Neurotensin interacts with the catecholamine neurotransmitters, particularly dopamine, and it is present in the substantia nigra, ventral tegmentum and locus coeruleus. Neurotensin can be released from neuronal tissue by a calcium-dependent process and radioligand binding studies have demonstrated

(a) p-Glu-Leu-Tyr-Glu-Asn-Lys-Pro-Arg-Arg-Pro-Tyr-Ile-Leu-COOH

(b) Asp-Arg-Val-Tyr-Ile-His-Pro-Phe-NH$_2$

(c) His-Ser-Asp-Ala-Val-Phe-Thr-Asp-Asn-Tyr-Thr-Arg-Leu-Arg-Lys-

Gln-Met-Ala-Val-Lys-Lys-Tyr-Leu-Asn-Ser-Ile-Leu-Asn-NH$_2$

(d) Asp-Tyr-Met-Gly-Trp-Met-Asp-Phe-NH$_2$
  |
  HSO$_3$

Figure 10.27 The amino acid sequences of (a) neurotensin, (b) angiotensin II, (c) vasoactive intestinal peptide (VIP) and (d) cholecystokinin octapeptide (CCK). Amino acids as in Figures 10.21 and 10.24

the presence of binding sites for neurotensin in regions of the brain which contain high levels of the peptide. Whether these sites are receptors for neurotensin remains to be established. It is possible that neurotensin may co-exist with dopamine in some nerve terminals and may be released together with dopamine, thus acting as a neuromodulator.

ANGIOTENSIN II

This is a highly active octapeptide (Figure 10.27b) that is produced by the action of angiotensin-converting enzyme on angiotensin I, a decapeptide having limited pharmacological activity. In turn, angiotensin II can be hydrolysed by amino-peptidase to yield a heptapeptide, angiotensin III, which also has some activity. However, only angiotensin II appears to have a role in the CNS. The brain contains a renin–angiotensin system which is independent of the peripheral renin–angio-tensin system in the kidneys. High levels of angiotensin II-like immunoreactivity have been found in the spinal cord, medulla, locus coeruleus and hypothalamus. The main effect of injections of angiotensin II into the brain is to produce increased drinking or compulsive thirst. It also causes the release of other hormones, such as vasopressin. However, there is as yet no definitive evidence for a neurotransmitter role for angiotensin II.

VASOACTIVE INTESTINAL PEPTIDE (VIP)

This peptide contains 28 amino acid residues (Figure 10.27c) and is found throughout the alimentary canal and associated organs, as well as in the lung, placenta and adrenal glands. It relaxes most smooth muscle, causing hypotension, bronchodilatation and relaxation of intestinal muscle, as well as inhibiting the secretion of gastric enzymes while stimulating the secretion of insulin, glucagon and somatostatin. It is co-released with acetylcholine from the terminals of the parasympathetic nerve fibres which innervate the salivary glands. However, the two substances are released under different conditions of stimulation, acetylcholine being released alone at low frequencies of stimulation and both acetylcholine and VIP at higher stimulus frequencies. Furthermore, whereas acetycholine stimulates the secretion of saliva, VIP does not stimulate directly but potentiates the action of acetylcholine.

In the CNS, VIP-like immunoreactivity has been found in the cerebral cortex, hypothalamus, amygdala, hippocampus and striatum. Vasoactive intestinal peptide is synthesized in neurones in the CNS and has been shown to be released by a calcium-dependent process. When applied by iontophoresis to single neurones, VIP causes excitation. Injected into the brain, it causes hypothermia and hypotension, as well as the release of other hormones such as prolactin and growth hormone. Binding sites for VIP have been demonstrated in the brain and the peptide is thought to co-exist with acetylcholine in interneurones in the cerebral cortex. While the evidence is as yet incomplete, it seems fairly certain that a neurotransmitter or neuromodulator role for VIP is likely to be established.

CHOLECYSTOKININ (CCK)

This is a hormone in the gut which causes contraction of the gallbladder. It has 33 amino acid residues; however, proteolysis of cholecystokinin gives rise to an octapeptide (CCK-8, Figure 10.27d), which is present in the gut, in the brain where high levels are found in the cerebral cortex, hippocampus, hypothalamus and amygdaloid nucleus, and in the spinal cord. It is also present in the periaqueductal grey matter of the brain stem. In the cerebral cortex, CCK-8 is more prevalent than other peptides.

Cholecystokinin octapeptide has been shown to co-exist with dopamine in the nigrostriatal fibres innervating the striatum and nucleus accumbens and it is thought that CCK-8 may control the release of dopamine. Although the functional role for CCK-8 in the CNS is not known, it has been shown that the level of CCK-8 in the blood rises after a meal and it is proposed that it may trigger a 'satiety' mechanism which causes the cessation of feeding. Thus, one possibility is that CCK-8 may be involved with the central control of feeding.

The peptides reviewed here represent some of the 40 or so peptides which have been found in the brain, other than in the hypothalamus. They have been chosen on the basis that some evidence exists to support a neurotransmitter or neuromodulator role. However, this is an area which is developing rapidly and it is quite possible that new peptides with important roles in the function of the CNS may yet be discovered. Some of those which have not been discussed are: bradykinin, luteinizing hormone, corticotropin (ACTH, which has been implicated in memory processes, see Chapter 20), bombesin and prolactin. In addition, there are the so-called sleep-inducing peptides.

Miscellaneous putative neurotransmitters

Adrenaline

Adrenaline (Figure 8.1d, Chapter 8) is important for its peripheral actions, particularly on the sympathetic nervous system, after its release as a local hormone from the adrenal medulla. Although it has been known for some time that small quantities of adrenaline are present in the brain, suitable methods for measuring the levels of adrenaline and also for detecting the activity of the enzyme responsible for its synthesis from noradrenaline, phenylethanolamine-N-methyl transferase, have only recently become available. It is now known that adrenaline-containing neurones are present in the brain stem (Figure 10.28), mainly in two groups: one,

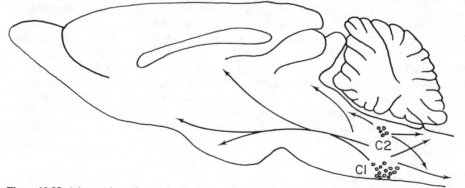

Figure 10.28 Adrenergic pathways in the brain, shown on a sagittal section of the brain of the rat. C1 and C2 represent the two groups of adrenaline-containing neurones in the rostral medulla (modified from Hökfelt *et al.*, 1974)

C_1, intermingles with noradrenaline-containing neurones of the lateral tegmental system; the other, C_2, in the dorsal medulla, is also in a region where noradrenaline-containing cells are found. The axons of these adrenaline-containing cells project into the hypothalamus. They also innervate the dorsal nucleus of the vagus nerve, the nucleus of the solitary tract and the locus coeruleus. In addition, there are descending adrenergic fibres projecting to the central grey matter of the spinal cord. Adrenaline-containing neurones have not been found in other regions of the brain.

The synthesis of adrenaline in neurones in the CNS is similar to the process which occurs in the adrenal medulla. The release of adrenaline from nerve terminals has been shown to be calcium dependent and its removal from the synaptic cleft is by a high-affinity uptake process. It is not clear, however, whether there is a separate transport system for adrenaline, or whether it is taken up into nerve terminals by the same process as that responsible for the re-uptake of noradrenaline.

Many of the drugs which affect noradrenaline-containing neurones also act on adrenergic neurones. Thus, the release of adrenaline is suppressed by clonidine and increased by yohimbine (Chapter 8). In addition, the indirectly acting sympatho-mimetic amine, amphetamine, causes the release of adrenaline from presynaptic terminals and monoamine oxidase inhibitors increase the level of adrenaline. However, as no drugs which act selectively on adrenergic mechanisms are available, it is not possible to establish how far adrenaline in the CNS may be involved in the actions of drugs such as clonidine and yohimbine. However, on the basis of its distribution in the brain, adrenaline is thought to be involved in cardiovascular and respiratory control mechanisms, the regulation of body tempera-ture and the regulation of food and water intake. It is possible that adrenaline may also be involved in certain neuroendocrine mechanisms, e.g. the control of secretions from the pituitary gland.

Some specific inhibitors of the enzyme phenylethanolamine-N-methyltransferase have been developed. The effects of one of these, 2,3-dichloro-α-methylbenzylamine (DCMB), provides support for a role for adrenaline in the central control of blood pressure.

Histamine

Peripherally, histamine is an important hormone, being stored in mast cells and in blood platelets. It is also present in the gastric mucosa, lungs and skin. Histamine is released from mast cells and platelets in response to tissue damage and allergic reactions, and from other sites by hormonal and neural signals. Histamine is present in the brain, although in smaller amounts than in other tissues. However, as it does not cross the blood–brain barrier, it is assumed that the histamine in brain is synthesized there from histidine, which can readily enter the CNS. Histamine is unevenly distributed in the brain, the highest levels being found in the hypothalamus.

The conversion of histidine to histamine requires the enzyme histidine decarboxylase, which utilizes pyridoxal phosphate (vitamin B_6) as cofactor (Figure 10.29). This enzyme is present in the brain, the largest concentration being in the hypothalamus. It is present in the cytoplasm of nerve endings and histamine can be released from these nerve endings, at least *in vitro*, by a calcium-dependent process. The release of histamine from the cerebral cortex has also been demonstrated *in vivo*. Histamine-containing neurones are present in the brain stem, with ascending

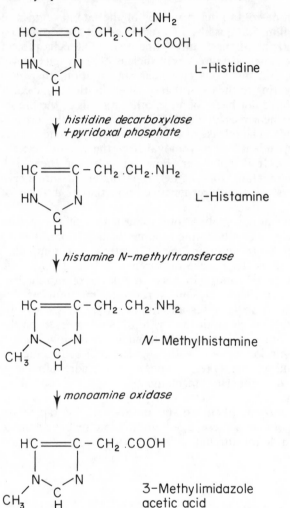

Figure 10.29 The synthesis and metabolism of histamine. The enzymes involved in each step are shown in italics

axons passing through the median forebrain bundle to project to the cerebral hemispheres. Nerve terminals containing histamine are found throughout the cerebral cortex and also in the hippocampus.

No high-affinity transport system for histamine has as yet been found and enzymatic transformation seems to be the most likely mode of inactivation. *N*-Methylation by the enzyme histamine *N*-methyltransferase, followed by oxidative deamination by monoamine oxidase to 3-methylimidazole acetic acid (Figure 10.29), is the most probable pathway through which histamine is metabolized in the brain, although other mechanisms are present peripherally.

A number of drugs which act selectively at histamine receptors are known and the development of antagonist drugs has demonstrated the existence of two types of histamine receptor, H_1 and H_2, although more is known about their roles in peripheral mechanisms than in the CNS. The H_1 receptors, which mediate the contraction of smooth muscle, are blocked by classic antihistaminic drugs such as mepyramine (Figure 10.30a), diphenhydramine (Figure 10.30b), promethazine (see Chapters 12 and 20, and Figure 20.4c) and chlorpheniramine (Figure 10.30c). These drugs are used in the treatment of hay fever and other allergic conditions. They are effective in the treatment of urticaria and influence vascular headache and so are useful in the treatment of migraine. These drugs are sedative and also anti-emetic and are used to relieve motion sickness (see Chapter 20). It is likely that the sedative and anti-emetic effects are due to central actions.

(a)

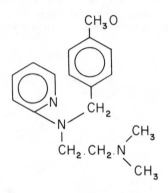

(b)

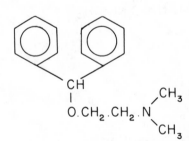

(c)

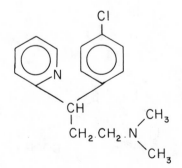

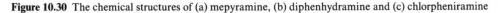

Figure 10.30 The chemical structures of (a) mepyramine, (b) diphenhydramine and (c) chlorpheniramine

The H_2 receptors mediate the peripheral actions of histamine in inducing gastric secretion and are selectively blocked by drugs such as metiamide (Figure 10.31a) and cimetidine (Figure 10.31b). These drugs block the stimulation of gastric secretion induced by activity in the vagus nerve or by the hormone gastrin and effectively reduce the acidity of the stomach, thus promoting the healing of gastric or duodenal ulcers. Cimetidine was the first H_2 blocker to be used for this purpose but, as it crosses the blood–brain barrier, it can cause confusion as a side-effect. Ranitidine (Figure 10.31c), which has similar actions to those of cimetidine on gastric secretion, has been claimed to have fewer side-effects but whether this is due to lack of penetration into the brain is not clear.

Both H_1 and H_2 receptors are present in the brain. The existence of an ascending histaminergic pathway from the brain stem to the cerebral cortex correlates with the sedative property of the H_1 antagonists and indicates a possible role for histamine in the brain in the control of wakefulness and sleep. Histamine is also involved in central mechanisms controlling nausea and vomiting (see Chapter 20).

(a)

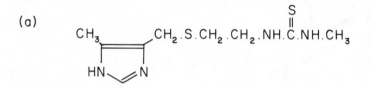

(b)

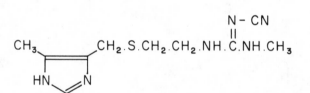

(c)

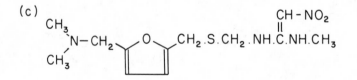

(d)

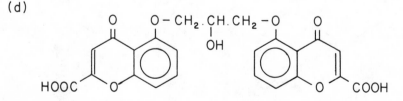

Figure 10.31 The chemical structures of (a) metiamide, (b) cimetidine, (c) ranitidine and (d) chromoglycate

Many drugs can induce the release of histamine; reserpine, which causes depletion of catecholamines and 5-HT (see Chapters 8 and 12) also depletes stores of histamine. A drug which prevents the release of histamine, although not from nerves, is disodium chromoglycate (DSCG; Figure 10.31d); it is useful in the treatment of asthma associated with allergic conditions, but must be given prophylactically as it is not effective once the release of histamine has started.

It seems possible that a third type of histamine receptor, designated H_3, may exist in the CNS. This appears to be located presynaptically on histamine-containing nerve terminals and to act as an autoreceptor, enabling histamine to control its own release.

Purines

It has long been known that adenosine nucleotides can have effects on smooth muscle. For example, if the smooth muscle of the intestinal wall is stimulated electrically, in the presence of atropine (to block parasympathetic effects) and either an adrenergic neurone blocker or both α- and β-adrenoceptor blockers (to block sympathetic transmission), then the muscle relaxes. It has been suggested that this effect is mediated by a non-cholinergic, non-adrenergic neurotransmitter, such as adenosine or adenosine triphosphate (ATP). The nerves which utilize adenosine or ATP as a neurotransmitter would form a 'purinergic' system. Peripherally, adenosine also has cardiovascular effects as, for example, in regulating the coronary vasodilatation associated with myocardial hypoxia.

In the CNS, the involvement of cyclic AMP as a second messenger mediating the actions of neurotransmitters and drugs at many receptors, is well established (see Chapter 3). Cyclic AMP is formed from ATP by the enzyme adenylate cyclase, which is an integral part of many receptor systems. However, there is some evidence that, in addition to its second messenger role, ATP or adenosine may be a neurotransmitter in the CNS, as well as peripherally. It has not been possible to demonstrate conclusively that purines are released from nerve terminals in response to stimulation. However, ATP is present in the intraneuronal storage complexes for catecholamines and may be released together with them, thus possibly acting as a co-transmitter (see below). Adenosine receptors have been identified in the CNS, mainly from binding studies, and they appear to be of two types:

P_1 receptors

These are more sensitive to adenosine and cyclic AMP than to ATP and are antagonized by theophylline. Stimulation of P_1 receptors leads to activation of adenylate cyclase which results in an increased intracellular concentration of cyclic AMP. These receptors appear to be widely distributed and they mediate purinergic effects on smooth muscle.

P_2 receptors

These are more sensitive to ATP than to adenosine or cyclic AMP and are antagonized by 2,2-pyridylisatogen tosylate. Activation of these receptors leads to increased synthesis of prostaglandins. They are less widely distributed than P_1 receptors.

It seems likely that presynaptic purinergic receptors may be present on cholinergic and adrenergic nerve terminals where their function is to control the release of the neurotransmitters. Autoreceptors, i.e. presynaptic receptors on purinergic nerve terminals, are also thought to exist. There is evidence that some primary afferent fibres release ATP to excite neurones in lamina II of the spinal cord. The receptors on these neurones would therefore be of the P_2 type. These receptors have also been found in the trigeminal nucleus.

Some central stimulant drugs, such as the methylxanthines, caffeine and theophylline (see Chapter 16), act as selective antagonists at adenosine receptors and it is possible that this is the mechanism responsible for their stimulant effect. However, they also inhibit the enzyme phosphodiesterase, which is responsible for the breakdown of cyclic AMP, and this provides an alternative mechanism for their action.

Unfortunately, the classification of purine receptors into P_1 and P_2 is not universally accepted and alternative classifications, e.g. A_1 and A_2, based on the potency of purine compounds to modify the activity of adenylate cyclase, have been proposed.

Prostaglandins

These are lipid acids, derived from a common precursor, arachidonic acid, which have well-defined biological activity. Although they were at one time considered to be putative neurotransmitters, it is now generally accepted that the prostaglandins and related substances act as autacoids or local hormones. The prostaglandins are endogenous substances but are synthesized and released as the occasion demands, rather than being stored.

The synthesis of prostaglandins and the related substances, prostacyclin and thromboxane, takes place in two stages (Figure 10.32). The first stage is catalysed by cyclo-oxygenase, an enzyme which is found in almost every cell in the body, to form the cyclic endoperoxides, PGG_2 and PGH_2 (Figure 10.32), which are very unstable. The second stage utilizes enzymes which are specific for different tissues and leads to the formation of either prostaglandins, prostacyclin or thromboxane. An alternative pathway from arachidonic acid, catalysed by lipoxygenases, leads to the formation of leukotrienes. However, of the various endogenous substances derived from arachidonic acid, only the prostaglandins have any actions which are relevant to the nervous system. It is important to note that the anti-inflammatory actions of the non-steroidal anti-inflammatory drugs, such as aspirin, are mainly attributable to the fact that they inhibit cyclo-oxygenase and so depress the formation of prostaglandins (and related substances); it is possible that this action may account for the analgesic properties of these substances (see Chapter 15).

The classification of the prostaglandins is both complicated and confusing, partly because the early classification into the 'E' and 'F' series was based on their solubility in ether. However, only two prostaglandins, PGE_2 and $PGF_{2\alpha}$, are important for their actions in the nervous system. Both PGE_2 and $PGF_{2\alpha}$ are released from the autonomic nervous system and PGE_2 has been shown to modulate the release of noradrenaline from sympathetic nerve endings (see Chapter 8), thus acting as a neuromodulator. Prostaglandins are also released from postsynaptic sites and may affect the interaction between the neurotransmitter and the postsynaptic receptor. Prostaglandins of the E and F series are found in the brain where they have a widespread but uneven distribution. In the hypothalamus they have been shown to be involved in the production of fever by bacterial pyrogens and toxins.

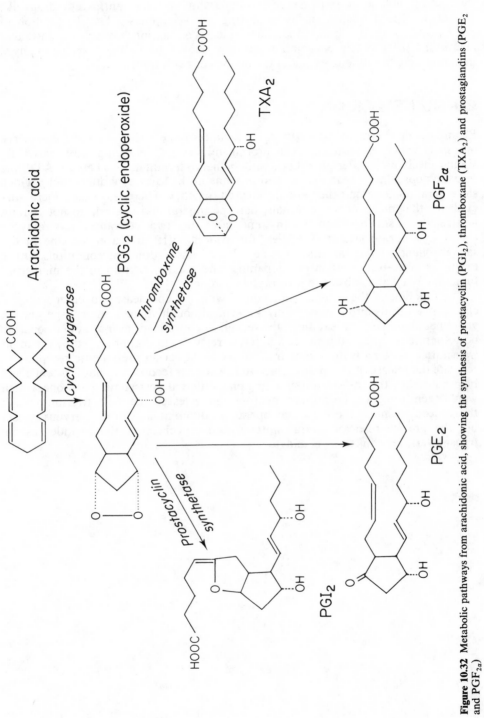

Figure 10.32 Metabolic pathways from arachidonic acid, showing the synthesis of prostacyclin (PGI$_2$), thromboxane (TXA$_2$) and prostaglandins (PGE$_2$ and PGF$_{2\alpha}$)

Pyrogens stimulate the synthesis of prostaglandins, whereas antipyretic drugs like aspirin depress the synthesis by inhibiting cyclo-oxygenase. The distribution of prostaglandins in the brain does not indicate a relationship to any particular neurotransmitter system or neuronal pathway. Nevertheless, they may be involved in modulating both the release and the actions of neurotransmitters.

CO-TRANSMISSION

Examples have already been given of peptides 'co-existing' in the same nerve terminals which contain classic neurotransmitters and of being 'co-released' by similar mechanisms. Peripheral sympathetic nerve terminals also contain ATP, the enzyme dopamine-β-hydroxylase, and proteins in the same synaptic vesicles which store noradrenaline and they are all released together. There is, in fact, increasing evidence that many nerve terminals, both peripheral and central, do not contain and release a single substance. In some cases, the two 'co-transmitters' may be stored in separate synaptic vesicles, for example VIP and acetylcholine in the salivary gland of the cat, and may be released under different conditions. Other examples of co-transmission are dopamine and cholecystokinin in the nigrostriatum, and 5-HT and substance P in raphe neurones.

The function of the second 'transmitter' which is co-released together with the classic neurotransmitter is not fully known, although there is much speculation about possible roles. For example, the second or co-transmitter may act on separate postsynaptic receptors to mediate a different response to that produced by the main transmitter. Alternatively, the co-transmitter could act on presynaptic receptors to regulate the release of the main transmitter; a similar feedback control system could be produced by the co-transmitter acting on a different postsynaptic neurone, which would then influence the primary neurone that released the main transmitter. All these mechanisms, and others, may operate at different sites in the nervous system but the precise roles of co-transmitters, and especially of the peptides as co-transmitters, remains to be elucidated.

Chapter 11

Anaesthetics, hypnotics and sedatives

The drugs in these three categories all have a depressant action on the central nervous system, leading to depression or loss of consciousness, the difference between them being largely one of degree. Thus, many sedative or hypnotic drugs will produce anaesthesia if given in sufficiently large doses. Nevertheless, different drugs are normally used for these different purposes. A sedative is a drug which reduces activity and moderates excitement, having a calming effect rather than making the subject sleepy. Sedatives are used to relieve anxiety (see Chapter 13) and tension and, in so doing, they may make sleep more likely. Hypnotic drugs are usually more potent than sedatives but, when given in small doses, they may be used as sedatives. Hypnotic drugs produce drowsiness and facilitate the onset and maintenance of a state of sleep which resembles natural sleep and from which the subject can be roused. Anaesthetics are drugs which, when given in adequate doses, cause complete but reversible loss of consciousness, such that loss of all sensations, and in particular the sensation of pain, occurs. This type of anaesthesia is known as general anaesthesia, as opposed to local or regional anaesthesia (see Chapter 9) which does not involve the loss of consciousness.

Drugs which produce generalized depression of the central nervous system, resulting in loss of consciousness or stupor, are also known as 'narcotic' drugs, a term derived from the Greek word 'narkotikos'. However, misuse of this term has resulted in drugs which produce dependence (e.g. cocaine) being called 'narcotics', even though they do not induce narcosis. The use of this term for depressant drugs is therefore best avoided.

General anaesthetics

Anaesthetic drugs can be divided into two main categories, according to their physical properties and the method of administration, i.e. inhalation or volatile anaesthetics, and intravenous or non-volatile anaesthetics.

Inhalation anaesthetics

These drugs are interesting historically as the first anaesthetics to be used for the relief of pain in surgery during the nineteenth century were administered by inhalation; the drugs were ether and chloroform. Before this, few surgical operations were attempted unless of an emergency nature. The ideal inhalation anaesthetic must be free from unwanted and/or toxic effects and should have a wide margin of safety in use. It should be non-irritant, be free from unpleasant taste or smell, and induction and recovery should be rapid and not associated with unpleasant effects such as nausea and vomiting. The anaesthetic should be non-flammable, chemically stable and also inexpensive. Unfortunately, none of the inhalation anaesthetics currently available satisfies all these criteria.

The inhalation anaesthetics include hydrocarbons, alcohols and ethers, together with their halogenated derivatives. These substances are absorbed through the lungs in the vapour phase and pass into the blood in which they are transferred to the tissues, where they will be taken up into fat, depending upon their lipid solubility. Because anaesthesia is produced by drugs entering the brain, the loss of the anaesthetic to other tissues will tend to reduce the anaesthetic action. The solubility of the anaesthetic in the blood is also important, low solubility resulting in a rapid action on the brain and hence fast induction and recovery.

Diethyl ether (Figure 11.1a)

Generally known as 'ether', this substance was one of the first anaesthetics to be discovered. It is a clear volatile liquid with a pungent smell, its boiling point being 36.5°C. The vapour forms an inflammable mixture with air or oxygen and special precautions were needed when ether was used in operating theatres to avoid the build-up of static electricity. It is highly lipid soluble and therefore highly soluble in the blood, causing the onset of action (induction) and recovery to be slow. Ether has an irritant action on the respiratory mucosa and produces increased salivation and bronchial secretion. The irritant effect leads to a high incidence of nausea and vomiting during induction and recovery, and also postoperatively. The increase in secretions can be prevented by premedication with atropine. Because of the unpleasant and unwanted effects, together with the danger of explosions, ether is rarely, if ever, used. Its advantage is that it has no cardiac effects and can be used in conjunction with the infiltration of adrenaline.

Chloroform (Figure 11.1b)

This anaesthetic was discovered at about the same time as ether but is also seldom used. It is a heavy, colourless liquid with a characteristic sweet and sickly odour and taste; it boils at 61°C. It is not highly inflammable and does not form explosive mixtures with air. Chloroform has a rapid onset of action but it is very toxic, sensitizing the heart to circulating catecholamines and increasing the risk of cardiac arrhythmias during anaesthesia. It is also hepatotoxic.

Halothane (Figure 11.1c)

This is a colourless sweet-smelling liquid which boils at 50°C. It is not inflammable and is relatively non-toxic. It was introduced in 1956 after the search for a non-flammable agent and it is now the most widely used of the inhalation anaesthetics. Its advantages are that it is potent and non-irritant and induction is, therefore, smooth and not unpleasant. It seldom induces coughing and the incidence of postoperative vomiting is low. Halothane, mixed with oxygen or with nitrous oxide/oxygen mixtures, is used for induction and also for maintenance anaesthesia. However, it is not a good analgesic and muscle relaxation may be poor, although

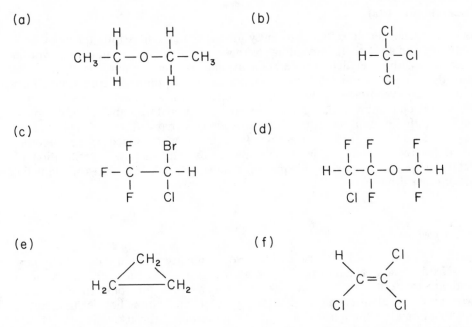

(a)

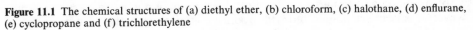

Figure 11.1 The chemical structures of (a) diethyl ether, (b) chloroform, (c) halothane, (d) enflurane, (e) cyclopropane and (f) trichlorethylene

both can be compensated for by administering other drugs, i.e. analgesics and muscle relaxants, in what is known as 'balanced anaesthesia'.

Halothane causes cardiorespiratory depression. The respiratory depression can lead to increased concentrations of carbon dioxide in the arterial blood and, because responsiveness to carbon dioxide is reduced, spontaneous ventilation cannot be safely used and respiration has to be controlled mechanically or manually. The myocardial depression induced by halothane can cause bradycardia. There is also some peripheral vasodilatation so that hypotension results. The cardiac depression can also result in arrhythmias. Because halothane sensitizes the myocardium to catecholamines, the use of infusions of adrenaline requires extreme care or is best avoided. There is evidence that repeated use of halothane can result in disturbances of liver function, including hepatitis. This complication is extremely rare and may be associated with a previous history of liver disease. Nevertheless, when repeat anaesthesia is required within a period of 4–6 weeks, an alternative anaesthetic agent may be preferred. There are also reports of adverse effects on operating theatre personnel caused by exposure to low levels of halothane over prolonged periods of time, but such reports are controversial. However, it is generally accepted that environmental contamination with halothane is best avoided. Halothane is one of the drugs which can trigger malignant hyperthermia, a rare inherited disease, which is characterized by intense and sustained muscle spasm and a sudden rise in body temperature. Although the condition is rare, the mortality rate is high. Treatment is with dantrolene, a drug which acts directly on skeletal muscle by interfering with the efflux of calcium from the sarcoplasmic reticulum and so blocking contraction.

Enflurane (Figure 11.1d)

This is an inhalation anaesthetic, recently introduced as a substitute for halothane. Its actions as an anaesthetic are similar to those of halothane, i.e. induction is rapid and smooth, with no evidence of excitement, and recovery is more rapid. It is less potent than halothane. Enflurane produces cardiorespiratory depression which results in the development of hypotension, but it does not appear to sensitize the heart to catecholamines; therefore infusions of adrenaline can be safely given during anaesthesia induced with enflurane. It is likely that enflurane does not cause liver dysfunction as only a small fraction of the drug is metabolized; it can therefore be used for repeat anaesthesia. Enflurane causes some degree of relaxation of skeletal muscle which may be adequate for some surgical procedures without the need for other drugs.

Nitrous oxide (N₂O)

In contrast to the substances described above, which are all highly volatile liquids, nitrous oxide is a gas at normal temperatures. It was, in fact, the first general anaesthetic to be discovered but was not used as such for some time after its discovery. It is a colourless gas with a faintly sweet smell and is heavier than air. It is not inflammable although it can support combustion. Nitrous oxide is relatively insoluble in blood and tissues and therefore both induction and recovery are rapid. However, it is not very potent and will produce complete anaesthesia only when the pure gas is inhaled. The person who has inhaled nitrous oxide to the point of unconsciousness is anoxic and cyanosed. Because even a brief period of anoxia can result in brain damage, nitrous oxide is given only when mixed with oxygen, in concentrations of 50–70% of the gas. Because of its low potency, nitrous oxide is rarely used on its own but is given in combination with other inhalation or intravenous anaesthetics. For example, nitrous oxide, mixed with oxygen, is commonly used for the maintenance of anaesthesia after induction with a rapidly acting barbiturate. It is an effective analgesic and, because of its rapid onset, it can be used to produce analgesia without loss of consciousness by self-administration, e.g. in obstetrics; in this case a mixture of 50% nitrous oxide with oxygen is used. Prolonged exposure of patients (and of anaesthetists) to nitrous oxide can lead to the development of megaloblastic anaemia.

Cyclopropane (Figure 11.1e)

This is a colourless sweet-smelling gas which is heavier than air. It is a potent anaesthetic but is inflammable and forms explosive mixtures with air and oxygen; it must therefore be used in a closed-circuit system. It produces rapid pleasant induction and rapid recovery, although there may be vomiting and restlessness. There is good muscle relaxation and a wide safety margin, even when used with spontaneous respiration. Cyclopropane causes cardiorespiratory depression but the arterial blood pressure is usually well maintained, possibly because peripheral vasodilatation is absent. However, it sensitizes the heart to catecholamines. Although cyclopropane is a useful anaesthetic, it is no longer used because of the risk of explosions.

Trichlorethylene (Figure 11.1f)

This is a colourless liquid which boils at 87°C and has an odour similar to that of chloroform. It is a weak anaesthetic and has poor muscle-relaxant properties but it is a potent analgesic; this latter attribute is made use of in obstetrics where trichlorethylene is used in subanaesthetic doses by self-administration from a vaporizer to relieve pain in labour. The toxic effects of trichlorethylene are similar to those of chloroform but are less marked. However, cardiac arrhythmias can occur. It is rarely used as an anaesthetic on its own but can be used to supplement nitrous oxide/oxygen mixtures. Used in this way, it is without serious side-effects, particularly cardiovascular effects. However, recovery is slow because metabolites of trichlorethylene are active and vomiting may occur.

Intravenous anaesthetics

These are drugs which are injected intravenously to produce a rapid loss of consciousness. They may be used alone for short surgical procedures but are more commonly used for induction only, after which, following tracheal intubation, anaesthesia is maintained with an inhalation anaesthetic.

Barbiturates (Figure 11.2)

The most important, and also the most widely used, intravenous anaesthetics are the barbiturates. They are all derivatives of barbituric acid which itself lacks central depressant properties. Substitution of alkyl or aryl groups for the hydrogen atoms on the carbon atom at position 5 (see Figure 11.2) confers sedative, hypnotic properties on the molecule. Barbiturates in which the oxygen at carbon atom 2 is replaced by sulphur are thiobarbiturates. The barbiturates are almost insoluble in water but, as they are weak acids, they can form sodium salts which dissolve in water. The thiobarbiturates are more lipid soluble than the 'oxybarbiturates' (i.e. with oxygen at carbon atom 2). The larger the aliphatic group at carbon atom 5, the greater the potency, but the duration of action is reduced; however, this is mainly due to differences in lipid solubility. Increasing lipid solubility decreases the duration of action and latency to onset of action, but usually increases the potency. Thus, the main differences between the sedative barbiturates are pharmacokinetic. In order to produce rapid loss of consciousness for the induction of anaesthesia, a high concentration of the drug in the brain must be attained quickly; therefore high lipid solubility is required and drugs such as thiopentone, hexobarbitone and methohexitone (Figure 11.2) are used. To produce sedation a slower onset of action is acceptable, if not desirable, and drugs which are absorbed when given orally, with reduced lipid solubility and hence longer duration of action, are used. Examples are phenobarbitone, barbitone, amylobarbitone, butobarbitone and pentobarbitone (Figure 11.2). However, some qualitative differences between different barbiturates exist. Drugs with a phenyl group at carbon atom 5 possess anticonvulsant properties (see Chapter 14) and some barbiturates, e.g. phenobarbitone, have been used in the treatment of anxiety (Chapter 13). The substitution of groups with more than seven carbon atoms at carbon atom 5 can result in compounds with convulsant activity.

The barbiturates possess no analgesic activity and when they are used as anaesthetics on their own, therefore, the loss of response to pain is solely attributable to the loss of consciousness. The main toxic effect is respiratory

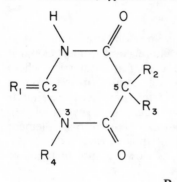

	R_1	R_2	R_3	R_4
Barbituric acid	O	H	H	H
Short-acting:				
Thiopentone	S	Ethyl	1-Methyl-butyl	H
Hexobarbitone	O	Methyl	1-Cyclohexen-1-yl	Methyl
Methohexitone	O	Allyl	1-Methyl-2-pentynyl	Methyl
Long-acting:				
Phenobarbitone	O	Ethyl	Phenyl	H
Barbitone	O	Ethyl	Ethyl	H
Amylobarbitone	O	Ethyl	*iso*-Amyl	H
Butobarbitone	O	Ethyl	*sec*-Butyl	H
Pentobarbitone	O	Ethyl	1-Methyl-butyl	H

Figure 11.2 The structure of barbituric acid, showing the substituent groups at R_1, R_2, R_3 and R_4 for some typical barbiturates

depression which can readily occur with a slight overdose. Cardiovascular toxic effects can also occur but are rare and the barbiturates do not sensitize the heart to catecholamines.

The most widely used barbiturate anaesthetic is thiopentone sodium. However, it is unstable in aqueous solution, especially when exposed to air. Furthermore, the solution is alkaline and therefore irritant to tissues, so that extravasation must be avoided. Accidental injection into an artery is particularly dangerous as intense vasoconstriction and thrombosis can occur and, unless immediately reversed by the injection of procaine, gangrene of the limb may result. The onset of anaesthesia with thiopentone is extremely rapid due to the high lipid solubility of the drug and the rich blood supply to the brain, resulting in the rapid transfer of a large part of the intravenous dose to the brain. However, because of its high lipid solubility the drug is taken up by other tissues, including adipose tissue, but this process is slower, due to the relatively poor blood supply. Thus, after a high initial concentration is reached in the brain, leading to loss of consciousness, the drug redistributes to other tissues and this lowers the concentration in the blood and causes rapid recovery of consciousness. Consciousness is therefore regained while there are still large amounts of the anaesthetic in the body and the duration of anaesthesia is dependent upon the process of 'redistribution' and not upon the metabolism or excretion of the drug. In fact, thiopentone is not metabolized particularly quickly in the liver. The fraction of drug which redistributes to tissues other than the brain is released slowly into the bloodstream; therefore, although the period of unconsciousness is short with a drug like thiopentone, the persistence of the drug in the bloodstream will result in sedation occurring for some hours after recovery of consciousness and 'hangover' effects may persist for 24 h or more, especially if more than one intravenous dose has been given.

Methohexitone is more potent than thiopentone and therefore smaller doses can be used and the duration of anaesthesia is shorter. However, involuntary muscle movement can occur with methohexitone, together with postanaesthetic pain at the injection site.

The metabolism of the barbiturates is discussed below under 'Hypnotics and sedatives' (page 187).

Propanidid (Figure 11.3a)

This is a non-barbiturate short-acting anaesthetic that has been used for minor dental and surgical procedures. The duration of action, which is about 6 minutes, is due to rapid hydrolysis of the drug by serum cholinesterase. Respiration is stimulated, at least initially, but numerous side-effects including nausea, vomiting and abnormal muscle movements can occur. Furthermore, propanidid has a depressant action on the myocardium resulting in hypotension, and cardiovascular collapse has been known to occur.

Etomidate (Figure 11.3b)

This is a short-acting potent anaesthetic agent which is used for the induction of anaesthesia. Its effects are similar to those of the short-acting barbiturates but it is considered to have a greater margin of safety because it has minimal cardiorespiratory effects. The short duration of action due to rapid metabolism in the liver means that hangover effects are less likely to occur. However, etomidate can cause pain on injection and there is a high incidence of extraneous muscle movements so that it cannot be used for prolonged anaesthesia. There is also evidence that prolonged use of etomidate can suppress adrenocortical function, causing loss of the response to stress.

Ketamine (Figure 11.3c)

This drug, which is 2-(o-chlorophenyl)-2-(methylamino)cyclohexanone, produces a state known as 'dissociative anaesthesia'. It is characterized by sedation, immobility, amnesia, analgesia and a feeling of dissociation from the environment. In this state, the patient may appear to be awake but does not respond to sensory stimuli. Ketamine is highly lipid soluble and is rapidly distributed to organs with a rich blood supply, such as the brain. It is subsequently redistributed to less well-perfused tissues from which it is slowly released, thus resulting in slow recovery. Ketamine is metabolized in the liver and some of the metabolites possess anaesthetic activity although they are less potent than ketamine itself. Muscle relaxation with ketamine is poor and muscle tone may be increased. Besides being a powerful analgesic, ketamine is the only intravenous anaesthetic which produces cardiovascular

(a)

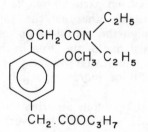

(b)

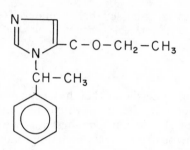

(c)

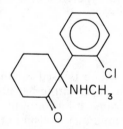

(d)

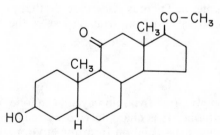

Figure 11.3 The chemical structures of (a) propanidid, (b) etomidate, (c) ketamine and (d) alphaxalone

stimulation. Arterial blood pressure and cardiac output are increased and there may be tachycardia.

The principal disadvantage with the use of ketamine is the high incidence of psychic phenomena which occur, mainly during recovery. These consist of disagreeable dreams or even hallucinations and they may recur at a later time. It is believed that these psychic disturbances occur less frequently in children and ketamine is used in paediatric anaesthesia. The drug is contra-indicated in patients with hypertension and those with a history of mental illness. The incidence of adverse psychic effects can be reduced by premedication with the benzodiazepine diazepam.

Ketamine is related chemically to phencyclidine which was also tested as a dissociative anaesthetic but abandoned because of its potent psychotomimetic action (see Chapter 18).

Alphaxalone (Figure 11.3d)

This is a steroid which is formulated with a closely related compound, alphadalone, to improve its solubility, although alphadalone is less potent as an anaesthetic than alphaxalone. The mixture has the proprietary name Althesin. An effective intravenous dose produces unconsciousness within 30–60 s, with a duration of 5–10 min; it is therefore useful for short procedures. Muscular relaxation is good and the drug does not affect the heart rate, although hypotension can occur. Recovery, which is rapid and complete, does not depend upon redistribution but upon metabolism in the liver. Alphaxalone therefore has some advantages over thiopentone for the induction of anaesthesia and for minor surgery. However, adverse effects, including severe sensitivity reactions resulting in cardiovascular collapse, can occur and have led to the drug being withdrawn from use.

Benzodiazepines

These drugs were first introduced for the treatment of anxiety and their use for this purpose is discussed in Chapter 13. However, they also possess sedative, anticonvulsant and muscle-relaxant actions. Unconsciousness can be produced with large doses of certain benzodiazepines, e.g. diazepam and midazolam. The onset of action is slower than that of the barbiturates and recovery is also slower. For example, the half life ($t_\frac{1}{2}$) of diazepam in plasma is 30 h. There is amnesia but no analgesia and muscle relaxation is poor. On the other hand, cardiorespiratory depression is moderate and diazepam has an application in patients who cannot tolerate the cardiovascular or respiratory depression associated with the barbiturates. However, the major problem with the use of benzodiazepines such as diazepam for anaesthesia is the marked variation in the effective dose in different individuals.

DIAZEPAM (Figure 11.4a)

Like most benzodiazepines, diazepam is insoluble in water and has to be dissolved in organic solvents. Intravenous injections are painful and venous thrombosis may occur with a delayed onset. Intramuscular injections are also painful and absorption is erratic. These problems can be overcome to some extent by special formulations, e.g. an emulsion of diazepam which is less painful on intravenous injection and less likely to cause thrombosis; however, the onset of action is slower.

MIDAZOLAM

This is one of the few benzodiazepines which is soluble in water and is therefore less irritant to veins. Recovery is faster than with diazepam but respiratory depression and hypotension with intravenous administration have been reported.

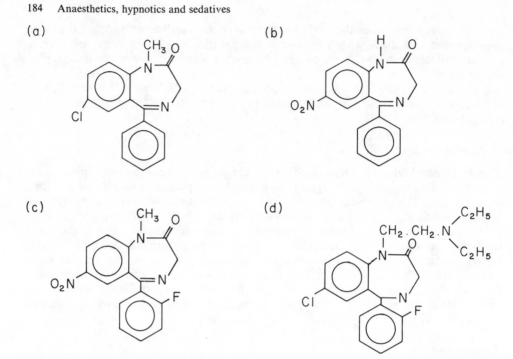

Figure 11.4 The chemical structures of the long-lasting benzodiazepines (a) diazepam, (b) nitrazepam, (c) flunitrazepam and (d) flurazepam

The benzodiazepines are used less as anaesthetics than as sedatives for minor or unpleasant procedures which do not require analgesia, e.g. bronchoscopy and cardiac catherization, or for operations under local anaesthesia, including dentistry. Because of their anti-anxiety action and also the amnesia which they produce, the benzodiazepines are often used for premedication before the administration of a general anaesthetic.

Neuroleptanalgesia

Strictly speaking, this should not come under the heading of anaesthesia as it is a state of complete disinterestedness and detachment from the environment, without loss of consciousness or the ability to communicate and respond to instructions. It is achieved by combining a neuroleptic drug (Chapter 12) with a potent opioid analgesic (Chapter 15), the drugs most commonly used being droperidol and fentanyl. It is a relatively safe and simple procedure which is useful in elderly or seriously ill patients, or for minor procedures. The drugs are mixed and infused intravenously, the onset of neuroleptanalgesia being 3–4 min. Droperidol has a prolonged duration of action (3–6 h), whereas the analgesic action of fentanyl lasts for only 30 min. Thus, supplementary doses of fentanyl must be injected at intervals. Cardiovascular effects are minimal but respiratory depression is marked, although predictable, and assisted or controlled ventilation may be necessary.

The combination of droperidol and fentanyl can be supplemented with a general anaesthetic, such as nitrous oxide, resulting in a state sometimes called 'neuroleptanaesthesia'. Because this state involves loss of consciousness, it can be used for major surgery. Cardiovascular stability is maintained, although respiratory depression occurs, and postoperative recovery is rapid.

Opioids

The detailed pharmacology of the opioid drugs is discussed in Chapter 15. These drugs are not anaesthetics as they do not depress consciousness to the extent of producing unconsciousness. However, because many anaesthetic drugs have no analgesic action, or are only weakly analgesic, potent opioid analgesics such as morphine are often used to supplement general anaesthesia, usually in combination with a nitrous oxide/oxygen mixture. In addition, premedication with a small dose of an opioid analgesic will reduce the dose of the general anaesthetic required to produce anaesthesia. Respiratory depression can be a problem, particularly when repeated doses of the opioid have been given, and it may persist postoperatively when artificial ventilation may be more difficult to provide. The use of respiratory stimulants or of opioid antagonists, such as naloxone, may therefore be required. Nevertheless, the opioid analgesics are widely used.

The signs and stages of anaesthesia

Ever since the introduction of general anaesthetics, attempts have been made to correlate their observable effects or signs with the depth of anaesthesia. This can readily be done when the induction of anaesthesia is slow, but with rapidly acting intravenous anaesthetics the earlier stages are passed through very quickly and may not be observed. Many of the signs refer to effects on respiration, reflex activity and muscle tone and originate from observations on the effects of ether, which is slow in onset. Traditionally, the effects of anaesthetics are divided into four stages:

I   *Stage of analgesia.*   The patient is conscious and can talk and obey commands but awareness of pain is reduced.
II   *Stage of excitement.*   This stage extends from the loss of consciousness to the beginning of surgical anaesthesia. The patient may appear delirious and excited and there may be involuntary movements. The pupils dilate, muscle tone increases and respiration becomes irregular. There may be incontinence and vomiting. For obvious reasons, efforts are made to limit the duration and severity of this stage of anaesthesia, which ends with the establishment of regular breathing.
III *Stage of surgical anaesthesia.*   This stage extends from the beginning of regular respiration through to complete cessation of spontaneous respiration. The excitement and irregular breathing of Stage II disappear, the pulse slows and reflexes progressively disappear. The reflexes controlling voluntary muscles are lost first, followed by loss of conjunctival and eyelid reflexes, and then the cough and vomiting centres in the medulla. This stage of anaesthesia is often divided into four planes, described in terms of the character of the respiration, the nature of eyeball movements, the presence or absence of certain reflexes and the size of the pupils.
IV   *Stage of medullary depression.*   This stage is present when spontaneous respiration ceases. Between Plane 4 of Stage III and Stage IV the respiration becomes

shallow and irregular; there is a rapid pulse and a fall in blood pressure, together with dilatation of the pupils. Stage IV represents severe depression of the respiratory centre and vasomotor centre in the medulla. Unless reversed by full circulatory and respiratory support, coma and death will ensue.

The early stages of anaesthesia may be missed when rapidly acting intravenous anaesthetics are used and the drugs used for premedication may also obscure the signs. For example, neuromuscular blocking agents such as tubocurarine and succinylcholine will affect muscle tone and therefore eliminate muscular indices of the depth of anaesthesia. Atropine, used to reduce secretions, also dilates the pupils, while opiate analgesics depress respiration and constrict the pupils. Under these circumstances, loss of the eyelash reflex (blinking of the eyelids when the eyelashes are stroked) and the establishment of a pattern of respiration that is regular in terms of rate and depth are used to indicate that Stage III (surgical anaesthesia) has been reached. In some cases the electroencephalogram (see below) has been used to monitor the depth of anaesthesia.

Theories of anaesthesia

Many theories have been advanced to explain the mechanism of action of anaesthetic drugs. One of the principal problems in arriving at a common theory is that so many different substances, ranging from inert gases (e.g. xenon) and simple inorganic (nitrous oxide) and organic (chloroform) compounds to complex organic molecules (e.g. alphaxalone), all produce anaesthesia. In fact, no one theory satisfactorily explains how all these diverse agents produce their anaesthetic effects.

A common property of anaesthetic agents is depression of excitatory transmission in the CNS without affecting nerve conduction. However, in the absence of a common chemical structure or of any structure–activity relationships for anaesthetic drugs, the possibility of a specific interaction with a receptor seems remote and most theories of anaesthesia are based on the physicochemical characteristics of anaesthetic drugs. The most striking of these is lipid solubility and this property has been shown to correlate well with anaesthetic potency. Molecules such as those of general anaesthetics are hydrophobic: they are non-polar and cannot form a significant number of hydrogen bonds. They therefore distribute to sites in which they are removed from an aqueous environment, i.e. in oil or lipid. For this reason, and because of the good correlation between anaesthetic potency and lipophilicity (lipid solubility), it is thought that anaesthetics are incorporated into membrane lipids, resulting in distortion of the membrane structure so causing occlusion of the pores through which ions pass, e.g. the sodium channel. Support for this theory has come from the observation that anaesthesia in animals can be reversed by the application of high barometric pressure. This has been shown to increase the ordering of lipids in the membrane, which would tend to remove any distortion present and so open the ion pores.

While this theory is attractive, it does not allow for the fact that not all lipid-soluble substances are anaesthetics. It is therefore likely that a unitary theory for the mechanism of action of general anaesthetics may not be achievable and it is quite possible that different types of anaesthetics may have different mechanisms of action, although the end result, i.e. the state of anaesthesia, is the same. For example, barbiturates are known to interact with γ-aminobutyric acid (GABA) receptors (see below) and ketamine acts on opiate receptors (see Chapter 15).

Similarly, it is not known whether all neurones in the brain are equally sensitive to anaesthetic drugs, or whether the neurones in some regions, e.g. the brain stem reticular formation, are more sensitive.

Hypnotics and sedatives

These are drugs which produce mild depression of the CNS when given in appropriate doses. A sedative will reduce tension and anxiety, having a calming effect and making sleep more possible, without actually inducing sleep. Hypnotics, on the other hand, should produce drowsiness and encourage the onset and maintenance of a state of sleep, from which the subject can be roused and which resembles natural sleep, as far as possible. However, the same drugs are used both as sedatives and hypnotics, the state produced depending mainly on the dose administered. They are used for the treatment of insomnia and sleep disturbances, for example those associated with air travel.

Barbiturates

Most barbiturates will produce sedation or induce sleep if administered in suitable doses; however, because rapid loss of consciousness and a short duration of action is not required, and may even be undesirable, different barbiturates to those used as anaesthetics are employed as sedatives and hypnotics.

The barbiturates were the traditional choice as sedative-hypnotics for many years, but have now been almost completely replaced by the benzodiazepines (see below). They are included here partly for historical reasons but also because, as they are still available for use as anaesthetics and for the treatment of epilepsy (Chapter 14), they may be self-administered as sedatives. The main derivatives of barbituric acid which have been used as sedatives and hypnotics are phenobarbitone, barbitone, amylobarbitone, butobarbitone and pentobarbitone (Figure 11.2). All are relatively long acting and are effective when taken by mouth. The principal adverse effect of these drugs is depression of respiration in overdose: death from poisoning with barbiturates can usually be attributed to respiratory failure. As they have a low therapeutic index, poisoning can occur with a relatively moderate overdose. Another adverse reaction to barbiturates is the development of tolerance with chronic use. Tolerance to the sedative effect develops more rapidly than to the lethal effects (respiratory depression) and thus the therapeutic index decreases and acute poisoning can occur readily in chronic barbiturate users. In addition, dependence can develop with the chronic use of barbiturates, leading to addiction; the sudden withdrawal of the drug in an addicted individual can have serious consequences. Mild withdrawal symptoms are insomnia, anxiety and EEG abnormalities. However, in severe cases, convulsions, delirium, hypotension, hypothermia and cardiovascular collapse resulting in death can occur with withdrawal of barbiturates. The abstinence syndrome can usually be aborted by the administration of a barbiturate, or a related sedative drug, provided that it is given when the signs of withdrawal first appear.

Other adverse effects of barbiturates result from interactions with other drugs, especially other sedatives. The major route of inactivation of the barbiturates is metabolism by the hepatic microsomal enzymes. The oxybarbiturates are metabolized only in the liver, whereas the thiobarbiturates are also transformed to some extent in other tissues (kidney and brain). Those with a high lipid solubility are not excreted in appreciable amounts, but those with low lipid solubility, e.g. phenobarbitone, are excreted largely unchanged and the renal excretion can be increased by alkalinization of the urine. An important aspect of the metabolism of the barbiturates is their ability to induce the hepatic drug-metabolizing enzymes and this action contributes significantly to the development of tolerance. Secondly, the drug-metabolizing enzymes in the liver are relatively non-specific and therefore the induction of enzymes produced by the barbiturates affects the metabolism of a wide variety of other drugs, i.e. those which are metabolized by the same enzyme system. Examples of such drugs are oral anticoagulants, digitoxin, β-blockers, oral contraceptives, phenytoin and tricyclic antidepressants. Increased metabolism of these drugs will necessitate the use of larger doses, but overdose will then occur if the administration of the barbiturate is terminated. For example, the response to the anticoagulant drug coumarin will be diminished by the chronic administration of a barbiturate, due to the induction of the hepatic microsomal enzymes and the increased metabolism of coumarin. This effect can be compensated for by increasing the dose of coumarin but, if the administration of the barbiturate is then discontinued, the drug-metabolizing enzymes rapidly return to their normal level of activity and the anticoagulant will be metabolized more slowly, resulting in an overdose such that bleeding may occur. Another consequence of the induction of microsomal liver enzymes by barbiturates is in cases of acute intermittent porphyria, because the enzyme which controls the synthesis of porphyrin will be induced, resulting in higher levels of porphyrins in the blood; this can precipitate an acute attack of porphyria.

One of the most serious examples of the interaction between barbiturates and other drugs is that with ethanol (ethyl alcohol). Not only are the depressant effects of the two drugs on the CNS additive but ethanol can inhibit the metabolism of barbiturates, thus increasing the depressant action and so leading to coma and death. As already mentioned, because of their low therapeutic index, overdosing can readily occur with the barbiturates and, when they were used for the treatment of insomnia, fatalities often occurred due to (1) ignorance of the dangers of consuming alcohol when taking barbiturates, and (2) some degree of amnesia or confusion after taking one dose of the sedative: this may induce sleep but, on waking, the patient has no memory of taking the first dose and consequently consumes a further dose or doses.

Benzodiazepines

Although the benzodiazepines were introduced originally for the treatment of anxiety states (see Chapter 13), they were found to have a useful sedative action and, because they are relatively safe even in overdose, these drugs have almost completely replaced the barbiturates as sedatives. The properties of the benzodiazepines as a group are dealt with in detail in Chapter 13 and only those which are used as sedatives are considered here. They are qualitatively similar in their properties, the main differences between individual drugs being in the duration of action. Thus, nitrazepam, flunitrazepam and flurazepam (Figure 11.4b,c,d) have a prolonged action and significant amounts may be present in the blood the following day, resulting in 'hangover' effects. With the regular use of such drugs, taken at bedtime to induce sleep, this effect will increase. These drugs are, therefore, used only when some daytime sedation can be tolerated (see below). Other benzodiazepines, such as temazepam, lormetazepam and triazolam (Figure 11.5a,b,c), have a shorter duration of action and are almost entirely eliminated by the next day, thus not producing 'hangover' effects. For example, the half-life ($t_{\frac{1}{2}}$) of temazepam in the blood is 8 h whereas that of nitrazepam is 30 h or more.

The benzodiazepines are well absorbed after oral administration and, due to their high lipophilicity, they rapidly enter the CNS from the bloodstream. They are metabolized by the hepatic microsomal enzymes and, in many cases, the metabolites are pharmacologically active. One of these, desmethyldiazepam, is formed from a number of different benzodiazepines. Thus, measuring the half-life of the drug which has been administered may not be relevant for the duration of action. There is some evidence that, because of their high lipid solubility, the benzodiazepines may undergo redistribution and that this, rather than metabolism, determines the duration of action.

The benzodiazepines have a high therapeutic index and are therefore relatively non-toxic. Because they are relatively safe they have become very popular and are widely used, having replaced the more dangerous barbiturates as sedatives. However, although fatalities as a result of overdose are extremely rare, some adverse effects have been reported, particularly those associated with excessive depression of the CNS, i.e. confusion, impairment of memory, reduced motor coordination and loss of intellectual function. These are more likely to occur in elderly patients or where hepatic function is impaired. In addition, an increase in

(a)

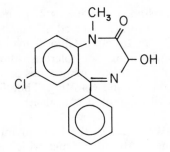

(b)

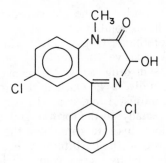

(c)

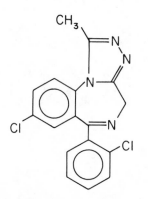

Figure 11.5 The chemical structures of the short-acting benzodiazepines (a) temazepam, (b) lormetazepam and (c) triazolam

the incidence of nightmares can occur during the first week of use. Paradoxical effects have also been known to occur with the use of benzodiazepines: for example, hypomanic and aggressive behaviour, anxiety, irritability and tachycardia have been reported, although the incidence of paradoxical effects is extremely low. Reports of tolerance and dependence developing with the chronic use of benzodiazepines are conflicting, although 'psychological' tolerance is not uncommon and rebound insomnia can occur if the drug is withdrawn suddenly. However, reports of adverse effects with the benzodiazepines are very often associated with the consumption of large doses and, although these drugs are relatively non-toxic, it is recognized that the use of doses larger than are needed is best avoided.

Although the benzodiazepines do not induce the liver enzymes and, therefore, interactions with other drugs due to enzyme induction are less likely to take place, some interactions do occur. For example, the benzodiazepines can interact with other CNS depressants and the depressant effect will be additive. This can be particularly important with ethanol, resulting in excessive depression of the CNS with the symptoms outlined above. However, the consequences of combining the consumption of alcohol with a benzodiazepine are less likely to be fatal than in the case of alcohol and barbiturates.

Other sedative drugs

Chloral hydrate

This is probably the oldest sedative drug in existence and it is still in use. It is crystalline, soluble in water and oil, and it is rapidly reduced in the body to trichlorethanol (Figure 11.6) which is the active metabolite. Chloral hydrate is a useful sedative for children and the elderly who may not tolerate other CNS depressant drugs so well. However, it is irritant to mucous membranes and, when taken orally, it can cause gastric irritation with nausea and vomiting. Therefore, for oral administration, chloral hydrate must be well diluted. It can also be administered rectally, in the form of suppositories.

Chloral hydrate stimulates the metabolizing enzymes in the liver in much the same way as the barbiturates. It therefore interacts with other drugs which are also metabolized by these enzymes. Chloral hydrate also inhibits alcohol dehydrogenase

(a)

(b)

Figure 11.6 The conversion of chloral hydrate (a) to trichlorethanol (b)

and therefore retards the breakdown of ethanol. Thus, the combination of chloral hydrate and ethanol is more than additive and this combination provides the basis for 'knockout drops' (also known as a 'Mickey Finn').

Paraldehyde (Figure 11.7a)

Like chloral hydrate, paraldehyde has been in use as a sedative for a considerable length of time. It is a polymer of acetaldehyde and on exposure to light and air it decomposes to form acetaldehyde. It also oxidizes to acetic acid. It is a colourless liquid with a strong odour and unpleasant taste. In spite of this it can be taken by mouth, but it needs to be well diluted as it has an irritant action on the mucous membranes; it can also be administered rectally or intramuscularly. Paraldehyde acts rapidly, sleep being produced in 10–15 min. In normal doses it does not possess any analgesic action and it has little effect on respiration or blood pressure; however, large doses can cause respiratory depression and hypotension. Paraldehyde has some anticonvulsant activity and has been used for the emergency treatment of convulsions arising from various causes, e.g. tetanus, eclampsia, status epilepticus and poisoning with convulsant drugs.

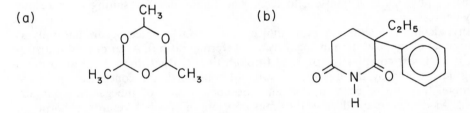

Figure 11.7 The chemical structures of (a) paraldehyde and (b) glutethimide

Most of the drug is metabolized in the liver but a proportion of the unchanged drug is excreted through the lungs and imparts an unpleasant odour to the breath.

Because of its unpleasant odour and taste, paraldehyde is rarely abused. Nevertheless, poisoning can occur, characterized by severe CNS depression, laboured breathing and hypotension. Paraldehyde has been used successfully to suppress the ethanol-withdrawal syndrome in alcoholics, but chronic alcoholics have been known to develop a desire for paraldehyde and to become paraldehyde addicts. Because of its toxicity and the toxic breakdown products (acetaldehyde and acetic acid) formed by its decomposition, paraldehyde is now little used.

Glutethimide (Figure 11.7b)

This drug, together with the related sedative thalidomide, was introduced as a non-barbiturate sedative. Thalidomide, which is more potent than glutethimide as a sedative, was withdrawn because of its teratogenic effects. Glutethimide is not teratogenic but it does produce addiction and an abstinence syndrome similar to that of the barbiturates; it is therefore little used. However, unlike most other sedatives, glutethimide possesses atropine-like properties and causes dilatation of the pupil, dry mouth and inhibition of intestinal motility. It also has an anti-emetic action which is probably related to its central atropine-like action.

Promethazine

This is a phenothiazine (see Chapter 12 and Figure 12.2c) which has antihistaminic properties and is also sedative. It is useful for treating occasional insomnia in children, as it is relatively safe.

Ethanol

Ethyl alcohol, or ethanol, which is present in varying amounts in alcoholic beverages, is a CNS depressant and, in general, the effects on the CNS are proportional to the concentration of alcohol in the blood. The apparent excitatory effects which are sometimes observed with the consumption of alcohol are due to depression of inhibitory pathways in the brain and the consequent release of cortical activity. The first mental processes to be affected are those which depend upon training and previous experience, i.e. those which make for sobriety and self-restraint. This results in behavioural activation, characterized by euphoria, talkativeness, aggressiveness and loss of behavioural control. As the concentration of ethanol in the blood increases, the individual passes from a stage of relaxation and decreased social inhibition to slurred speech, ataxia, decreased mental activity, decreased physical coordination, to coma and finally death resulting from respiratory depression.

Ethyl alcohol is a simple organic molecule (C_2H_5OH) which occurs naturally as the product of the oxidation of sugar by yeast (fermentation). After oral administration, it is almost completely absorbed through the GI tract, the rate of absorption being determined by the quantity of ethanol consumed, the concentration in the beverage, the rate of consumption and the composition of the gastric contents. Eating food before or during the consumption of alcohol retards absorption, especially if the food has a high lipid content. Because it is volatile, ethanol can be absorbed by inhalation; however, the concentration in the atmosphere would have to be very high for this to occur to any appreciable extent.

After absorption, ethanol is distributed throughout the body water, the rate of distribution to different parts depending upon the degree of vascularization. Thus, in organs with a high blood flow, such as the brain, liver, lungs and kidney, equilibration will occur quickly; in tissues with a low blood flow, such as muscle, equilibration will be slower. Ethanol readily crosses the placental barrier into the fetal circulation. Although the concentration of alcohol in the blood can be quite predictable, measurements of blood levels, especially when they are rising, can lead to erroneous conclusions because the values obtained can underestimate the concentration in the brain. The principal metabolic pathway for ethanol is breakdown in the liver by the enzyme alcohol dehydrogenase to acetaldehyde, which is then metabolized further to acetate by the enzyme acetaldehyde dehydrogenase; the acetate itself is then metabolized to carbon dioxide and water. The first step, i.e. conversion of ethanol to acetaldehyde, involves nicotinamide adenine nucleotide as cofactor to alcohol dehydrogenase. The reaction is linear with time and is independent of the concentration of ethanol. Because the metabolism is slow, continued ingestion of ethanol will result in its accumulation and hence its intoxicating effect. The additive and, in some cases, potentiating effects of combined consumption of ethanol with other CNS depressants, which can result in coma and death, have already been referred to.

The chronic consumption of ethanol over a long period of time can lead to the development of tolerance and physical dependence. This is associated with increased metabolism but there is no evidence that the enzyme alcohol dehydrogenase is induced as a result of chronic consumption. Nevertheless, withdrawal symptoms occur when the consumption of alcohol is discontinued and they can be severe (e.g. delirium tremens). The drug disulfiram (see Chapter 8 and Figure 8.6d) has been used successfully to treat alcoholism by producing an aversion to alcohol. Taken on its own, disulfiram causes no untoward effects; however, when ethanol is consumed after the administration of disulfiram, increased concentrations of acetaldehyde appear in the blood and cause a number of unpleasant symptoms, including vasodilatation, resulting in flushing and a pulsating headache, nausea and vomiting, sweating, thirst, chest pains and hypotension. There may also be blurred vision, vertigo and weakness. All these symptoms can be attributed to the increased blood levels of acetaldehyde due to inhibition of the enzyme acetaldehyde dehydrogenase. The facial flush is replaced by pallor as the blood pressure falls. After these symptoms wear off, exhaustion usually follows.

The main action of ethanol is depression of the CNS, the precise mechanism of which is not known. However, ethanol is a small molecule, which can penetrate the fluid space of most tissues, and it has been proposed that ethanol exerts its actions by entering the lipid bi-layer of neuronal membranes and, because it has a polar hydroxyl group, it is restricted to the lipid–water interface, thus causing increased fluidity of the membrane at the surface of the bi-layer. Thus, ethanol may produce its effects by 'disordering' the membranes.

There are also some peripheral effects: for example, moderate doses of ethanol cause peripheral vasodilatation, especially of cutaneous vessels, which can lead to flushing and a fall in body temperature. Ethanol can stimulate salivary and gastric secretions, which is why the consumption of alcohol with a meal aids digestion. It has a diuretic effect which is partly due to the increased fluid intake and partly to inhibition of the release of antidiuretic hormone from the posterior pituitary gland. It is this diuretic action which makes ethanol an unsatisfactory sedative. Ethanol can also reduce levels of testosterone in the blood, resulting in sexual dysfunction.

Although ethanol is of little use as a sedative because of its diuretic action, it does have some therapeutic uses, for example in liniments and as a disinfectant for the skin. It can be taken orally in low concentrations, to stimulate the appetite in illness or in convalesence and for anorexia. Ethanol can also be injected close to nerves to relieve long-lasting pain, such as in trigeminal neuralgia and inoperable carcinomas.

Methanol or methyl alcohol (wood alcohol) is the simplest aliphatic alcohol (CH_3OH). It is mainly used as an industrial solvent but, because its properties are similar to those of ethanol, it is sometimes consumed either accidentally or as a substitute for ethanol, with disastrous consequences (blindness, coma and death). The initial effects are similar to those of ethanol. Methanol is metabolized by the same enzyme, alcohol dehydrogenase, which breaks down ethanol, but the metabolic products of methanol, formaldehyde and formic acid, are neurotoxic and cause blindness by selectively attacking the optic nerve. As ethanol has a higher affinity for alcohol dehydrogenase than does methanol, the administration of ethanol in cases of methanol poisoning will retard the metabolism of methanol, thus reducing the concentrations of the toxic products. Other agents which inhibit alcohol dehydrogenase, e.g. 4-methyl-pyrazole, have similar actions and may be given in combination with ethanol for poisoning with methanol.

There is a theory that the 'hangover' caused by the consumption of alcoholic drinks may be due to the presence of traces of methanol in some drinks. If this theory is correct, then the traditional remedy for a 'hangover', i.e. of taking a small quantity of alcohol (ethanol) the next day (the 'hair of the dog'), could have a rational basis.

Mechanisms controlling sleep and wakefulness

It is generally accepted that the level of consciousness is controlled by a region of the brain stem known as the reticular formation. Anatomically, this region is ill defined and consists of the tegmental parts of the medulla, pons and midbrain, excluding the cranial nerve nuclei, the relay nuclei of the lemniscal system and the cerebellar relay nuclei. The region has been defined more satisfactorily on the basis of physiological criteria, as electrical stimulation of the reticular formation using suitable stimulus parameters produces increased wakefulness or arousal, which can be observed in terms of behaviour and changes in the electroencephalogram (see below). Furthermore, lesions of the reticular formation not only block the responses to stimulation, but result in the appearance of chronic somnolence or coma, in which sensory stimuli are ineffective in eliciting arousal. These observations, together with many others, led to the concept of the 'brain stem reticular activating system' and the proposal that a tonic facilitatory influence – arising from the reticular formation of the brain stem and influencing other regions of the brain, especially the cerebral cortex, through diffuse ascending pathways – was responsible for the maintenance of wakefulness (Figure 11.8). Thus, the presence of the ascending facilitatory influence is thought to produce increased wakefulness or alertness, while its absence results in sleep or unconsciousness. Sensory influences on wakefulness and sleep, i.e. arousal to sensory stimuli, are thought to be mediated through collaterals from the main sensory pathways into the reticular formation and

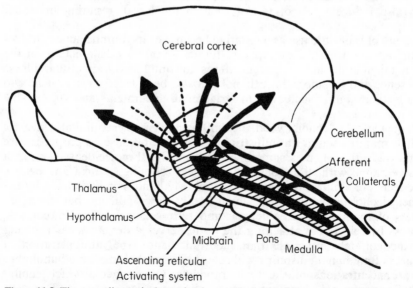

Figure 11.8 The ascending reticular activating system, shown diagrammatically on a sagittal section of the brain of the cat (modified from Starzl, Taylor and Magoun, 1951)

it has been found that many neurones in the reticular formation can be influenced by more than one afferent modality, i.e. they show convergence.

However, the somewhat simple idea of levels of consciousness and sleep being controlled by the brain stem reticular activating system, and of sleep being the passive state and wakefulness the active state, has had to be modified in the light of other observations. For example, experimental animals with chronic lesions of the reticular formation, although showing somnolence initially, eventually recover consciousness and some patients in coma due to damage to the brain stem may eventually regain consciousness. Thus, it seems possible that, although in normal circumstances the forebrain is dependent upon the ascending influence from the brain stem for the maintenance of consciousness, when the brain stem influence is no longer available the forebrain can become independent, in terms of wakefulness and sleep. Secondly, electrical stimulation of certain regions of the reticular formation has been found to induce sleep, provided that suitable stimulus parameters are used. There is, therefore, the possibility that a 'sleep' centre may also exist in the brain stem and that both sleep and wakefulness might be active states, the level of consciousness being determined by a balance between the activities of the 'sleep' and 'wakefulness' centres.

A number of neurotransmitter systems appear to be concerned with sleep and wakefulness. The ascending pathway, originating from 5-hydroxytryptamine-containing neurones in the raphe nuclei of the brain stem (see Chapter 10 and Figure 10.7), appears to be of prime importance in sleep, particularly in 'slow-wave' sleep (see below). Not only do increased levels of 5-hydroxytryptamine promote sleep but melatonin, which is synthesized from 5-hydroxytryptamine in the pineal gland and may also occur in other parts of the brain, also has a role in sleep and is a potent inducer of sleep in man. On the other hand, noradrenaline promotes waking and inhibits slow-wave sleep. Thus, there appears to be a reciprocal relationship between noradrenergic and 5-hydroxytryptaminergic systems, in so far as the control of sleep and wakefulness is concerned. Other neurotransmitters, such as acetylcholine and γ-aminobutyric acid, also play a part and there is evidence that peptides may be important. In fact, a sleep-inducing peptide has been isolated and found to induce sleep in experimental animals.

The electroencephalogram

As indicated above, the state of the organism in terms of wakefulness and sleep can be observed both in the behaviour and also by the pattern of activity recorded in the electroencephalogram (EEG). The EEG is usually recorded by means of electrodes placed on the scalp, although an electrocorticogram (ECoG) can also be recorded from the surface of the cerebral cortex in experimental animals and also in man during neurosurgical operations. The EEG or ECoG consists of an oscillatory electrical potential with an average amplitude of about 50 microvolts, the frequency of the oscillations varying between 1 and 30 Herz. The oscillations consist of complex rhythmic waves, the pattern of which never repeats precisely and they are therefore usually traced on a moving strip of paper. The rhythmic activity is thought to be generated by the synchronized activity of the dendrites which make up the superficial layers of the cerebral cortex. The most characteristic rhythm of the EEG in normal awake humans is the alpha rhythm, which has a frequency range of 8–13 Hz (Figure 11.9). This rhythm is present in most people in the occipital regions of the cerebral cortex (visual area) when the eyes are closed and the subject is relaxed, and it disappears when the eyes are opened or the subject engages in mental activity. When the eyes are open the EEG potentials are very small and irregular, with components in the frequency range 14–30 Hz. With the onset of drowsiness and sleep there is a further slowing of the EEG rhythms, the alpha activity being replaced by slower irregular potentials on which are superimposed 'sleep spindles' which consist of short bursts of faster waves at a frequency of 8–14 Hz (see Figure 11.9). Eventually the sleep spindles disappear and the EEG consists of large irregular slow waves in the frequency range 0.5–3 Hz. However, this stage represents only moderately deep sleep; in the deepest sleep the slow waves in the EEG disappear and low-voltage fast activity, very similar to that seen in the fully alert state, appears. This state of deep sleep with a desynchronized EEG was originally called 'paradoxical' sleep but it was noted that, in man, this stage of sleep was characterized by regular rapid movements of the eyes, and it was subsequently termed Rapid Eye Movement (or REM) sleep. In REM sleep, muscle tone is considerably diminished and it is the stage of sleep in which dreaming most frequently occurs.

During a normal night's sleep in an adult, the EEG will show fluctuations between slow-wave sleep and REM sleep, the bouts of REM sleep lasting for 5–20 min and appearing on average every 90 min. Four or five such bouts normally occur during the night and, towards morning, the periods of REM sleep lengthen (Figure 11.10). If the subjects are awakened during REM sleep they tend to show irritability. Furthermore, on subsequent nights a greater percentage of REM sleep occurs, to compensate for that lost. It is thought that both types of sleep, i.e. slow-

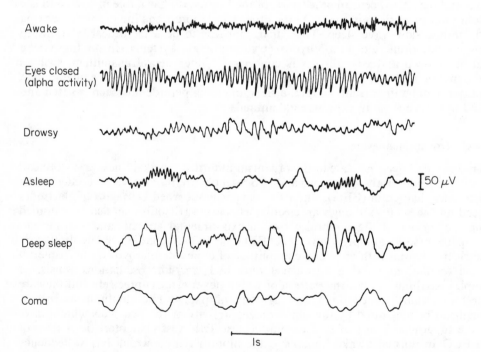

Figure 11.9 Characteristic EEG patterns associated with different states of wakefulness and sleep (modified from Penfield and Jasper, 1954)

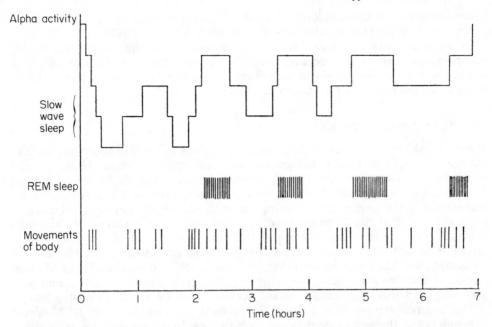

Figure 11.10 Cyclical changes in the EEG during sleep, showing the alternating periods of REM and slow-wave sleep and the relationship of REM sleep to body movements (modified from Dement and Kleitman, 1957)

wave sleep and REM sleep, are necessary and that both subserve restorative functions. There is some support for the hypothesis that long-term memory traces are consolidated during REM sleep. Although there are considerable variations between different individuals in the amount of time spent in REM sleep and, in fact, in total sleep time, it is relatively stable for any one individual. Sedative and hypnotic drugs have marked effects on these parameters.

Mechanisms of action of sedative drugs

Although the barbiturates are distributed, and also probably act, throughout the CNS, the induction of sleep, and probably of anaesthesia as well, is due to a depressant action on the brain stem reticular formation. These drugs have been shown to depress preferentially polysynaptic neuronal pathways and it is probable that the reticular formation, with its network of short-axon neurones, is more sensitive to this depressant action than are other regions of the brain. The benzodiazepines, on the other hand, appear to act more selectively on the limbic system, although effects on the thalamus and midbrain reticular formation have been found. They are not general neuronal depressants, as are the barbiturates, and this may account for their lower toxicity. At the synaptic level, both the barbiturates and the benzodiazepines have been found to modify synaptic transmission mediated by γ-aminobutyric acid (GABA). In both cases there is facilitation of transmission which, because GABA is an inhibitory transmitter, will result in increased inhibition. The effects produced are related to changes in chloride conductance, although there are differences in the way the barbiturates and benzodiazepines affect the chloride channels. This action is discussed in more detail in Chapter 13 where the benzodiazepines are dealt with more fully.

Of the other sedative drugs, little is known about their precise mechanisms of action except that they all depress neuronal activity. Ethanol, for example, as a solvent, affects the fluidity of cell membranes (see above) and this, in turn, is likely to influence the receptors for neurotransmitters.

The effects of drugs on the EEG

Sedative and hypnotic drugs induce patterns in the EEG which resemble those of natural sleep. They mostly reduce the time of onset of sleep. However, the relationship between the periods of slow-wave sleep and REM sleep may be disturbed. For example, barbiturates reduce the proportion of REM sleep and this occurs even if the drug is taken during the day, i.e. the amount of REM sleep at night is reduced. If the drugs are used regularly, this effect is cumulative although eventually, even with continued use of the drug, the amount of REM sleep may return to normal. Thus, tolerance develops to the effects on the EEG. However, if consumption of the barbiturate is discontinued, a rebound increase in REM sleep can occur and this may persist for some time. Since REM sleep is associated with dreaming (and also nightmares), the subject may think he or she is sleeping badly.

The benzodiazepines also reduce the amount of time spent in REM sleep, although not to the same extent as the barbiturates. In some cases, e.g. with short-acting benzodiazepines such as temazepam, administered in small doses, the overall amount of REM sleep may not be changed. Thus, REM sleep lost during the early hours of sleep is made up later.

The treatment of insomnia

Insomnia embraces a number of different sleep problems, including difficulty in falling asleep, frequent awakenings, short duration of sleep and 'unrefreshing' sleep. It can be a serious condition which needs careful evaluation to uncover the possible causes, which may be organic, e.g. pain, psychiatric, such as anxiety or depression, or extraneous factors such as noise, shift work or jet lag. Other causes can include the consumption of food or stimulant drinks near bedtime and excessive consumption of alcohol. If the cause of the insomnia can be identified and eliminated, then recourse to treatment with sedative or hypnotic drugs may be avoided.

It is generally recognized that transient or short-term insomnia can be treated successfully with hypnotic drugs. Thus, transient insomnia which may be caused by a minor situational stress or jet lag can be relieved by the administration of a short-acting benzodiazepine such as temazepam. The drug is administered only once or twice at the most and is rapidly eliminated. Short-term insomnia may be associated with an emotional problem or serious illness and may last for a few weeks and may recur. Again, a benzodiazepine is usually prescribed, starting with a small dose, to be increased if necessary or discontinued if one or two nights of acceptable sleep are obtained. The drug used here can also be a short-acting one unless daytime sedation is required. The period of treatment should not exceed three weeks and, when it is no longer needed, the drug must be withdrawn gradually.

In cases of insomnia associated with psychiatric states it is better to treat the psychiatric condition first, although the anti-anxiety properties of the benzodiazepines (Chapter 13) make them useful drugs for relieving the insomnia associated with anxiety states. Sleep disturbances often occur in depressive illness, with early awakening a common sign. However, treatment of the depression, particularly with an antidepressant drug which is also sedative (see Chapter 17), eliminates the need for a hypnotic drug.

Hypnotic drugs, used for the treatment of transient or short-term insomnia, apart from being short-acting should have a high therapeutic index so that they are safe in overdose (accidental or intentional) and they should preferably provide a fairly rapid onset of sleep which is of adequate duration, with minimal 'hangover' effects such as drowsiness, or mental or motor depression. The short-acting benzodiazepines, such as temazepam, triazolam and lormetazepam (Figure 11.5), are currently the drugs of choice.

The long-term treatment of insomnia with drugs is controversial and it is generally accepted that the continued use of hypnotic drugs should be avoided. The reason for this is the rebound insomnia and other withdrawal symptoms that may occur when administration of the drug is discontinued. When the administration of a hypnotic drug such as a benzodiazepine cannot be avoided, it should be given every second or third night and should be discontinued as soon as possible. It should be withdrawn gradually but, even so, normal sleep may not be re-established for some days.

Chapter 12

Neuroleptic drugs

The drugs in this category are also known as antipsychotics, major tranquillizers or antischizophrenic drugs. They are effective in alleviating the symptoms of certain psychotic disorders, such as schizophrenia, and can be used both in the acute phase and also for maintenance therapy, to reduce the risk of relapse. Before their discovery the only drugs available for dealing with the violent, sometimes self-destructive, behaviour associated with psychotic states were the barbiturates, which often had to be given in doses which depressed consciousness and were therefore unsuitable for long-term treatment. One characteristic of the antipsychotic drugs, which distinguishes them from other types of central depressant drugs such as the barbiturates, is that they are non-sedative or only weakly sedative in the doses needed to control the symptoms of psychosis. However, most are sedative if given in sufficiently large doses.

The term psychosis is used to describe severe psychiatric disorders, which are usually of unknown origin ('functional') and in which there are not only disturbances of behaviour but an inability to think coherently and to comprehend reality. The most important psychoses are schizophrenia and the affective disorders (depression and mania, see Chapter 17). However, some psychoses are organic in origin, being associated with morphological, metabolic, toxic or endocrinological disturbances. The neuroleptic drugs are effective in alleviating the symptoms of psychoses of both functional and organic origin. Neuroses are usually less severe and may be acute and transient, although they can recur. They are often regarded as an abnormal reaction to the environment and may include mood changes (e.g. anxiety, see Chapter 13) or abnormalities of thought (e.g. phobias).

The neuroleptic drugs are used primarily for the treatment of schizophrenia, although some have other uses. Schizophrenia is a disorder of the brain which is manifested by the appearance of abnormal thoughts, behaviour and affect. There may also be delusions, hallucinations and changes in motor behaviour in either direction, i.e. lowering towards a stuporous state or over-excitement and violent activity. However, the symptomatology can be so variable that the concept of a 'disease entity' has been questioned. Nevertheless, the drugs are effective in treating the various symptoms, both acutely and for long-term maintenance therapy. However, it has been suggested that the neuroleptics are more effective in abolishing the positive symptoms of the disease than in treating the negative symptoms.

The discovery of neuroleptic drugs is usually attributed to a French surgeon, Laborit (1952), who was examining the effectiveness of various antihistaminic drugs in relieving stress in his patients. He used a 'lytic' cocktail, which contained two phenothiazines for premedication. However, it was two psychiatrists, Jean Delay and Pierre Deniker (1952), who described the antipsychotic action and coined the term 'neuroleptic' which literally means 'to clasp the neurone'. The drug that they used was chlorpromazine, a phenothiazine and the 'prototype' for many other neuroleptic drugs. It was one of a number of phenothiazine derivatives that were being tested for antihistaminic activity. One of these, promethazine, had good antihistaminic properties but was also sedative. When it was tested in schizophrenic patients it was found to be no more effective than other sedatives, such as the barbiturates. However, another derivative, chloro-phenothiazine, or chlorpromazine, had less antihistaminic activity but was found to be very effective in the treatment of schizophrenia and was therefore the first of the phenothiazine neuroleptics.

The classification of neuroleptic drugs

Although all the neuroleptics, by definition, have similar actions on psychotic states, they are diverse chemically. Furthermore, they have only certain pharmacological properties in common. They are therefore best classified according to their chemical structure.

Rauwolfia alkaloids and related substances

The shrub *Rauwolfia*, which is indigenous to India, Africa and S. America, is an abundant source of alkaloids and extracts of its root were used in folk medicine for many centuries for the treatment of mania and also for snake bites. However, the effects were ignored in Western medicine until the active constituent, reserpine, was isolated in 1952.

Reserpine (Figure 12.1a)

This is an indole. Its most important pharmacological action is to deplete tissue levels of amines, an action which is manifested both peripherally and centrally. Thus, noradrenaline, dopamine and 5-hydroxytryptamine are depleted in the brain.

As reserpine is highly lipid soluble, it rapidly penetrates cell membranes and it binds to the granular membranes of the amine-containing synaptic vesicles in nerve terminals. This prevents the uptake of the amines into the intracellular storage vesicles, so that depletion occurs and, ultimately, there is a failure of transmission, as it is the bound transmitter in the granular vesicles that is released synaptically. This action is thought to be due to inhibition of the ATPase-dependent uptake mechanism in the vesicular membranes. Thus any amine which diffuses out of the vesicles will not be pumped back in again and will be degraded by the enzyme monoamine oxidase in the cytoplasm (see Chapters 8 and 10). Doses of reserpine which are just sufficient to cause failure of transmission produce a reversible impairment of the storage vesicles but function can be restored by the administration of exogenous amine or its precursor. However, larger doses of reserpine cause damage to the vesicles and the effects are much less easily reversed. Chronic administration of reserpine has been shown to cause increased activity of the enzymes tyrosine hydroxylase and tryptophan hydroxylase, leading to a compensa-

(a)

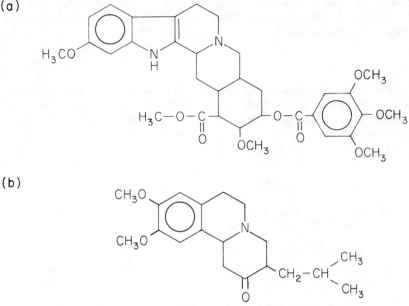

(b)

Figure 12.1 The chemical structures of (a) reserpine and (b) tetrabenazine

tory increase in amine synthesis; there is a similar effect on choline acetyltransferase, thus increasing the levels of acetylcholine in the brain.

The clinical effects of reserpine are similar to those of chlorpromazine (see below)
but with a slower onset. However, there is a high incidence of side-effects
associated with the use of reserpine: these are sedation, extrapyramidal symptoms,
a lowering of seizure thresholds and impairment of autonomic function. The latter
can be related to reduced sympathetic activity, due to depletion of catecholamines
and consequent parasympathetic 'release'. Thus, all the symptoms associated with
parasympathetic overactivity can occur, e.g. excess salivation, nausea, diarrhoea,
nasal congestion, flushing, bradycardia, etc. In addition, there may be hormonal
effects due to a disturbance of hypothalamic function. Probably the most important
side-effect, which has resulted in reserpine no longer being used as a neuroleptic, is
the tendency for mental depression, closely resembling endogenous depression, to
occur even with relatively small doses. In addition, the advent of other, more
effective, neuroleptic drugs with fewer or less pronounced side-effects has
influenced the popularity of reserpine in psychiatry.

Because of the reduction in sympathetic activity which results from the depletion
of catecholamines, both peripherally and centrally, reserpine still has a place in the
treatment of hypertension (Chapter 8).

Tetrabenazine (**Figure 12.1b**)

This is a benzoquinolizine derivative and therefore not related to reserpine
chemically. However, its pharmacological properties are very similar as it causes
depletion of amines by disrupting storage mechanisms, although the effect is mainly
on the CNS and is less marked peripherally. The side-effects, however, are just as
marked and include depression and extrapyramidal symptoms. Thus tetrabenazine,

too, is no longer used as a neuroleptic, although it has an application in the treatment of movement disorders associated with Huntington's chorea, senile chorea and related neurological conditions (see Chapter 19).

Phenothiazines

These are tricyclic ring compounds (Figure 12.2) and include the dye methylene blue, and also compounds with antiseptic and anthelminthic properties. Interest in phenothiazine derivatives as drugs appeared after it was found that they had an antihistaminic action and the interest increased further when their antipsychotic properties were discovered.

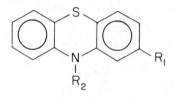

	R_1	R_2
(a)	H	$CH_2.CH_2.N(C_2H_5)_2$
(b)	H	$CH_2.CH_2.CH_2.N(CH_3)_2$
(c)	H	$CH_2.CH(CH_3).N(CH_3)_2$
(d)	Cl	$CH_2.CH_2.CH_2.N(CH_3)_2$

Figure 12.2 The chemical structures of some substituted phenothiazines: (a) diethazine, (b) promazine, (c) promethazine and (d) chlorpromazine

The derivatives of phenothiazine are obtained by substitution on the carbon atom in one of the benzene rings at position 2 (R_1) and on the nitrogen atom in the pyridine ring at position 10 (R_2). The substitution at R_1 is essential for neuroleptic activity and can be a halogen atom, e.g. chlorine (chlorpromazine), trifluoromethyl ($-CF_3$), which increases the potency, or methyl-mercapto ($-SCH_3$). Thus, in Figure 12.2, only chlorpromazine (Figure 12.2d) is a neuroleptic, possessing weak sedative and antihistaminic properties, while promazine (Figure 12.2b) and promethazine (Figure 12.2c) are potent antihistamines and potent sedatives, but lack neuroleptic actions. Note that the only difference between promazine and chlorpromazine is the presence of the chlorine atom at R_1 on the chlorpromazine molecule. The fourth compound, diethazine (Figure 12.2a), is weakly antihistaminic but is a potent antimuscarinic, anticholinergic drug. It was used at one time in the treatment of Parkinson's disease (see Chapter 19).

The phenothiazine neuroleptics can be divided into three groups according to the type of substitution on the aromatic nitrogen (R_2; Figure 12.3). This side-chain can be aliphatic or it can contain piperidine or piperazine moieties. The nature of this side-chain determines the potency and pharmacological actions.

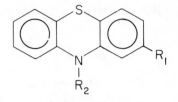

R_1	R_2	
		Aliphatic
Cl	$CH_2.CH_2.CH_2.N(CH_3)_2$	Chlorpromazine
CF_3	$CH_2.CH_2.CH_2.N(CH_3)_2$	Triflupromazine
		Piperidine
$S-CH_3$	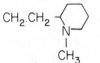	Thioridazine
CN	$CH_2.CH_2.CH_2.N$ ⟩-OH	Pericyazine
		Piperazine
Cl	$CH_2.CH_2.CH_2.N$ ⟩N.CH_3	Prochlorperazine
CF_3	$CH_2.CH_2.CH_2.N$ ⟩N.CH_3	Trifluperazine
Cl	$CH_2.CH_2.CH_2.N$ ⟩N.$CH_2.CH_2.OH$	Perphenazine
CF_3	$CH_2.CH_2.CH_2.N$ ⟩N.$CH_2.CH_2.OH$	Fluphenazine

Figure 12.3 The chemical structures of some phenothiazine neuroleptics

Aliphatic

The optimum length for neuroleptic activity is a three-carbon atom chain separating the nitrogen atom in the side-chain from that in the central ring, e.g. chlorpromazine and triflupromazine (Figure 12.3). Of these, triflupromazine is more potent than chlorpromazine as a neuroleptic because of the $-CF_3$ group at

R_1. Phenothiazines with shorter side-chains at R_2 are not neuroleptics (promethazine, Figure 12.2c).

Piperidine

Although a number of neuroleptic drugs with piperidine side-chains at R_2 have been developed, only a few are now used, the main ones being thioridazine and pericyazine (Figure 12.3). These are roughly equipotent to the corresponding phenothiazines with aliphatic side-chains, but are more sedative and are therefore used where anxiety and agitation are prominent. In addition, thioridazine has greater antimuscarinic potency than chlorpromazine and it is thought that this property might explain the reduced tendency for the appearance of extrapyramidal symptoms with this drug (see below).

Piperazine

Phenothiazine neuroleptics with piperazine side-chains (Figure 12.3) represent some of the most powerful neuroleptic drugs. They are less sedative than the other phenothiazine neuroleptics and cause fewer side-effects related to disturbances of autonomic function. They have marked anti-emetic actions and readily produce extrapyramidal side-effects.

CHLORPROMAZINE

As the first of the modern neuroleptic drugs to be discovered, chlorpromazine (Figure 12.2d and 12.3) has been very extensively studied and more is known about its pharmacology than that of any other neuroleptic. It may therefore be regarded as the 'prototype' neuroleptic.

Peripherally, chlorpromazine has a wide range of pharmacological actions, mostly as an antagonist of different neurotransmitter systems. The antihistaminic properties of the phenothiazines as a group have already been referred to, together with the fact that chlorpromazine is relatively weak as an antihistamine. It is also a weak antagonist of the actions of acetylcholine and 5-hydroxytryptamine. The most marked peripheral action of chlorpromazine is as an antagonist at α-adrenergic receptors. This action causes a loss of vasomotor tone and is probably responsible, at least in part, for the postural hypotension which sometimes accompanies the use of therapeutic doses of the drug. Although chlorpromazine appears to have little, if any, ganglionic blocking activity, the hypotensive action appears to be complex and involves central as well as peripheral actions, i.e. depression of the vasomotor control centre in the hypothalamus and medulla. Chlorpromazine has a local anaesthetic action but this does not appear to have been exploited.

The same antagonist properties of chlorpromazine are also present centrally. Thus, the drug antagonizes the actions of acetylcholine, noradrenaline, 5-hydroxytryptamine and histamine at receptors in the brain and it is clear, from the widespread distribution of the receptors for these neurotransmitters (Chapter 10), that chlorpromazine must have actions at many sites in the CNS. However, in addition to the actions described above, the phenothiazine neuroleptics, including chlorpromazine, are all antagonists at dopamine receptors, as are, in fact, all the neuroleptic drugs. This antidopaminergic action explains many of the central effects, e.g. the anti-emetic effect (see Chapter 20). An antidopaminergic action can also explain some of the endocrinological effects of the neuroleptics. For example, neuroleptics cause increased release of prolactin and, as dopamine receptors in the tubero-infundibular tract normally inhibit the release of prolactin, an antagonist action at these receptors can account for the increased release. Other endocrinological effects which can be related to a depressant action on the hypothalamus include inhibition of growth hormone and reduced release of gonadotropin. Whereas large doses of chlorpromazine have been found to inhibit the release of adrenocorticotrophic hormone (ACTH) in stress, moderate doses stimulate release. These effects have been correlated with an action of chlorpromazine (and of other neuroleptic drugs) to increase the ability of living organisms to resist stress, or stressful stimuli.

An increase in appetite is often associated with the administration of neuroleptic drugs to psychotic patients and this effect is thought to be due to depression of the satiety centre in the hypothalamus. One of the first effects of chlorpromazine to be discovered was that it caused hypothermia and Laborit devised a 'lytic cocktail', which contained both promethazine and chlorpromazine, to produce a state of artificial hibernation due to the lowering of body temperature. However, chlorpromazine acts by interfering with temperature regulation and this is thought to be due to an action on the hypothalamus, although the precise mechanism is not known. Thus, the disturbance of temperature regulation can result in either hypo- or hyperthermia, depending upon the ambient temperature, and in climates where the ambient temperature is high, patients taking phenothiazine medication may suffer episodes of hyperthermia.

Thioxanthenes

These are also tricyclic compounds and they are structurally very closely related to the phenothiazines, the thioxanthene nucleus differing from the phenothiazine only in that the aromatic nitrogen is replaced by carbon (Figure 12.4). Thus, the side-chain R_2 is attached to a carbon, instead of a nitrogen atom.

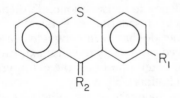

	R_1	R_2
(a)	Cl	$CH.CH_2.CH_2.N(CH_3)_2$
(b)	Cl	$CH.CH_2.CH_2.N\quad N.CH_2.CH_2.OH$
(c)	CF_3	$CH.CH_2.CH_2.N\quad N.CH_2.CH_2.OH$

Figure 12.4 The chemical structures of thioxanthene drugs: (a) chlorprothixene, (b) clopenthixol and (c) flupenthixol

Chlorprothixene is the thioxanthene analogue of chlorpromazine (Figure 12.4a). It resembles chlorpromazine in most of its pharmacological properties but is more potent in its anticholinergic, atropine-like activity. Thus, as with the phenothiazine thioridazine, the incidence of extrapyramidal side-effects with chlorprothixene is less than with chlorpromazine and it is thought that this is due to the greater antimuscarinic potency. On the other hand, there is an increased tendency for anticholinergic side-effects, e.g. cardiovascular symptoms, to occur with chlorprothixene. The drug is a potent anti-emetic, is less sedative than chlorpromazine and possesses some antidepressant activity. It is the least potent of the thioxanthene neuroleptics.

The other members of this group, clopenthixol (Figure 12.4b) and flupenthixol (Figure 12.4c), have piperazine side-chains at R_2. Thus, clopenthixol is the thioxanthene analogue of perphenazine and flupenthixol is the analogue of fluphenazine (Figure 12.3). However, flupenthixol exists in two stereoisomeric forms, which have been isolated and tested both for pharmacological and for clinical activity. The α- or cis-isomer has been found to be active, whereas the β- or trans-isomer is inactive.

Butyrophenones and diphenylbutylpiperidines

These drugs differ from the previous two groups in not possessing a tricyclic structure. They are related chemically to the analgesic drug pethidine, and were discovered accidentally when a series of derivatives of norpethidine were being screened for analgesic activity. They were found to be devoid of analgesic activity but closely resembled chlorpromazine in many ways. The first butyrophenone to be used was haloperidol (Figure 12.5a) and it is still widely used as an antipsychotic. Others are benperidol (Figure 12.5b) and droperidol (Figure 12.5c). They all have similar pharmacological properties. They are potent antipsychotics but lack some of the other properties of the phenothiazines. Thus, they have little or no anti-histaminic, anticholinergic or anti-adrenergic activity and they are therefore non-sedative and have a reduced tendency to cause autonomic disturbances compared with the phenothiazines. The lack of sedation is noticeable, although it is less marked with droperidol, and haloperidol has been known to cause insomnia. All the butyrophenones have a very marked propensity to cause extrapyramidal symptoms and this has been attributed to a greater affinity for the extrapyramidal system, but it may also be due to the low anticholinergic potency.

Benperidol is more potent than haloperidol but otherwise does not have any advantage over the latter; it has been used to suppress antisocial sexual behaviour. Droperidol is relatively short acting and is the drug of choice, in combination with the potent analgesic drug fentanyl, to induce neuroleptanalgesia (Chapter 11). Droperidol has also been used for premedication, when it produces a quiet relaxed state. The most potent member of this group of compounds is spiroperidol; however, this substance is not used clinically but is a useful tool in experimental studies, especially in receptor-binding assays.

The diphenylbutyropiperidines (Figure 12.6) are very similar in chemical structure to the butyrophenones. The best-known drug of this group and also the first to be used is pimozide (Figure 12.6a). It is a derivative of the butyrophenone, benperidol. Pimozide is not sedative even when given in large doses and, compared with other neuroleptic drugs, has a reduced tendency to cause extrapyramidal symptoms; however, these can still be observed when large doses are used.

(a)

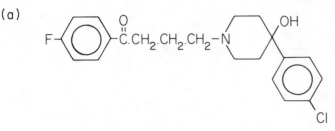

(b)

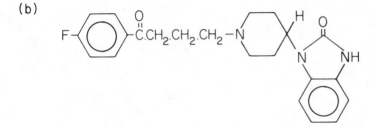

(c)

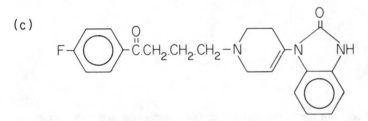

Figure 12.5 The chemical structures of clinically important butyrophenones: (a) haloperidol, (b) benperiodol and (c) droperidol

Epileptiform convulsions have been known to occur following the withdrawal of pimozide.

Two other drugs in this group are penfluridol (Figure 12.6b) and fluspirilene (Figure 12.6c); these are longer acting than pimozide. Penfluridol, which is active when given orally, can be administered at weekly intervals.

Dibenzazepine derivatives

These are drugs with a tricyclic structure, although the central ring differs from that of the phenothiazines and thioxanthenes as it is seven-membered (see Figure 12.7). There are also important differences in the positions of the substituent groups. The principal drug in this class is clozapine (Figure 12.7), which has a piperazine side-chain. Clozapine is strongly sedative and has muscle-relaxant properties. It has been reported not to produce extrapyramidal symptoms in patients and this may be due to a potent anticholinergic action. Clozapine interacts with other neurotransmitter systems in the CNS, e.g. 5-hydroxytryptamine and histamine.

(a)

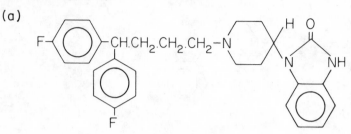

(b)

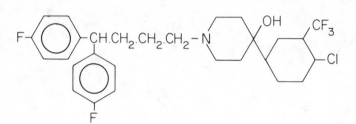

(c)

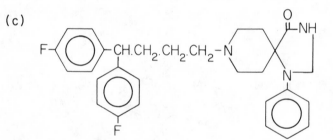

Figure 12.6 The chemical structure of some clinically important diphenylbutyropiperidines: (a) pimozide, (b) penfluridol and (c) fluspirilene

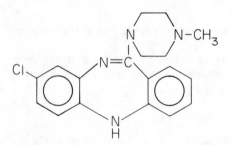

Figure 12.7 The chemical structure of clozapine

Because of the absence of extrapyramidal side-effects, clozapine has been referred to as an 'atypical' neuroleptic. Unfortunately, because of a high incidence of agranulocytosis in patients being treated with clozapine, the drug is no longer used. It is, however, of interest as the first 'atypical' neuroleptic drug to be developed.

Substituted benzamides

This is a relatively new class of neuroleptic drugs, which are chemically related to the anti-arrhythmic agent procainamide. Modification of the structure of procainamide led to metoclopramide (5-chloro-2-methoxy procainamide, Figure 12.8a), which is an anti-emetic and also reduces gastric motility; it shows some neuroleptic activity, but is not very potent. A related drug, sulpiride (Figure 12.8b), was at first used in gastroenterology, but was soon found to be a useful neuroleptic. However, like clozapine, sulpiride lacks some of the properties of the older neuroleptic drugs and is also classed as 'atypical'. At first it was thought that sulpiride was unlikely to produce extrapyramidal side-effects; however, this has not proved to be the case.

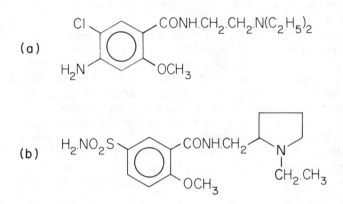

Figure 12.8 The chemical structures of (a) metoclopramide and (b) sulpiride

Effects of neuroleptic drugs on behaviour

Animals which have been given neuroleptic drugs show reduced motor activity and diminished responses to external stimuli and they appear to have little interest in their environment. However, there is no reduction in motor power or coordination, nor is there a tendency for excessive somnolence, unless very large doses are administered. Cats treated with neuroleptic drugs show increased sociability and reduced hostility and, in those species which are normally aggressive or defensive, the drugs have a 'taming' effect; this property has been utilized in veterinary practice. In general, the changes observed in animals parallel those in man, and animal models for studying neuroleptic drugs and for screening new drugs for possible neuroleptic activity have been used extensively.

Conditioned responses in animals have been used for studying and screening neuroleptic drugs. The drugs are particularly active in suppressing conditioned avoidance behaviour, i.e. blocking a conditioned response without affecting the unconditioned response, whereas a sedative drug such as a barbiturate will block both responses. They also have effects on more complex conditioned responses involving discrimination. For example, chlorpromazine has been found to delay the acquisition of conditioned responses and to enhance extinction and habituation.

Many neuroleptic drugs antagonize the increased locomotor activity and stereotyped behaviour produced by small and large doses, respectively, of the central stimulant, amphetamine, (Chapter 16) and also by apomorphine. However, thioridazine and clozapine do not antagonize the effects of amphetamine and as these two drugs have a lower tendency than other neuroleptics to produce extrapyramidal side-effects in man, it is thought that antagonism of the effects of amphetamine might be unrelated to the antipsychotic action.

The mechanism of action of neuroleptic drugs

The neuroleptic drugs, and especially the phenothiazines, interact with a number of neurotransmitter systems in the brain and these actions can account for many of the pharmacological properties of the drugs. However, in many cases there is no clear correlation with the clinical antipsychotic action.

There is no correlation between the central effects of the phenothiazine neuroleptics and their antihistaminic potency, as measured peripherally. Furthermore, as this property is minimal in some of the most potent neuroleptic drugs, it is unlikely that the antihistaminic action contributes to the therapeutic effect. It is possible that the antihistaminic action may contribute to the sedative action of the drugs, especially as the most potent antihistamine phenothiazines, e.g. promethazine, are useful as sedatives. Similarly, there is no clear relationship between antiserotoninergic properties and the clinical effects of neuroleptic drugs, although drugs which affect serotoninergic systems in the brain can have profound effects on mental function, e.g. tricyclic antidepressants (Chapter 17) and psychotomimetic drugs (Chapter 18). Again, there might be a link between the antiserotoninergic action of neuroleptic drugs and sedation.

Most of the neuroleptic drugs have an anticholinergic action that is atropine-like, i.e. antimuscarinic and, in the case of some of these drugs, e.g. thioridazine and clozapine, this action can be very marked. Antimuscarinic drugs are used successfully in the treatment of Parkinson's disease (see Chapter 19) and it is thought that this property of thioridazine and clozapine may be responsible for the low incidence of extrapyramidal side-effects with these drugs (see below).

By far the most important actions of the neuroleptic drugs are their interactions with catecholamines and, in the brain, especially with dopamine. The most marked peripheral action of chlorpromazine is as an antagonist at α-adrenergic receptors. This action causes a loss of vasomotor tone and is probably responsible, at least in part, for the postural hypotension which can occur with this drug. The first clue that effects on catecholamines in the brain might be important for the therapeutic actions of neuroleptic drugs came from the observation that reserpine, which has clinical effects similar to those of the other neuroleptic drugs, causes depletion of monoamine stores in brain. However, neuroleptic drugs, apart from reserpine, do not affect the levels of catecholamines in the brain but alter their metabolism, increasing the quantities of the metabolites formed. For dopamine, the metabolite is homovanillic acid (see Chapter 10), and the increase produced by neuroleptic drugs correlates well with their clinical potency. Thus, the therapeutic effectiveness of the neuroleptic drugs is correlated with their effect on dopaminergic systems in the brain (increased turnover, leading to increased production of metabolite) and not with effects on other neurotransmitter systems. The action of the neuroleptics at dopamine receptors is an antagonist action and all known neuroleptic drugs are dopamine antagonists. This action explains not only the therapeutic action of the drugs, leading to the current hypothesis of 'the dopamine theory of schizophrenia', but also many of their other effects, including some side-effects.

Associated with the increased production of the metabolite of dopamine (homovanillic acid) by the neuroleptic drugs is an increase in the activity of the neurones which release dopamine. Thus, it seems that there may be an increase in the release of transmitter to compensate for the reduced dopaminergic transmission due to the blockade of postsynaptic dopamine receptors by neuroleptic drugs. There are two possible mechanisms by which the increased release of transmitter, and hence increased production of metabolite, could come about. One is through feedback from the postsynaptic to the presynaptic neurone and a pathway is known to exist from the striatum to the substantia nigra which is inhibitory, as the transmitter released is γ-aminobutyric acid (see Figure 19.1). A reduction in activity in this inhibitory feedback pathway would result in increased activity in the dopaminergic neurones which it influences. The second mechanism is a blocking of presynaptic receptors (autoreceptors) on the dopamine-containing nerve terminals. Dopamine released from nerve terminals, and also dopamine agonists, act on the autoreceptors to reduce the further release of transmitter; an antagonist (neuroleptic) action would therefore increase transmitter release.

However, there is more than one subtype of dopamine receptor in the brain (see Chapter 10): there are D_1 receptors, which are coupled to adenylate cyclase as the second messenger, and the precise functional role of which is not yet clear, and D_2 receptors, which are characterized by either no effect on levels of cyclic AMP or a decrease. The postsynaptic actions of dopamine are mediated by D_2 receptors. The presynaptic autoreceptors are also of the D_2 type but, as they are more sensitive to dopamine agonists than the postsynaptic D_2 receptors, it has been suggested that they be designated as a third subtype of dopamine receptor, D_3. Both D_1 and D_2 dopamine receptors are present in the main dopamine-containing regions of the brain, the nigrostriatal pathway and the mesolimbic system (Figure 10.5).

Although the classification of subtypes of dopamine receptors was made initially on the basis of biochemical data, i.e. activation of adenylate cyclase, D_1 and D_2 receptors have also been found to differ pharmacologically (Table 12.1). Thus, dopamine itself shows a different potency at the two sites, being effective in micromolar concentrations at D_1 receptors and in nanomolar concentrations at D_2 sites. Apomorphine, which is a dopamine agonist, has different effects at the two receptors: at D_2 receptors it mimics the action of dopamine with a similar potency; however, at D_1 receptors, apomorphine can act as either a partial agonist or an antagonist, depending on the concentration. Similar effects are shown by some

Table 12.1 The pharmacological characteristics of dopamine D_1 and D_2 receptors

	D_1 receptor	D_2 receptor
Adenylate cyclase activity	Stimulated	Unaffected or inhibited
Dopamine	Agonist (μM potency)	Agonist (nM potency)
Apomorphine	Partial agonist or antagonist	Agonist (nM potency)
Bromocriptine	Antagonist (μM potency)	Agonist (nM potency)
Thioxanthenes	Antagonists	= Antagonists
Phenothiazines	Antagonists	< Antagonists
Butyrophenones	Weak antagonists	≪ Potent antagonists
Sulpiride	No effect	Antagonist

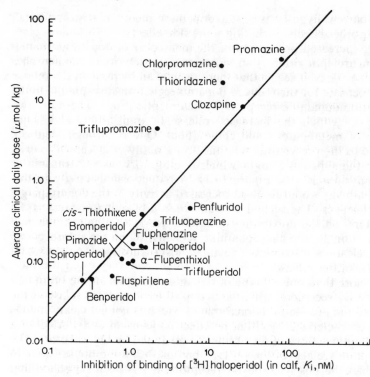

Figure 12.9 The correlation between the clinical potencies of some neuroleptic drugs, in terms of the average daily dose, and their affinity for the dopamine D_2 receptor (as measured by competition with the binding of [^{3}H]haloperidol) (redrawn from Creese, Burt and Snyder, 1978)

ergot derivatives with dopaminergic agonist activity, e.g. bromocriptine. The 'classic' neuroleptic drugs, such as the phenothiazines and thioxanthenes, are effective antagonists at both D_1 and D_2 dopamine receptors, whereas the butyrophenones have only weak activity at D_1 receptors and the substituted benzamides, e.g. metaclopramide and sulpiride, are selective, being antagonists at D_2 sites but almost inactive at D_1 receptors (Table 12.1). Furthermore, it has been shown that the clinical efficacy of a range of neuroleptics correlates with their affinity for D_2 receptors (Figure 12.9) and not with their ability to stimulate adenylate cyclase. In fact, sulpiride does not influence the activity of dopamine-stimulated adenylate cyclase. Thus, it is generally accepted that the central actions, and especially the antipsychotic action, of neuroleptic drugs are related to an antagonist action at dopamine D_2 receptors.

As D_2 dopamine receptors are present in both the dopaminergic nigrostriatal pathway and the mesolimbic system, the question arises as to which of these sites is reponsible for mediating the therapeutic effects of the neuroleptics. The nigrostriatal pathway is part of the extrapyramidal system of the brain which is involved in the coordination and fine control of movements. Furthermore, degeneration of this region is responsible for the symptoms of Parkinson's disease in which motor activity is disrupted and rigidity and tremor occur (see Chapter 19). The mesolimbic dopamine system, on the other hand, projects to those areas of the brain which are involved with emotional behaviour. Thus, it is currently thought that the antipsychotic effects of the neuroleptics are due to an antagonist action at dopamine D_2 receptors in the mesolimbic forebrain system, whereas the extrapyramidal side-effects are attributable to a similar action in the nigrostriatal system. There is some experimental evidence which supports this hypothesis. Although an exclusively postsynaptic action of the neuroleptics can account for most of their effects, it is not clear at present whether or not presynaptic actions are involved and it is possible that an action at both sites is important.

The antagonism by the neuroleptic drugs of the stereotyped behaviour induced in experimental animals by amphetamine and apomorphine, although indicating an action on dopamine receptors, because apomorphine is a dopamine agonist and amphetamine releases dopamine from presynaptic nerve terminals, is probably related to an action on the nigrostriatal system as the drugs which produce this effect are the ones which cause extrapyramidal side-effects in man. Thioridazine and clozapine, which have a lower tendency to produce these side-effects, do not antagonize the stereotyped behaviour induced by amphetamine or apomorphine.

Most experimental studies of the actions of neuroleptic drugs have been performed with acute administration of the drug, whereas clinically the drugs are administered on a chronic basis, often over long periods, and very often the full therapeutic effect does not appear immediately. Some studies using chronic administration of neuroleptic drugs to experimental animals have been carried out and a supersensitivity of dopamine receptors has been reported which can account for some of the long-term side-effects of these drugs, such as tardive dyskinesia (see below). It has been found that the increase in the activity of dopaminergic neurones that occurs with acute administration of neuroleptic drugs is not maintained when they are given chronically. In addition, an increase in the numbers of dopamine receptors has been noted after long-term administration of neuroleptics. So far, the interpretation of these findings remains obscure but the adaptive changes in the CNS produced by prolonged administration of drugs needs further study.

The clinical uses of neuroleptic drugs

The tranquillizing property of the neuroleptic drugs, which produces a calming effect and a reduction in hyperactivity without impairing consciousness and without paradoxical excitement, means that these drugs can be used to quieten disturbed patients whatever the underlying psychopathology, which may be due to trauma, toxic delirium, agitated depression, mania or an acute behavioural disturbance. However, the principal use for these drugs is in the treatment of psychosis, particularly schizophrenia.

The treatment of schizophrenia

The neuroleptics are very effective in relieving the florid or 'positive' symptoms of schizophrenia, such as thought disorders, hallucinations and delusions, together with paranoia and aggressive behaviour. They are less effective on the 'negative' symptoms, such as apathy, withdrawal and reduction in speech, although an activating effect can sometimes occur. For example, large doses of chlorpromazine have been known to restore acutely ill schizophrenics, who are withdrawn, mute and akinetic, to normal activity and social behaviour. In previously untreated patients, the sedative action of the neuroleptic appears immediately while the antipsychotic action may take 2–3 weeks to develop. However, patients with psychosis are less sensitive to the sedative actions of neuroleptics than are non-psychotics and can often tolerate large doses without any signs of sedation being apparent.

It has not proved possible to distinguish between different neuroleptic drugs in terms of their effectiveness on specific symptoms, syndromes or subtypes of schizophrenia. In fact, there is no evidence that any one drug is better than another or can influence, more selectively, a given symptom. The choice of neuroleptic is therefore made on the basis of the patient's medical history in relation to the side-effects associated with the use of a particular neuroleptic. As the side-effects are considerable and may be severe (see below), such considerations may be very important.

Although patients with acute schizophrenia respond well to treatment with neuroleptics, which will arrest the development of new symptoms, long-term treatment may be necessary to prevent the illness from becoming chronic. Long-term treatment is also needed in chronic schizophrenic patients to prevent relapse. Problems with compliance can be avoided by the use of long-acting depot preparations of neuroleptic drugs for maintenance therapy. These are administered by deep intramuscular injection at intervals of 1–4 weeks.

As neuroleptic drugs can both depress symptoms of hyperactivity in some schizophrenic patients and 'activate' patients who are withdrawn, it is considered that these drugs have a specific antipsychotic or antischizophrenic action, although whether this action is against the disease state itself, or simply against the symptoms, will not be known until the aetiology of schizophrenia is more fully understood.

Side-effects of neuroleptic drugs

The neuroleptic drugs are relatively non-toxic and can often be tolerated in very large doses; however, side-effects occur readily. Some of these have already been referred to; they are numerous and vary from one drug to another, thus influencing the choice of drug for a particular patient. The side-effects of the phenothiazines, for example, can be largely accounted for by their pharmacological actions: thus, anticholinergic activity can result in blurred vision, dry mouth and nasal stuffiness, slight constipation and urinary retention with therapeutic doses of those drugs which possess this action, i.e. aliphatic and piperidine phenothiazines and clozapine. Postural hypotension resulting from blockade of α-adrenoceptors can also be troublesome, but again is associated mainly with the aliphatic and piperidine phenothiazines. Thus, a phenothiazine of the piperazine type, or a different type of neuroleptic, should be used when these side-effects are to be avoided. Changes in body temperature can occur due to interference with temperature regulation and the possible occurrence of hypothermia in elderly patients has to be avoided.

With the introduction of chlorpromazine as the first widely used neuroleptic, many side-effects due to idiosyncratic or hypersensitive reactions were noted. These included jaundice, the incidence of which was low, the effects being mild and resembling obstructive jaundice; the effect disappeared quickly if the drug was withdrawn. Blood dyscrasias, such as agranulocytosis, are also very rare but are potentially fatal and the incidence of this side-effect with clozapine has restricted the use of the drug. Skin reactions to phenothiazines are common: first, urticaria can occur during the first few weeks of treatment but usually clears up even when administration of the drug is continued; secondly, contact dermatitis can occur in personnel handling chlorpromazine; thirdly, photosensitive reactions, which resemble severe sunburn, can occur. Prolonged use of chlorpromazine can also result in abnormal skin pigmentation. Fortunately, the above side-effects are mainly associated with the phenothiazines (with the exception of clozapine) and the newer, non-phenothiazine neuroleptics tend to have fewer side-effects.

The increased secretion of prolactin can cause inappropriate lactation in females and gynaecomastia can occur in males. Decreased libido in both sexes and impotence in males is associated with the phenothiazines. The neuroleptic drugs can cause changes in appetite, and weight gain can occur and may even be troublesome. It is possible that the improvement in appetite may, at least in part, be due to the improved mental state.

Probably the most prevalent and most troublesome side-effects associated with the therapeutic use of neuroleptic drugs are those due to stimulation of the extrapyramidal system. These effects are produced by all known neuroleptic drugs, although the incidence may vary with different agents and they may not be seen at all in some patients. It has been claimed that the incidence of extrapyramidal symptoms is less with the 'atypical' neuroleptic drugs, such as sulpiride. The symptoms closely resemble those of Parkinson's disease (see Chapter 19) and it has been suggested that the parkinsonian syndrome, associated with the administration of neuroleptic drugs, is indistinguishable from idiopathic Parkinson's disease. Three syndromes can be distinguished: (1) dystonia, characterized by facial grimacing and abnormal body movements; (2) akathisia, or motor restlessness; (3) tardive dyskinesia, which takes longer to develop and may not appear until years after treatment with the drug was initiated. The characteristic rigidity and tremor at rest, seen in patients with Parkinson's disease, are frequently observed. The acute parkinsonian symptoms remit if the drug is withdrawn or sometimes if the dose is reduced. Alternatively, antiparkinson drugs of the anticholinergic type, such as benztropine (Figure 19.6c), can be used.

Tardive dyskinesias appear late, as the name implies; they occur less frequently than the acute extrapyramidal symptoms and are present mainly in elderly patients. The condition worsens if the neuroleptic is withdrawn and is unresponsive to treatment. Tardive dyskinesia usually appears as stereotyped involuntary orofacial movements, such as sucking and smacking the lips, lateral movements of the jaw and darting of the tongue ('fly-catching'). Although it is the subject of extensive study, the pathophysiology of tardive kyskinesia is still obscure. 'Drug holidays' in which the administration of the drug is discontinued for a short period, perhaps one month in six, have been advocated but it is not clear whether such holidays are likely to prevent the condition. However, 'drug holidays' could serve to provide a warning of patients who are at risk, i.e. those who might develop tardive dyskinesia at a later stage. Drugs used to treat acute parkinson-like symptoms can exacerbate tardive dyskinesias.

Although all neuroleptic drugs are able to produce extrapyramidal symptoms as side-effects, their potency varies. Thus the butyrophenones, such as haloperidol, are the most potent in this respect but have a few other side-effects; the piperazine phenothiazines are also fairly potent, whereas the other phenothiazines are only moderately potent at producing extrapyramidal effects, and drugs which are potent anticholinergics, such as thioridazine and clozapine, have a very low potency in this regard, as would be expected.

Because all neuroleptic drugs produce extrapyramidal disturbances, and as all are dopamine antagonists, it is reasonable to conclude that these side-effects are attributable to an action on dopamine receptors in the basal ganglia. An antagonist action at this site would depress dopaminergic transmission and this is exactly what occurs in idiopathic parkinsonism (see Chapter 19), the symptoms of which closely resemble those of the drug-induced state. Furthermore, it is the D_2 receptors which appear to be defective in this disease. Tardive dyskinesia, on the other hand, is thought to be due to adaptive changes taking place in the postsynaptic dopamine receptors in the basal ganglia over a long period of time, such that supersensitivity develops. According to this hypothesis, unmasking of the supersensitive dopamine receptors, for example by reducing the amount of neuroleptic, would result in the appearance of tardive dyskinesia. There is, in fact, some evidence from studies on animals, given neuroleptic drugs over long periods of time, to support this theory.

Other uses of neuroleptic drugs

Some of these have already been referred to: for example, the use of phenothiazines in premedication for surgical operations and in the 'lytic' cocktail of Laborit. Benzodiazepines are now usually preferred, however. Another use for chlorpromazine was as an adjunct to the induction of hypothermia, again for surgical procedures, due to the loss of temperature regulation which is produced. One of the butyrophenones, usually droperidol, is used in combination with the potent analgesic fentanyl, in neuroleptanalgesia (see Chapter 11).

One of the main uses for the neuroleptic drugs, other than as antipsychotics, is in the control of nausea and vomiting from various causes (see Chapter 20). Chlorpromazine will relieve nausea and vomiting in pregnancy but drugs are no longer used for this purpose because of the risk of teratogenic effects. Chlorpromazine does not appear to be effective in the control of motion sickness, although other antihistaminic phenothiazines (non-neuroleptic) are. The mechanism for the anti-emetic effect can be attributed to antagonism of dopamine receptors in the hypothalamus (see Chapter 20). Neuroleptics, e.g. pimozide, have also been used in the treatment of Huntington's chorea (see Chapter 19).

The dopamine hypothesis of schizophrenia

Over the years there have been numerous hypotheses that have attempted to provide a rational explanation for schizophrenia; most are now only of historical interest. The latest theory, and the one which currently fits the observed facts, is the dopamine theory, which has its origin in the observation that the common property of all the drugs used to treat the symptoms of psychosis is that they are dopamine antagonists. The hypothesis is very simple: it is that the symptoms of schizophrenia are due to overactivity of dopamine systems in the brain. Thus, any influence which tends to increase dopaminergic activity will exacerbate the symptoms, whereas an influence which reduces dopaminergic activity will ameliorate the symptoms. The following observations support the theory:

1. The consumption of large doses of amphetamine in man can induce a state, known as the 'amphetamine psychosis', the symptoms of which are indistinguishable from those of schizophrenia. It has been proposed that amphetamine provides a model of paranoid schizophrenia. Amphetamine is an indirectly

acting sympathomimetic amine (see Chapter 8) which releases the catecholamines, noradrenaline and dopamine, from presynaptic nerve terminals. Evidence from studies in animals suggests that the release of dopamine is probably responsible for the 'amphetamine psychosis'.
2. The administration of modest doses of amphetamine to schizophrenic patients was found to precipitate or intensify their psychotic symptoms (although not all the subjects tested responded to the amphetamine challenge).
3. All neuroleptic drugs are dopamine antagonists, their antipsychotic potency closely paralleling their affinity for dopamine D_2 receptors (Figure 12.9)
4. Neuroleptic drugs effectively block the 'amphetamine psychosis'.

Some arguments against the dopamine hypothesis are:

1. Much of the data obtained from animal studies have been related to acute administration of the drugs whereas, in man, the drugs are administered chronically and there may be a delay of 2–3 weeks before a therapeutic effect is seen.
2. The administration of amphetamine to schizophrenic patients [see (2) above] has been found in some cases to lead to an improvement in their condition.
3. Studies of autopsy material from the brains of schizophrenic patients have not yielded any consistent or conclusive evidence to support the dopamine hypothesis. Changes in the turnover of dopamine have been found in some cases but these changes were not consistent. Changes in the affinity of dopamine receptors have also been found in material obtained *post mortem*, but it is thought that this effect is more likely to be associated with previous treatment with neuroleptic drugs than with the disease itself.

The dopamine hypothesis of schizophrenia probably represents a useful working hypothesis to explain how the symptoms of the disease may be produced but helps little in improving our understanding of the aetiology of schizophrenia.

Chapter 13

Anti-anxiety drugs

These are drugs which are used to treat neuroses, the most common of which is anxiety. A state of emotional tension and unease about what may or may not happen is a common experience and a moderate level of anxiety or of being 'keyed up' may, in fact, be beneficial and may improve the performance of certain tasks. However, sometimes the symptoms of anxiety can be severe and discomforting and may interfere with sufferers' ability to manage their lives. Feelings of fear, panic, apprehension and foreboding can all occur and are often accompanied by somatic components which are the consequence of overactivity of the sympathetic nervous system: these are tachycardia and increased blood pressure, increased tension of voluntary muscles, which may result in tremor or pain, e.g. headaches or back pain, gastrointestinal disturbances such as dry mouth, nausea and diarrhoea, and respiratory difficulties which, although subjective, can result in rapid breathing, making the patient dizzy or even causing loss of consciousness; excessive sweating can also occur.

Anxiety is a ubiquitous symptom which may be associated with medical as well as psychiatric disorders, in which case diagnosis and effective treatment will remove the cause of the anxiety, an example being the anxiety which may accompany depression (see Chapter 17). Some anxiety states are clearly related to situations, e.g. agoraphobia (fear of open spaces); other phobias may be more specific, e.g. fear of spiders. However, in some cases no primary illness or cause is present and the anxiety appears to have no origin. In such cases treatment with drugs can be very successful and the principal use for the drugs known as minor tranquillizers is as 'anti-anxiety or anxiolytic' drugs.

Almost any drug with a depressant action on the central nervous system will relieve anxiety; however, this will often occur at doses which produce noticeable sedation. The newer anti-anxiety drugs, e.g. the benzodiazepines, are effective in relieving the symptoms of anxiety without inducing undue sedation.

There are three main groups of drugs with an anti-anxiety action: barbiturates, benzodiazepines and a group of miscellaneous compounds.

Barbiturates

These are drugs which produce a generalized depression of the central nervous system, resulting in sedation, sleep or loss of consciousness, depending on the dose and the type of compound administered. Their actions and uses are described in

Chapter 11. Long-acting barbiturates, such as phenobarbitone (see Figure 11.2), are effective in relieving the symptoms of anxiety without producing marked sedation. However, the dangers involved in the use of barbiturates (see Chapter 11), together with the availability of safer effective anti-anxiety drugs (benzodiazepines), has resulted in the barbiturates no longer being used for the treatment of anxiety.

Benzodiazepines

These are currently the most important anti-anxiety drugs. Although they are sedative when given in large doses (see Chapter 11), the anti-anxiety action is present at non-sedative doses and they are regarded as having a selective anxiolytic action. Thus, it appears that anti-anxiety actions can be separated from sedative effects by the careful selection of dose. The benzodiazepines all share the same ring structure and can be divided into three classes according to the following substitutions.

Simple 1,4-benzodiazepines

This group includes chlordiazepoxide (Figure 13.1a), diazepam (Figure 13.1b) and lorazepam (Figure 13.1c).

(a)

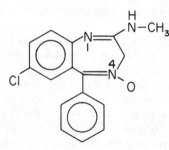

(b)

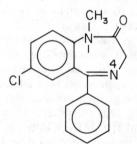

(c)

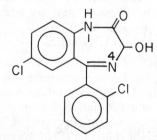

Figure 13.1 The chemical structures of the 1,4-benzodiazepines (a) chlordiazepoxide, (b) diazepam and (c) lorazepam

Heterocyclic 1,4-benzodiazepines

Examples are alprazolam (Figure 13.2a), triazolam (Figure 13.2b) and prazepam (Figure 13.2c).

(a)

(b)

(c)

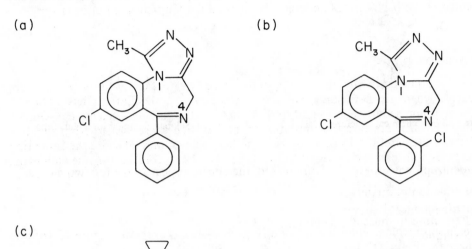

Figure 13.2 The chemical structures of the heterocyclic 1,4-benzodiazepines (a) alprazolam, (b) triazolam and (c) prazepam

1,5-Benzodiazepines

Examples of these are clobazepam (Figure 13.3a) and triflubazepam (Figure 13.3b).

Although all the benzodiazepines possess similar properties, i.e. reduction in anxiety, sedation and anticonvulsant properties, the 1,5-benzodiazepines have been found to be less sedative. In addition, the benzodiazepines produce a significant degree of muscle relaxation without impairment of coordination. As anxiety is often accompanied by increased muscle tone, the muscle-relaxant effects of the benzodiazepines add to the anti-anxiety action. It is thought that this effect may be due to depression of spinal and supraspinal motor reflexes; however, it must be noted that any degree of sedation will result in muscle relaxation. As the dose of a

(a)   (b)

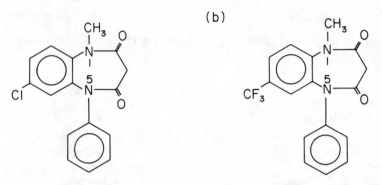

Figure 13.3 The chemical structures of the 1,5-benzodiazepines (a) clobazepam and (b) triflubazepam

benzodiazepine is progressively increased, the effects appear in the following order:

1. Reduction in anxiety;
2. Anticonvulsant effects;
3. Reduction in muscle tone and
4. Sedation.

Thus, only the most potent benzodiazepine drugs are likely to cause sedation.

In animals, the anti-anxiety action of the benzodiazepines is manifested in a reduction in aggression, or a 'taming' effect, allowing the animals to be handled more easily, together with an increase in social behaviour.

Effects on sleep and the use of benzodiazepines in the treatment of insomnia are discussed in Chapter 11 and the use of these drugs in the treatment of epilepsy, in Chapter 14.

The pharmacological properties of the benzodiazepines enables them to be readily distinguished from other groups of centrally acting drugs, such as the neuroleptics and antidepressants. They are also characterized by a low toxicity, even when used as sedatives (see Chapter 11), and there is a wide margin between the smallest dose which is pharmacologically active and the dose which produces undesired or toxic effects. They were originally thought to have no actions on peripheral tissues, but binding sites for benzodiazepines have been found on blood platelets and in the heart and kidney, although it is not known what pharmacological effects, if any, are mediated at the peripheral sites.

The mechanism of action of benzodiazepines

For a number of years after the discovery of their actions, little was known about the mechanism of action of the benzodiazepines. However, it was found that radio-labelled 1,4-benzodiazepines bound with a high affinity to specific sites in the brain. Other benzodiazepines were found to inhibit this binding competitively, with affinities that corresponded roughly to their pharmacological potency. However, these binding sites did not correspond to those of any known neurotransmitter receptor, although their distribution in brain was found to coincide with that of receptors for γ-aminobutyric acid (GABA). In fact, the benzodiazepines were found to facilitate the actions of GABA at GABA$_A$ receptors in the CNS. They do not act directly on the GABA receptor or affect the chloride channel directly, but they modulate the action of GABA on its receptor, thus increasing the conductance to chloride ions and so producing inhibition. This action is known as 'allosteric modulation' and represents a relatively new phenomenon in receptor pharmacology. The benzodiazepines also oppose the actions of antagonists of GABA, such as bicuculline.

The binding sites for benzodiazepines are distributed unevenly in the CNS, the highest density being found in the cerebral cortex and limbic system, a moderate density in the cerebellar cortex and the lowest in the brain stem and spinal cord. This agrees roughly with the distribution of GABA receptors. In fact, the two binding sites, i.e. for GABA and the benzodiazepines, are now known to be present on the GABA$_A$ receptor. The protein which represents the GABA receptor in the neuronal membrane has been extracted and purified, and the amino acid sequence has been determined. From this it has been shown that there are two subunits, α and β, there being two of each subunit in each receptor (Figure 13.4a), i.e. the receptor consists of $2\alpha,2\beta$. The benzodiazepines act on the α-subunit and GABA on the β-subunit. How the two subunits interact is not known but binding studies have shown that the benzodiazepines and GABA increase each other's binding. However, the benzodiazepines do not open the chloride channel (Figure 13.4b) but simply facilitate the action of GABA and it is possible that this is due to the increase in the affinity of GABA for the receptor. The enhancement of the action of GABA by the benzodiazepines has been found to be due to an increase in the number of ion channels opened rather than to a change in the length of time for which they are open.

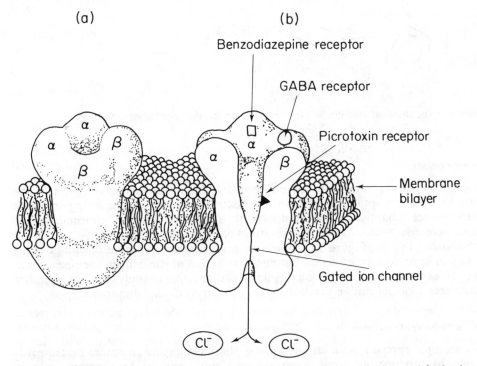

Figure 13.4 Diagrammatic representation of the GABA receptor, showing (a) the α- and β-subunits and (b) the chloride channel (redrawn from Costa, 1988)

Benzodiazepine antagonists

Substances which act as competitive antagonists at benzodiazepine receptors have been made. The first, and probably the best-known, of these is flumazenil (which is ethyl 8-fluoro-5,6-dihydro-5-methyl-6-oxo-4H-imidazo[1,5-a][1,4]benzodiazepine-3-carboxylate and is known by the code number Ro 15-1788; Figure 13.5a). This compound blocks all the known actions of the benzodiazepines and binds well to the benzodiazepine receptor in the CNS but not to peripheral benzodiazepine-binding sites. As competitive antagonists, flumazenil and other benzodiazepine antagonists would be expected to lack intrinsic activity. However, some actions, albeit weak, have been found and flumazenil has been shown to be a weak anticonvulsant, which is consistent with a partial agonist action. This drug has also been found to possess an anxiogenic action, i.e. it increases anxiety, which is more characteristic of an 'inverse agonist' action (see below).

(a)

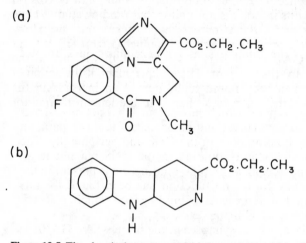

(b)

Figure 13.5 The chemical structures of (a) flumazenil and (b) ethyl β-carboline-3-carboxylate

Inverse agonists

During the search, which proved unsuccessful, for an endogenous ligand of the benzodiazepine receptor (analogous to the discovery of enkephalins acting on opiate receptors, see Chapter 10), substances with a different kind of pharmacological action were discovered. They are derivatives of β-carboline, e.g. ethyl β-carboline-3-carboxylate (β-CCE; Figure 13.5b), which bind to benzodiazepine receptors in the brain and have an agonist action but opposite to that of the benzodiazepines. Thus, they increase anxiety, i.e. are 'anxiogenic', and are also convulsant. The effects of the inverse agonists can be blocked by antagonists such as flumazenil.

The benzodiazepine receptor

This receptor appears to be unique among pharmacological receptors because it is unable to produce a response on its own and appears to function only in collaboration with the GABA receptor which it modulates. Thus, the benzodiazepine receptor influences the efficiency with which the GABA receptor is coupled to its effector mechanism and, hence, the opening of chloride channels in the neuronal membrane. To explain the actions of agonists (benzodiazepines) and inverse agonists (β-carbolines), it has been proposed that the benzodiazepine receptor exists in two conformational states which are normally in equilibrium. The presence of an agonist (benzodiazepine) shifts the equilibrium in one direction, towards a conformational state which causes allosteric modulation of the GABA recognition site, facilitating the action of GABA in opening the chloride channel (as described above). The result is that the chloride channels are more readily opened by a given GABA stimulus than if the benzodiazepine receptor was not occupied by an agonist drug. However, if the benzodiazepine receptor is occupied by an inverse agonist, then the opposite is true: the equilibrium is shifted towards a conformational state in which the allosteric interaction with the GABA receptor results in a reduction of the influence of GABA on the chloride channel; thus, inhibition will be decreased. In this scheme, the antagonists, such as flumazenil, bind to both receptor conformations without disturbing the equilibrium, as they antagonize the actions of both the agonists and inverse agonists. There is no direct evidence for this model but it currently fits the experimental data and appears to be widely accepted.

There are some indications that the binding sites for benzodiazepines are not homogeneous, although whether this indicates the existence of subtypes of receptors, as for most other pharmacological receptors, is debatable. For example, a close derivative of diazepam, which is inactive in the CNS, binds to peripheral benzodiazepine receptors and clonazepam, which has potent CNS actions, shows only weak binding in the kidney, adrenal cortex and blood cells. Flunitrazepam, on the other hand, shows high-affinity binding both in the CNS and peripherally. The antagonist flumazenil also shows high-affinity binding in the CNS but not to all peripheral sites. The peripheral type of benzodiazepine-binding site is present in the CNS as well as on peripheral tissues. So far no function has been found for this binding site and it is possible that it represents a binding site which is not a functional receptor, i.e. an 'acceptor' (see Chapter 1).

A facilitatory action by benzodiazepines at synapses in the brain where GABA is the transmitter readily explains most of the pharmacological actions of these drugs, e.g. the anticonvulsant action, muscular relaxation and sedation. However, the association of GABA with the anti-anxiety action is less clear. There are anti-anxiety drugs which have no action on GABA mechanisms (see below) and the function of 5-hydroxytryptamine in brain, especially in the limbic system, has been implicated in anxiety states. In fact, the benzodiazepines do have effects on other neurotransmitter systems in the brain, including dopamine, noradrenaline and 5-hydroxytryptamine, but it is thought that these effects are indirect and may be mediated by GABA which then influences the other neurotransmitter systems. Thus, GABA has been shown to exert a tonic inhibitory influence on 5-hydroxytryptamine-containing neurones in the raphe nucleus and this action is potentiated by the benzodiazepines. The anti-anxiety action of the benzodiazepines may therefore be indirect.

The kinetics of benzodiazepines

Most benzodiazepines are administered orally, although they can also be given intravenously (e.g. diazepam in status epilepticus, see Chapter 14). They are readily absorbed from the gut and may be bound to plasma proteins. In addition, because of their lipid solubility, they may accumulate in body fat. However, many benzodiazepines are metabolized to active metabolites (Figure 13.6). The principal metabolite which is formed from both chlordiazepoxide and diazepam is desmethyl-diazepam (or nordiazepam), which has a half-life of about 60 h and therefore accounts for the long duration of action of these two drugs. It also accounts for the cumulative effects which appear if long-acting benzodiazepines are taken regularly. The short-acting benzodiazepines, which are preferred as sedatives (see Chapter 11), either have no active metabolite (e.g. lorazepam) or have metabolites with short half-lives (e.g. temazepam and oxazepam). All the benzodiazepines are excreted in the urine as inactive glucuronide conjugates.

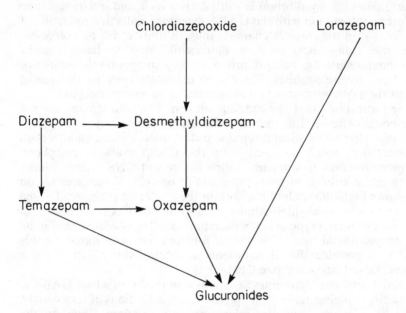

Figure 13.6 The metabolism of the benzodiazepines

Miscellaneous anti-anxiety drugs

Before the discovery of the anti-anxiety action of benzodiazepines, and because of the dangers associated with the use of barbiturates, a number of other compounds were investigated for possible use in relieving anxiety. Most of these are no longer used, although some new drugs have been developed.

Meprobamate

This is a propanediol carbamate (Figure 13.7a) which was introduced in the 1950s as a long-acting muscle relaxant. Its anti-anxiety action was soon recognized and the drug became very widely used, particularly in the United States, where it was marketed under the name 'Miltown'. It is sedative and drowsiness is the most common side-effect. With the advent of the benzodiazepines, meprobamate is now only rarely used as it is less effective than the benzodiazepines and is hazardous in

(a)

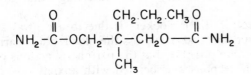
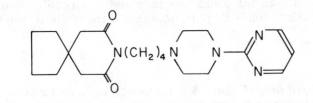

(b)

(c)

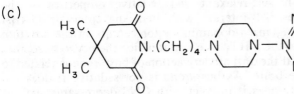

(d)

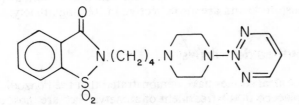

Figure 13.7 The chemical structures of (a) meprobamate, (b) buspirone, (c) gepirone and (d) ipsapirone

overdose; it can also produce dependence. Virtually nothing is known of the mechanism of action of meprobamate but it does not appear to act through GABA mechanisms. Meprobamate is related chemically to the muscle-relaxant drug mephenesin, which acts selectively on polysynaptic reflexes in the spinal cord and is used to relieve muscle spasm (see Chapter 19). It is quite possible that the combined sedative and muscle-relaxant properties of meprobamate account for its anti-anxiety effect.

β-Adrenoceptor antagonists

It is surprising that these drugs, the β-blockers (see Chapter 8), in addition to their cardiovascular actions, should act as anti-anxiety agents. They are particularly useful for relieving chronic anxiety, panic attacks and the debilitating anxiety that can occur in otherwise healthy individuals placed in a stressful situation (e.g. stage fright). Propranolol (Figure 8.16a) is the drug that has been chiefly used for this purpose and it is claimed that it reduces anxiety without affecting either physical or intellectual performance.

Whether the anti-anxiety effect of the β-blockers is due to a central action is debatable as practolol, a β-blocker that does not cross the blood–brain barrier, has been found to be effective. It is quite possible that the peripheral actions of the β-blockers, blocking the autonomic responses associated with anxiety, i.e. tremors, sweating, tachycardia, etc, may account for the reduction in anxiety. Certainly, these drugs are less potent than the benzodiazepines and it is possible that they produce an anti-anxiety effect simply by relieving some of the physical manifestations of anxiety.

Buspirone

This is a recently developed drug (Figure 13.7b), representing a new class of anti-anxiety agents. It is as effective as diazepam in the treatment of generalized anxiety but lacks the anticonvulsant, muscle-relaxant and sedative properties of the benzodiazepines. Buspirone does not interact with benzodiazepine or GABA receptors in the brain but it antagonizes dopamine autoreceptors in the striatum and it binds with a high affinity to the 5-HT$_1$ receptor at which the benzodiazepines show no activity. It is thought that the anti-anxiety action of buspirone is related to an interaction with 5-HT in the brain. As buspirone is not sedative it does not impair skills such as driving, nor does it interact with CNS depressants such as ethanol. It is also considered to have a low abuse potential. Related drugs are gepirone (Figure 13.7c) and ipsapirone (Figure 13.7d), which have similar pharmacological properties to buspirone and are also effective in treating anxiety.

The clinical uses of anti-anxiety drugs

A number of controlled clinical studies have demonstrated that the benzodiazepines are more effective than placebo in the treatment of anxiety. They are most effective in anxious patients showing high levels of emotional and somatic symptoms with low levels of depression, but they can also be used to treat the anxious, depressed patient. However, in depressed patients their use is limited to the extent to which the anxiety contributes to the depression. They can also be used to relieve anxiety associated with organic disease, although they do not, of course, affect the underlying pathology. Because of their low toxicity compared with barbiturates, the benzodiazepines have become very popular and there has been a tendency for them to be widely prescribed for any stress-related symptom, unhappiness or minor physical disease. This is now recognized as undesirable and it is considered that the use of benzodiazepines should be confined to patients in which the anxiety is a clear handicap which interferes with their work, leisure or family relationships. One of the reasons for this is that the benzodiazepines are not without adverse effects and, with long-term use, dependence can occur.

The main side-effects of the benzodiazepines are drowsiness, dizziness and ataxia. The impaired motor coordination results in the loss of manual skills. For this reason, the dose used for the treatment of anxiety should be limited to the smallest effective dose. In addition, tolerance can develop with long-term use, although the anti-anxiety action has less tendency to show tolerance. Administration of therapeutic doses of benzodiazepines for 6 months or longer can result in physical dependence, characterized by a withdrawal syndrome when administration of the drug is discontinued. With larger doses the physical dependence develops more rapidly. The symptoms associated with the sudden withdrawal of benzodiazepines are similar to those associated with the withdrawal of barbiturates or ethanol, but are usually less severe, i.e. confusion, agitation and irritability, insomnia, tremor, headache, dizziness, muscle twitches, nausea and vomiting. Convulsions are rare except in patients with a history of seizure disorders. Obviously, long-term use of these drugs must be avoided and withdrawal should be gradual.

As far as their anti-anxiety action is concerned, there appears to be little difference between the various benzodiazepines, provided that they are used in appropriate doses. The choice of drug may therefore be determined by the duration of action, a long half-life and therefore a sustained anti-anxiety action being usually preferred. The drugs shown in Figures 13.1, 13.2 and 13.3 are among those used for the treatment of anxiety, being mainly long-acting. Lorazepam (Figure 13.1c) is short acting and can be used for acute anxiety or for relieving phobic panic attacks. Diazepam or lorazepam, given either by mouth or intravenously, can be used to control severe panic attacks.

Certain of the antipsychotic drugs, e.g. chlorpromazine and flupenthixol, are occasionally used in small doses to alleviate severe anxiety. However their use is regarded as a short-term measure. It seems quite possible that buspirone and related drugs may become the anti-anxiety drugs of the future, particularly where depression of the CNS is undesirable.

Chapter 14

Anticonvulsant drugs

The principal use for anticonvulsant drugs is in the treatment of epilepsy, although not all seizures or convulsive states necessarily indicate the presence of epilepsy. Thus, seizures can occur as a toxic manifestation of central stimulant and other drugs; they may also be observed in eclampsia, uraemia, hypoglycaemia, hyperthermia (febrile seizures can occur in babies), pyridoxine deficiency and as part of the abstinence syndrome in individuals who are addicted to barbiturates. However, by far the largest number of convulsive disorders is associated with epilepsy, which affects approximately 0.5% of the population and is not restricted to humans but can occur in other species, such as dogs.

Epileptic seizures consist of spontaneous, paroxysmal and recurrent abnormal discharges of a group of neurones in the brain. The abnormal discharge may start at a localized site and then spread to other areas of the brain or it may remain localized. The symptoms produced depend upon the region of the brain involved in the seizure and range from a simple brief lapse of attention (*petit mal* epilepsy) to tonic–clonic convulsions with loss of consciousness (*grand mal* epilepsy). There is also a discontinuity of symptoms with widely varying periods between the seizures (interictal period). A notable feature of epilepsy, which in fact distinguishes epileptic seizures from other types of seizures, is that the neuronal discharge is reflected in a characteristic pattern in the electroencephalogram, the most striking of which is the 'spike and wave' pattern (Figure 14.1) seen in *petit mal* epilepsy.

Epilepsy can be idiopathic, having no known cause, or it may be symptomatic, being due to trauma to the head, to tumours, infections or cerebrovascular disease, etc. In all probability, epilepsy is not a single disease entity but a group of disorders having in common the clinical phenomenon of the seizure and the cellular phenomenon of an abnormal paroxysmal discharge of neurones. Thus, different drugs are effective in treating different types of epilepsy and the classification of the epilepsies is important in relation to their treatment.

The classification of epileptic seizures

Clinically, the epilepsies can be classified into two main types, i.e. partial, in which the seizure remains localized, and general, in which the seizure may start locally but rapidly spreads to involve most, if not all, of the brain.

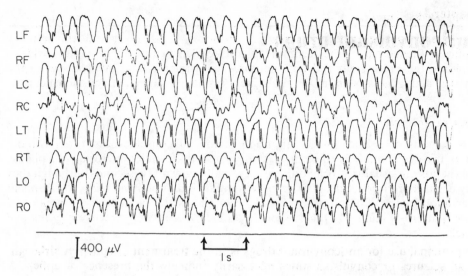

LF
RF
LC
RC
LT
RT
LO
RO

$\rceil$400 μV
I s

Figure 14.1 Electroencephalographic recordings from a child with a history of *petit mal* epilepsy showing generalized spike and wave activity during an attack. LF, left frontal; RF, right frontal; LC, left central; RC, right central; LT, left temporal; RT, right temporal; LO, left occipital; RO, right occipital (from Pincus and Tucker, 1974)

Partial seizures

These are focal seizures in which the epileptic discharge arises in a localized area of the brain, often the cerebral cortex, and its spread is limited. It can be due to the presence of a tumour or to damage to the brain at the site of origin.

Simple

These are localized seizures, with elementary symptoms depending on the area of the brain involved, and do not result in loss of consciousness. The seizure may consist of involuntary muscle contractions, abnormal sensory experiences or autonomic discharges. If the epileptic focus is in the motor cortex, the seizure may be confined to a single limb or group of muscles which show repetitive jerking; this is known as Jacksonian epilepsy. The neuronal discharge associated with simple partial seizures is usually seen as a pattern of spikes in the electroencephalogram and can often be localized by this means.

Complex

In this case there are attacks of confused behaviour, impairment of consciousness and amnesia. These seizures are often due to an epileptic focus in the temporal lobe which results in automatic patterns of behaviour with stereotyped movements, frequently accompanied by a strong emotional response. This is known as psycho-motor epilepsy. The localization of the focus to the temporal lobe can usually be clearly seen in the EEG.

Generalized seizures

Here the epileptic discharge originates subcortically, usually in the thalamus or midbrain (hence the name 'centrencephalic' epilepsy) and then spreads widely, involving the brain stem and both cerebral hemispheres. The involvement of the reticular activating system of the brain stem results in the loss of consciousness.

Absence (petit mal)

This consists of a brief loss of attention or loss of consciousness, often without motor involvement. It is therefore less dramatic than the other forms of epilepsy and the fits are usually of brief duration, typically only a few seconds, although they may occur more frequently. It often occurs in late childhood and tends to disappear after adolescence. The electroencephalogram shows the characteristic 'spike and wave' pattern (Figure 14.1). Occasionally, a petit mal fit may precede a grand mal attack.

Tonic–clonic seizures (grand mal)

These are major convulsions with loss of consciousness and the patient usually falls to the ground, sometimes uttering a cry. Initially, there is maximum tonic spasm of all the body musculature. This is the tonic phase which is followed by rhythmic clonic contractions of the muscles, thus producing the characteristic convulsive jerking. The seizure is followed by a period of prolonged depression, known as postictal depression, during which consciousness slowly returns but the patient is confused and weak for some time. During the tonic phase, the electroencephalogram shows high-voltage synchronous discharges arising over the whole cerebral cortex (Figure 14.2b) and in the clonic phase, intermittent synchronous discharges (Figure 14.2c). However, the electrical patterns may be obscured by artefacts due to the movements. Status epilepticus is a condition of continuous tonic–clonic seizures in which the patient fails to regain consciousness between the attacks. Although relatively rare, it is life-threatening and requires emergency intervention.

Myoclonic and akinetic seizures

Myoclonic seizures consist of isolated clonic jerks of the head, limbs or body which are associated with brief bursts of multiple spikes in the electroencephalogram. Myoclonic epilepsy is often associated with brain damage. In akinetic seizures there are no muscle movements but a sudden and transitory loss of tone in the postural muscles and the victim may fall to the ground. Normal muscle tone returns rapidly and usually there is no loss of consciousness.

Infantile spasms

Also known as 'hypsarrhythmia', this is characterized by attacks which begin in the early months of life and take the form of head nodding and body flexion. There may be progressive mental retardation and this form of epilepsy is usually associated with gross abnormalities of brain structure and function. However, infantile spasms can also result from pyridoxine (vitamin B_6) deficiency and can readily be cured if the deficiency is remedied.

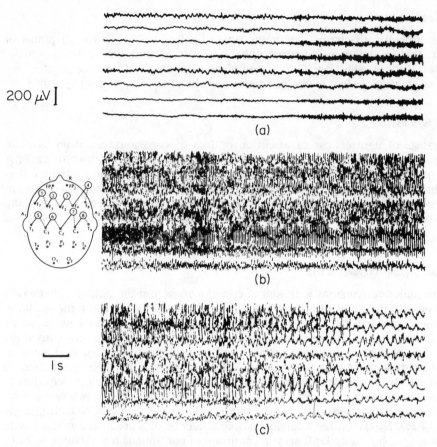

200 μV

1 s

Figure 14.2 Electroencephalographic recordings of a generalized seizure in a patient suffering from *grand mal* epilepsy: (a) the onset of the seizure; initially, the EEG is fairly normal but generalized spikes develop in all regions; (b) the tonic phase in which there are generalized high-voltage discharges mixed with movement artefact; (c) the clonic phase of the epileptic fit in which there are groups of spikes separated by slow waves (from Pincus and Tucker, 1974)

Drugs used in the treatment of epilepsy

Many agents have been used over the centuries for the treatment of epilepsy and before the development of more specific drugs, bromides and barbiturates were used. However, their side-effects and low level of activity severely limited their usefulness. Nevertheless, the barbiturate phenobarbitone is still used and many of the drugs in use today are derived from barbiturates.

Phenobarbitone (Figure 14.3a)

This is a barbiturate in which the anticonvulsant activity is greater in relation to the sedative action than that of other barbiturates (Chapter 11). It is probably the most effective anticonvulsant drug available but, because of the many adverse effects, it is no longer a drug of first choice but tends to be used only when other anti-epileptic

(a)

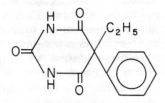

(b)

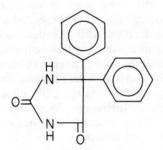

(c)

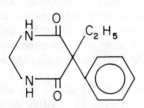

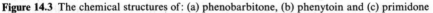

Figure 14.3 The chemical structures of: (a) phenobarbitone, (b) phenytoin and (c) primidone

drugs have been found to be ineffective. It seems to act against most types of seizures but is used mainly to control generalized tonic–clonic (*grand mal*) epilepsy and some focal seizures. Phenobarbitone is a long-acting barbiturate with a half-life in plasma of 50–140 h which means that, when given daily, there is a cumulative effect. Apart from causing sedation in adults, it suffers from all the disadvantages of the barbiturates described in Chapter 11, including the risks of overdosage, the development of tolerance and the induction of hepatic microsomal enzymes. Therefore, its use in combination with other drugs is severely restricted. Rebound seizures may occur if the drug is withdrawn or the dose reduced and, in children, it can cause behavioural disturbances and hyperkinesia. In spite of its many disadvantages, phenobarbitone is often effective where other drugs have failed.

Methylphenobarbitone is demethylated to phenobarbitone in the liver and offers no advantages over phenobarbitone.

Phenytoin (diphenylhydantoin, Figure 14.3b)

This is one of the most widely used anticonvulsant drugs and was the first anti-epileptic drug without sedative activity. It is effective against tonic–clonic and partial seizures where it is often the drug of first choice, but not against *petit mal* which may be exacerbated, or against akinetic and atonic seizures. Phenytoin is well absorbed when taken orally but is highly bound to plasma proteins (about 90%) and the relationship between the dose and plasma concentration is non-linear: thus, a small increase in dose can sometimes result in a large rise in plasma concentration with the consequent appearance of toxic or side-effects. Because phenytoin has a low therapeutic index, monitoring of the plasma concentration is often employed in order to adjust the dose level. The drug is metabolized in the liver to the *p*-hydroxyphenyl derivative and then conjugated with glucuronide which is excreted. The *p*-hydroxylation is a rate-limiting step and may become saturated. In addition, the drug causes induction of the microsomal hepatic enzymes, which can affect the metabolism of other drugs and this, in turn, can modify the metabolism of phenytoin. Thus, the kinetics of the elimination of phenytoin may be complicated.

The side-effects of phenytoin are numerous. However, as the drug has been used extensively and as patients suffering from epilepsy must take drugs over long periods, a high incidence of side-effects is perhaps not surprising. Mild effects are dizziness, nausea, skin rashes, insomnia and gastric disturbances. More serious are nystagmus, ataxia and diplopia, which are probably due to cerebellar malfunction, and they disappear if the drug is withdrawn or the dose reduced. Other side-effects are gingival hyperplasia (although the incidence can be reduced by the use of capsules so that the drug does not come into contact with the mouth), hirsutism, which is an unpleasant side-effect in young female patients, and megaloblastic anaemia. The latter is due to interference with folate metabolism and can be corrected by giving folic acid. Phenytoin has also been reported to cause fetal abnormalities when taken by the mother during pregnancy. Whether or not these are related to folate deficiency is not clear. It is now thought possible that the antifolate action may be involved, in some way, with the anti-epileptic action (see below).

Phenytoin has other therapeutic uses. It has been found to be effective in relieving trigeminal neuralgia and also in the treatment of cardiac arrhythmias. Given intravenously, phenytoin has been used to treat status epilepticus, although it may have a delayed action.

Primidone (Figure 14.3c)

Chemically, primidone is very similar to phenobarbitone, which it also resembles pharmacologically. It is adequately absorbed after oral administration and plasma protein binding is low, but the drug is metabolized to two active metabolites, phenobarbitone and phenylethylmalonamide. It seems likely that the anticonvulsant action is due to the formation of phenobarbitone and that both primidone itself and phenylethylmalonamide are relatively inactive. Thus, the side-effects are mainly those associated with barbiturates and the drug has no particular advantages over phenobarbitone.

Carbamazepine (Figure 14.4a)

This was the first anti-epileptic drug to be developed that is unrelated chemically to the barbiturates. In fact, in structure it resembles the tricyclic antidepressants (see Chapter 17). Its spectrum of activity closely resembles that of phenytoin: it is

(a)

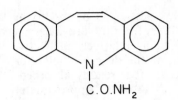

(b)

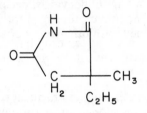

(c)

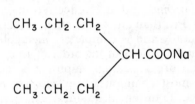

Figure 14.4 The chemical structures of: (a) carbamazepine, (b) ethosuximide and (c) sodium valproate

effective in generalized tonic–clonic seizures and partial seizures but not in *petit mal*, which can be made worse. It is well absorbed and some 70% is bound to plasma proteins. After a single dose the half-life is 30–50 h but with chronic administration this may be as short as 10–20 h, due to induction of enzymes. Only 2% is excreted unchanged, the rest being metabolized in the liver, one of the metabolites having anticonvulsant activity.

Carbamazepine has a higher therapeutic index than phenytoin. Its side-effects include dizziness, drowsiness, dry mouth and blurring of vision, all of which are dose related and can be prevented by reducing the dose and adjusting the timing of medication. With carbamazepine it is essential to initiate therapy with a small dose and to build up the dose over 1–2 weeks. Other side-effects which, although rare, can be more serious are blood dyscrasias such as agranulocytosis, thrombocytopenia and leukopenia, skin rashes and light-sensitive dermatitis. However, these are so rare as to be regarded as idiosyncratic responses.

It is not clear whether carbamazepine, with its tricyclic structure, has any antidepressant action. If so, then this might be an advantage in an anti-epileptic drug, most of which are depressant. Apart from its use in the treatment of epilepsy, it is the drug of choice for trigeminal neuralgia and can be used in combination with phenytoin in refractory cases.

Ethosuximide (Figure 14.4b)

Although this drug is not a barbiturate, it was developed by modifying the ring structure of barbituric acid (Figure 11.2). It differs from the drugs described above in being effective in *petit mal* epilepsy while being relatively ineffective in other types of epilepsy. Ethosuximide was at one time the drug of choice for *petit mal* but has now been replaced by sodium valproate. It is readily absorbed after oral administration and has a plasma half-life of 40–60 h. Approximately 20% is excreted unchanged and the rest is metabolized in the liver to inactive metabolites. The side-effects include gastrointestinal disturbances, drowsiness, dizziness, and ataxia, and are usually transient, occurring only initially. Rashes, liver disorders and haematological disorders, such as leucopenia and agranulocytosis, occur rarely. Ethosuximide can be combined safely with other anticonvulsant drugs for patients with multiple types of seizures, i.e. *petit mal* combined with other types of seizures.

Sodium valproate (Figure 14.4c)

This is a relatively new drug, with a different and much simpler chemical structure compared with other anticonvulsants, and it was developed on a rational basis (see below). It is also unique in being effective against most types of epilepsy; it is the drug of choice in the treatment of *petit mal* and it is effective in infantile spasms. Its mechanism of action is better known than any of the other anti-epileptic drugs. Sodium valproate is well absorbed orally and is completely metabolized in the liver to inactive compounds. The plasma half-life is of the order of 15 h.

Compared with most other anticonvulsant drugs, sodium valproate is relatively non-toxic and has fewer side-effects. The most common side-effects are nausea, vomiting, abdominal cramps and diarrhoea. Transient drowsiness can occur and loss of hair (alopecia) has been reported in about 5% of patients. Prolongation of the bleeding time, due to inhibition of platelet aggregation, and thrombocytopenia have also been observed. A few cases of impaired hepatic function, leading to fatal hepatic failure, have been reported and the drug is contra-indicated where there is any hepatic impairment. It is recommended that liver function should be monitored before and during the first 6 months of therapy.

Benzodiazepines

All the benzodiazepines possess anticonvulsant properties to some degree (see Chapter 13) and a number have been investigated for possible use in the treatment of epilepsy. However, only two, clonazepam (Figure 14.5a) and diazepam (Figure 14.5b), are used extensively. Clonazepam is effective against tonic–clonic seizures and partial seizures but its sedative effects are a disadvantage. It is used to treat *petit mal* epilepsy in children, drowsiness being the main side-effect. Unfortunately, with prolonged use, tolerance can develop to clonazepam and after 6 months some patients no longer respond to the drug. This phenomenon has also been observed with other benzodiazepines. Diazepam, given by slow intravenous injection or intramuscularly, is the drug of choice for interrupting the convulsions of status epilepticus. As it has a short half-life the seizures may return, but the diazepam can be repeated with slow intravenous infusion, or a longer-acting benzodiazepine, such as clonazepam or lorazepam, can be used instead. The main side-effect is depression of respiration, leading to apnoea; hypotension can also occur. Therefore,

(a)

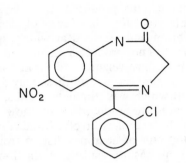

(b)

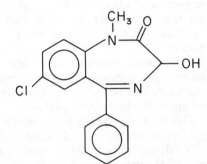

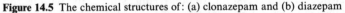

Figure 14.5 The chemical structures of: (a) clonazepam and (b) diazepam

resuscitation facilities must be on hand when these drugs are administered intravenously.

The mechanism of action of anticonvulsant drugs

There are two ways in which drugs can abolish or attentuate seizures: they can act on the pathologically hyperactive neurones directly, to reduce their excessive discharges, or they can prevent the spread of the discharges to other areas, i.e. to neurones which are otherwise normal. Most, if not all, anti-epileptic drugs at present in use appear to act, at least in part, through the second mechanism. However, the variety of chemical structures and pharmacological properties of the drugs makes a single theory for their mechanism of action unlikely and at, present, the mechanism of action of anti-epileptic agents is poorly understood.

Because of the difficulties inherent in analysing the underlying neuronal abnormality in humans, various experimental models of epileptic seizures have been produced in animals. These include the use of convulsant drugs, such as pentylenetetrazol, the application of alumina cream or penicillin to the surface of the cerebral cortex, the application of electric shocks to the brain and the use of genetically susceptible animals such as mice, which produce audiogenic seizures, and baboons, which show fits with intermittent photic stimulation. The usefulness of such models for studying epilepsy and for testing potentially useful anticonvulsant drugs is uncertain, although drugs which block the convulsions induced by pentylenetetrazol are effective in the treatment of *petit mal* epilepsy and drugs which block electrically induced convulsions have been found to be effective in controlling tonic–clonic seizures.

A potentially more informative model, that can be produced in a variety of species of animals, is that of 'kindling'. In this procedure, low levels of electrical stimuli are applied to certain regions of the brain and repeated at widely spaced intervals, e.g. once a day. Initially, the stimulus does not produce a seizure but after-discharges appear and these increase in intensity until seizures are evoked by the low-level stimulation. Ultimately, spontaneous seizures occur and these may appear at sites in the brain which are remote from that which was stimulated. Thus, while the precise mechanism by which 'kindled' seizures are produced is not known, it is clear that adaptive changes have occurred in the neurones involved and, further-more, that these changes have taken place in groups of neurones distant from the site of stimulation, through synaptic connections. Many aspects of the kindling model of epilepsy are congruent with observations made on epileptic patients, e.g. the delay, sometimes of many years, before the appearance of convulsions after a penetrating head wound and the need to remove large amounts of brain tissue in order to excise an epileptic focus due to trauma.

It seems likely that the seizures which occur in most patients with epilepsy begin with, and are sustained by, the synchronous high-frequency discharge of a relatively localized group of neurones. Epileptic attacks can arise from this primary focus (partial seizures), or may emerge from other areas in which functional abnormalities have been induced (generalized seizures). The neurones which comprise the focus from which the original epileptic discharge originates have been found to possess unusual electrical properties. The burst of neuronal activity arises from a sudden large depolarization, termed a 'paroxysmal depolarizing shift', in which the membrane remains depolarized for a few seconds, and which resembles a giant excitatory postsynaptic potential. Electrical events resembling the paroxysmal depolarizing shift have been produced by activation of the subtype of excitatory amino acid receptors which are selective for N-methyl-D-aspartic acid (NMDA) (see Chapter 10 and below).

Although there is as yet no definitive explanation for the production of the paroxysmal discharges in primary epileptic foci, both a reduction in inhibitory influences and stimulation of excitatory influences are likely candidates for involvement: there is evidence for both types of mechanism in the actions of anti-epileptic drugs.

Inhibitory mechanisms

As the principal inhibitory transmitter in the brain, γ-aminobutyric acid (GABA) is most likely to be involved in seizure activity, although other inhibitory substances, such as glycine and taurine, should not be ignored. As far as GABA is concerned, the following facts support its involvement: (1) lowering levels of GABA in the brain results in the appearance of convulsions; (2) convulsant drugs, such as bicucullin, picrotoxin and pentylenetetrazol are GABA antagonists; (3) certain anti-epileptic drugs enhance the synaptic actions of GABA. Thus, barbiturates, such as phenobarbitone, facilitate GABA-mediated synaptic transmission by binding to a site on the GABA receptor, and the benzodiazepines modulate the actions of GABA by binding to the GABA receptor (see Chapters 10, 11 and 13). However, phenobarbitone is more potent as an anticonvulsant than pentobarbitone, although both drugs are equally effective in potentiating the actions of GABA. It is possible that other actions of phenobarbitone may also be important: for example, it has been found to reduce the excitatory effects of glutamate and it may have direct depressant effects on neurones. Finally, sodium valproate, which is unrelated chemically to any of the other anticonvulsant drugs, interacts with the metabolism of GABA in brain. Valproate has been found to increase the level of GABA in the brain without affecting that of other amino acids. It is an inhibitor of the enzymes which inactivate GABA, GABA-transaminase and succinic semialdehyde dehydrogenase (Chapter 10). This action prevents the breakdown of GABA and leads to its accumulation. For some time it was thought that this mechanism was solely responsible for the anticonvulsant action of valproate, but it is now known that the concentrations reached with therapeutic doses would not produce appreciable inhibition of the enzymes. Although the precise mode of action of valproate is not known, it has been found to potentiate responses to GABA and a direct postsynaptic action at GABA receptors has been proposed.

Excitatory mechanisms

The activation of excitatory amino acid receptors by glutamate normally produces a fast excitatory postsynaptic potential (Figure 14.6a). However, of the three subtypes of excitatory amino acid receptors (see Chapter 10), that which is selective for N-methyl-D-aspartate produces long-lasting, burst-like activity similar to a paroxysmal

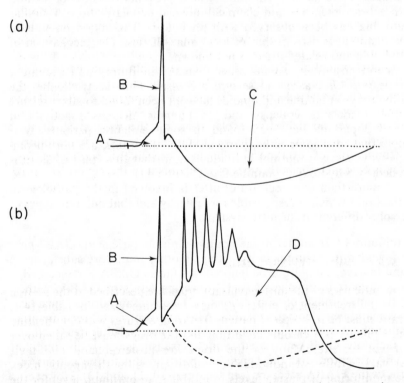

Figure 14.6 (a) A normal synaptic potential evoked by glutamate: A represents the excitatory postsynaptic potential (EPSP), B is the action potential and C is the inhibitory postsynaptic potential (IPSP). (b) Activation of an NMDA receptor by glutamate, with reduced extracellular magnesium concentration: A and B as in (a), but D represents prolonged depolarization, i.e. the paroxysmal depolarizing shift (redrawn from Anderson, 1987)

depolarizing shift, when activated by glutamate in a larger concentration than normal, and with a reduced concentration of magnesium ions (Figure 14.6b). This epileptiform discharge can be blocked with antagonists of N-methyl-D-aspartate, such as 2-amino-5-phosphonovalerate which also shows potent anticonvulsant effects on audiogenic, photogenic, chemically induced and kindled seizures in animals, as well as convulsions due to reduced levels of GABA. The inward membrane current responsible for the paroxysmal depolarizing shift is likely to be due to the movement of sodium and calcium ions and the extracellular concentration of calcium has been found to be reduced in various types of seizures. Furthermore, certain drugs which block calcium channels, e.g. flunarizine (see below), are anticonvulsants. Thus, excitatory as well as inhibitory synaptic mechanisms in the brain are probably important in the generation of seizure activity although, apart from flunarazine, there are no anti-epileptic drugs known to act on these mechanisms.

Other mechanisms

Not all the anti-epileptic drugs fit into the above categories. Thus, phenytoin and carbamazepine have a membrane-stabilizing action. This is due to the blocking of sodium ion channels in the nerve membrane, which prevents the flow of sodium ions during both action potentials and chemical-induced depolarization. A similar effect on calcium flux has been observed with phenytoin. The action on sodium channels can be distinguished from that of local anaesthetics. The mechanism of action of ethosuximide and related drugs is not known.

In addition, neurotransmitter systems other than the inhibitory and excitatory amino acids, appear to have a role in seizure processes. Thus acetylcholine, the monoamines, 5-hydroxytryptamine and opioids have all been found to affect seizure activity in animal models of epilepsy and, in humans, decreased activity of noradrenaline and dopamine has been found in some epileptic patients. It is interesting to note that myoclonic jerks, particularly of the limbs, are not uncommon during slow-wave sleep in normal individuals, and that this stage of sleep is probably controlled by 5-hydroxytryptamine (see Chapter 11).

It is likely that more than one neurotransmitter is involved in the pathological disturbance of the brain which is responsible for epilepsy and that different types of epilepsy may involve different transmitter systems.

The clinical uses of anticonvulsant drugs

Most of the therapeutic uses of the anticonvulsant drugs are described in the section on 'Drugs used in the treatment of epilepsy'; they are summarized in Table 14.1. The aim of therapy must be to keep the patient free from seizures without affecting normal function. Epilepsy is a chronic condition and the drugs must be taken over long periods, if not for life. Many of the drugs are protein-bound and their metabolism may vary in different individuals; in addition, as the therapeutic index may be low, the monitoring of plasma levels to establish an optimum level for the therapeutic effect is important and may help to avoid the incidence of unwanted side-effects. If the first drug prescribed fails to provide adequate control of the seizures in the maximum tolerated dose, then another drug may be substituted, but more often a second drug is added. This is known as polytherapy, which is now

Table 14.1 Drugs used in the treatment of epilepsy

Type of seizure	Drug
Partial	
Simple	Phenytoin
	Carbamazepine
	Valproate
Complex	Phenytoin
	Carbamazepine
	Phenobarbitone
	Valproate
Generalized seizures	
Absence (*Petit mal*)	Ethosuximide
	Valproate
Tonic–clonic (*Grand mal*)	Phenobarbitone
	Phenytoin
	Carbamazepine
	Valproate
Myoclonic attacks	Clonazepam
	Valproate
Infantile spasms	ACTH
	Clonazepam
	Valproate
Status epilepticus	Diazepam
	Clonazepam

regarded as undesirable and to be avoided if possible. Toxic effects may be enhanced rather than reduced in combinations of drugs and interactions may occur due to induction of liver enzymes, etc.

Little reference has been made above to infantile spasms. This is because treatment with adrenocorticotrophic hormone (ACTH, corticotropin) is often more effective than conventional anti-epileptic drugs. Benzodiazepines, such as clonazepam or valproate, can be used in infantile spasms which are refractory to treatment with ACTH.

New types of anticonvulsant drugs

In recent years, new drugs with anticonvulsant properties have been developed which may provide some different pharmacological approaches to the treatment of epilepsy. To some extent the new developments have been based on knowledge of the mechanism of action of existing drugs. For example, the increasingly important role of GABA in seizure mechanisms, the evidence for which has been outlined above, has led to the testing of drugs which modify GABA transmission as possible anti-epileptic agents.

Drugs which modify GABA-mediated neurotransmission

Increasing the amount of GABA available for synaptic transmission can be accomplished in a number of different ways:

1. By administering a GABA agonist, such as muscimol (Figure 10.17b). However, this drug is too toxic to be used clinically.

(a)

$$N.CH_2.CH_2.CH_2.\overset{\overset{O}{\|}}{C}.NH_2$$

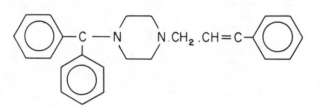

(b)

$$CH_2=CH.NH.CH_2.CH_2.CH_2.COOH$$

(c)

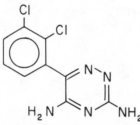

$$N.CH_2.CH=C$$

(d)

Figure 14.7 The chemical structures of: (a) progabide, (b) γ-vinyl-GABA, (c) flunarizine and (d) lamotrigine

2. By using a pro-drug which crosses the blood–brain barrier and is then converted to GABA. Such a compound is progabide (Figure 14.7a) which has an anticonvulsant potency equivalent to that of valproate. It has been found to be effective in controlling both partial and generalized seizures, but side-effects, such as drowsiness, dizziness and headache, have been reported.
3. Inhibition of the metabolism of GABA. Drugs which have this action include sodium valproate and γ-vinyl-GABA (Figure 14.7b), which inhibit GABA-transaminase by acting as a substrate for the enzyme. γ-Vinyl-GABA has an interesting profile of anticonvulsant activity, being effective against audiogenic and photically induced seizures, as well as against seizures induced by electric

shock, but less effective against seizures produced by bicuculline and picro-toxin, and the anticonvulsant effects do not always correlate with the level of GABA in the brain. However, it has been found to be effective in clinical trials in patients with partial seizures. Drowsiness and dizziness are the main side-effects.

Calcium ions

Calcium ions are known to have an important role in neuronal excitability. The voltage-dependent entry of calcium ions into nerve terminals is an important mechanism for the release of neurotransmitters (see Chapters 3 and 10) and the influx of calcium is also important in the generation of the paroxysmal depolarizing shift. Thus, drugs which block the entry of calcium through membranes, i.e. calcium channel blockers, while having other applications, may be considered as putative anticonvulsants. Most calcium-channel blockers do not cross the blood–brain barrier, but flunarizine (Figure 14.7c) is active in the CNS. The drug has antihypoxic properties and has been used in the treatment of migraine. It is effective as an anticonvulsant in various animal models of epilepsy with a similar profile of activity to phenytoin and carbamazepine. In clinical trials in which it was used to supplement existing therapy, flunarazine was found to be effective in generalized epilepsy in children, which had been resistant to the existing therapy. Few side-effects have been reported. However, trials in epileptics in which flunarazine is the sole medication are needed to demonstrate the effectiveness of this drug as an anti-epileptic.

Folic acid metabolism

Many anti-epileptic drugs interfere with the metabolism of folic acid, which is pteroylglutamic acid, although it has generally been assumed that this action is more likely to be responsible for side-effects than for the anticonvulsant action. However, folic acid, in large amounts, has been shown to counteract the anticon-vulsant effects of phenobarbitone, primidone and phenytoin and to increase the frequency of seizures in susceptible children. On this basis, compounds with antifolate actions have been screened as possible anticonvulsants and the drug lamotrigine (Figure 14.7d) has emerged. It has a high profile of anticonvulsant activity, similar to that of phenytoin and carbamazepine, but is more potent. So far, clinical trials with lamotrigine suggest that it controls partial and generalized seizures, but with drowsiness, ataxia, dizziness and headache as side-effects. It has also been found that lamotrigine inhibits the release of the excitatory neuro-transmitter glutamate, and this action may provide the main basis for its anticonvulsant activity, rather than inhibition of folic acid metabolism. However, this is an interesting area for future development and research.

Chapter 15

Analgesic drugs

Pain is an unpleasant experience which, because it is subjective, cannot be accurately defined, although the physiological responses associated with pain can be recorded and measured. It can be elicited by noxious stimuli in normal individuals, in which case it acts as a warning of impending damage to tissues, or it may indicate that damage has already occurred, e.g. in trauma. Pain is, of course, the outstanding symptom in many diseases. By drawing attention to potential danger, pain produces a protective response, e.g. the rapid reflex withdrawal of a limb in response to a pin-prick, a blow, or contact with a hot object, to limit the damage. Thus, persons who lack pain sensation are prone to burns and other injuries. Pain may also lead to appropriate action being taken to deal with certain pathological states and can be helpful in the diagnosis of disease. However, the protective value of pain is limited, as postoperative pain and the chronic pain associated with malignant disease appear to serve no useful purpose. Furthermore, some noxious agencies such as ultraviolet light and radiation, both of which can cause tissue damage, do not evoke pain at the time of exposure.

Free nerve endings have been identified as pain receptors in pain-sensitive tissues, e.g. skin, muscles and viscera. There is reason to believe that other types of sensory receptors may also take part in the detection and transmission of pain impulses and that intense stimulation of these can generate pain reactions. The peripheral afferent nerves which carry pain impulses are of small diameter and include myelinated A-delta fibres, which cause the sensation of sharp, localized pain, and unmyelinated C fibres, which are slower conducting and cause dull, burning pain. Most nociceptive receptors at the terminals of C fibres are polymodal receptors, i.e. they respond to different modalities of noxious stimulation. The cell bodies of the spinal nociceptive afferent fibres are in the dorsal ganglia and the fibres enter the spinal cord through the dorsal roots and terminate in the grey matter of the spinal cord, the substantia gelatinosa of the dorsal horn. The terminals of the primary afferent pain fibres in the dorsal horn of the spinal cord release substance P as their neurotransmitter (see Chapter 10 and Figure 10.22). The second-order neurones in the spinal cord give rise to ascending fibres, most of which cross the cord to form the contralateral ascending spinothalamic tract which projects to various sites in the brain. This pathway is polysynaptic and relays in the reticular formation of the brain stem before passing to the ventral and medial thalamus and thence to the sensory cortex. The pathway also connects with the limbic system and the hypothalamus where emotional responses and reactions of the autonomic nervous system can be evoked. The pain pathway is shown

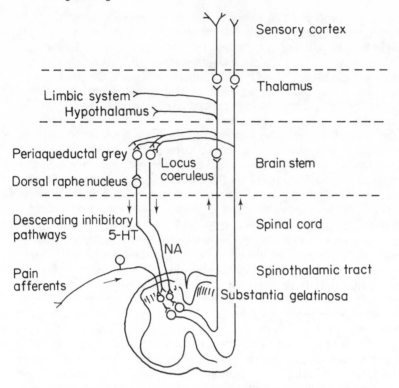

Figure 15.1 Simplified diagrammatic representation of the main neuronal pathways involved in the transmission of pain. NA, noradrenaline; 5-HT, 5-hydroxytryptamine

diagrammatically, in simplified form, in Figure 15.1. The first-order, primary afferent neurones (A-delta and nociceptor C fibres), as well as the second-order neurones of the spinothalamic tract, show specificity for noxious stimuli. In fact, sectioning of the spinothalamic tract abolishes pain from the lower part of the body. From the brain stem upwards, there is less specificity.

There is also a descending pathway which is involved in pain sensation. This is a polysynaptic pathway which arises from the periaqueductal grey matter of the midbrain, a small area surrounding the central canal; it passes through the dorsal raphe nucleus in the medulla and then in the dorsolateral funiculus in the spinal cord to terminate in the dorsal horn. This pathway also receives connections from other regions of the brain (Figure 15.1). The function of the descending pathway is mainly inhibitory, as electrical stimulation of either the periaqueductal grey or the dorsal raphe nucleus in experimental animals produces analgesia which outlasts the stimulus and, in patients with chronic pain, the analgesia resulting from electrical stimulation of these regions can last for 20 h. Analgesia can also be produced by the local injection of morphine into the region of the periaqueductal grey matter and this effect is reversed by the opiate antagonist, naloxone. The neurotransmitter released by the terminals of the descending pathway is 5-hydroxytryptamine. Opiate receptors and opioid peptides, particularly enkephalins (see Chapter 10 and below), are concentrated in the dorsal horn of the spinal cord, the periaqueductal grey matter and in the thalamus and it is thought that the enkephalins may function as neurotransmitters in these regions.

In some cases pain can be alleviated by removing the cause. Thus, the pain of peptic ulcer is relieved by antacids and that of angina pectoris by glyceryl trinitrate. Similarly, migraine is treated with vasoactive substances such as ergotamine, although analgesics are also used, and the pain of trigeminal neuralgia can be relieved with carbamazepine. Analgesic drugs relieve pain irrespective of its cause, i.e. they ameliorate the sensation of pain itself. They are useful in removing discomfort while the normal recuperative processes of the body continue to work or while other more specific measures are taken to correct the underlying cause. However, the indiscriminate use of analgesics can be dangerous, particularly if the sense of well-being they may induce prevents the patient from seeking treatment. There are two main types of analgesic drugs: (1) those used to relieve severe or deep pain, such as the pain originating in the viscera, or pain associated with trauma, e.g. postoperative pain, burns, etc, the prototype drug being morphine; (2) mild or moderate pain such as musculoskeletal pain, headache, etc, the prototype drug being aspirin. The drugs in this category, i.e. the 'weak' analgesics, also have other important actions: they show anti-inflammatory and antipyretic actions. The local anaesthetic drugs (Chapter 9) may be considered to be a third type of analgesic, but the relief of pain in this case is produced by virtue of the route of administration, rather than the mechanism of action of the drug.

Opioid analgesics

The term 'opioid' applies to any substance which has agonist activity at opiate receptors (see Chapter 10). It includes not only morphine and related drugs but also peptides. These drugs are also known as 'narcotic' analgesics because of their ability to produce dependence and addiction. Unfortunately, misuse of the term 'narcotic' by applying it to drugs which do not cause narcosis, i.e. generalized depression of the CNS resulting in stupor (see Chapter 11), has caused confusion.

Opioid agonists

Morphine

This is not only the prototype analgesic drug but probably the most widely used and also the first to be used therapeutically (see Introduction). It is an alkaloid (Figure 15.2a) which is present in the seeds of the opium poppy, *Papaver somniferum*. Opium, a word derived from the Greek name for juice, is an extract of the unripe seed capsules. However, opium contains many other alkaloids besides morphine, including codeine, papaverine, thebaine and noscapine. Papaverine has a relaxant action on smooth muscle and noscapine is used as an antitussive (see Chapter 20); thebaine is almost inactive as an analgesic and has no medicinal uses. Pure morphine was isolated from opium by a German pharmacist, Setürner, in 1803; its chemical structure was subsequently determined and a great many related substances were synthesized and tested for analgesic activity. Some of these are used as analgesics but there are also synthetic analgesics which are structurally unrelated to morphine.

(a)

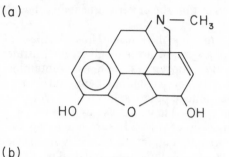

(b)

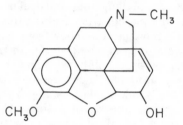

Figure 15.2 The chemical structures of (a) morphine and (b) codeine

Morphine is effective against all types of pain, although it is normally only used to relieve severe pain. There are two components to its action: it reduces the sensation of pain and it also affects the reaction to pain, i.e. the affective response. Both of these components are thought to be important as many patients treated with morphine report that they are still aware of the pain but are no longer troubled by it. The direct action of morphine, and probably of most other opiate analgesics, on the sensation of pain appears to be specific as other sensory systems, including vision, hearing and touch, etc., are unaffected. Besides analgesia, the mechanism for which is described below, morphine has a number of other pharmacological actions, some of which are central and others peripheral. In therapeutic doses, morphine produces sedation and drowsiness, although this is not as marked as with sedative–hypnotic drugs (Chapter 11) and the patient, although drowsy, can still be easily roused. However, large doses of morphine can cause excitement and even convulsions. Morphine also produces a feeling of contentment and well-being or euphoria and this action undoubtedly contributes to its abuse potential (see Chapter 18). It seems probable that both the drowsiness and the euphoria contribute to the analgesic action, especially the reaction to pain. Morphine also produces depression of respiration by a direct action on the respiratory centre in the pons and medulla and this occurs with normal therapeutic doses. This is due to a reduced responsiveness of the respiratory centre to increases in CO_2 tension. The respiratory depression increases with dose and is the usual cause of death from overdose. There is also an antitussive action (see below and Chapter 20) and, at one time, morphine was a constituent of cough mixtures. Morphine also produces nausea and vomiting. This effect is more prominent initially and may subside if therapy with morphine is continued.

The most important peripheral actions of morphine are on the gastrointestinal tract. The resting tone of the smooth muscle of the stomach and the small and large intestines is increased, resulting in decreased motility. Peristaltic contractions are reduced and this results in slower passage of material through the intestines and increased reabsorption of water from the contents of the bowel, leading to constipation, which can be severe. Morphine also causes spasm of the smooth muscle of the biliary tract, which results in increased pressure and epigastric distress resembling biliary colic. In normal therapeutic doses morphine has little direct effect on the cardiovascular system, but large doses can cause hypotension and bradycardia due to the action of the drug on the medulla. Morphine also causes miosis due to a stimulant action on the nucleus of the oculomotor nucleus, and 'pin-point' pupils are a characteristic diagnostic feature of morphine overdose. One of the most characteristic properties of morphine is its ability to produce tolerance and dependence, leading to addiction. This is discussed below.

Morphine is readily absorbed from the GI tract and also from other tissues, such as the nasal mucosa and lung when opium is smoked. The absorption from the gut can be variable and a significant amount fails to reach the general circulation due to the first-pass effect as the drug is metabolized in the liver. Morphine is therefore rarely given orally but is usually administered intramuscularly or, for a very rapid action, intravenously. It is mainly metabolized in the liver and excreted as inactive glucuronides. When morphine is administered by a route which avoids the bloodstream, e.g. intrathecally (see Chapter 9), it is effective in much smaller doses than are needed systemically and the side-effects are less pronounced.

Other opium alkaloids

Morphine is a phenanthrene derivative, related opioid alkaloids being thebaine, which lacks significant analgesic activity, and codeine, both of which are present in opium. Codeine (Figure 15.2b) which is methylmorphine, is a much less potent analgesic than morphine but is effective when administered by mouth. It does not cause euphoria, is not addictive and does not cause appreciable respiratory depression. Because of its low potency, it is used to treat mild pain, such as headache. Like morphine, it has an antitussive action and it causes constipation.

Drugs derived from morphine

These are synthetic or semisynthetic compounds and include the opioid antagonists (see pages 257–258).

HEROIN (Figure 15.3a)

This is diacetylmorphine, or diamorphine, which is made from morphine. It is more potent than morphine but this is probably due to the fact that it is more lipid soluble and therefore penetrates into the CNS more readily; however, heroin is converted to morphine in the body. It is more likely to produce euphoria and addiction than morphine but causes relatively less nausea and constipation. Heroin appears to have little advantage over morphine except, perhaps, that the greater solubility allows effective amounts to be injected in smaller volumes and this can be an advantage in relieving severe pain in terminal cancer. However, the drug is more popular than morphine as a drug of abuse (see Chapter 18) and for this reason its manufacture is banned in many countries.

(a)

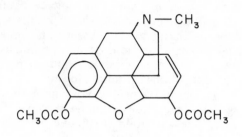

(b)

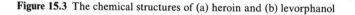

HO

Figure 15.3 The chemical structures of (a) heroin and (b) levorphanol

LEVORPHANOL (Figure 15.3b)

This drug resembles morphine in many ways but it is more potent as an analgesic and respiratory depressant; it has less sedative activity and is longer acting than morphine. It is used for the relief of severe pain in patients where the lack of sedation is an advantage.

Analgesics unrelated to morphine

This group includes a number of synthetic compounds with varying chemical structures.

PETHIDINE (Figure 15.4a)

This drug, a phenylpiperidine derivative, is known as meperidine in the United States. It resembles both morphine and atropine in its pharmacological properties. It has about one-tenth the analgesic potency of morphine but in equivalent doses produces the same degree of analgesia, sedation and respiratory depression; it also produces euphoria. However, pethidine has no antitussive action and it does not constrict the pupil or cause constipation, as it has less spasmogenic action. The antimuscarinic properties can cause dry mouth and blurring of vision. Pethidine has a shorter duration of action than morphine. It is demethylated in the liver to norpethidine, which has excitatory effects (see below); the norpethidine is subsequently conjugated and excreted.

(a)

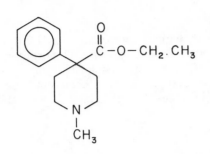

(b)

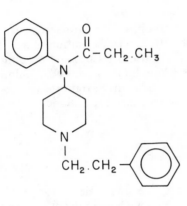

(c)

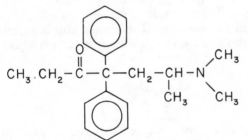

(d)

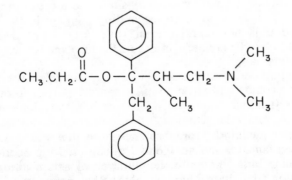

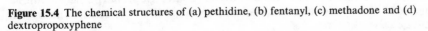

Figure 15.4 The chemical structures of (a) pethidine, (b) fentanyl, (c) methadone and (d) dextropropoxyphene

FENTANYL (Figure 15.4b)

This is also a phenylpiperidine derivative which is approximately 80 times more potent than morphine. Its actions are very similar to those of morphine but the duration of action is much shorter, the half-life in plasma being of the order of 20 min. The main use for fentanyl is in anaesthesia, e.g. in neuroleptanalgesia (see Chapter 11). Related compounds have been made, e.g. lofentanyl and sufentanyl, with even greater analgesic potency.

METHADONE (Figure 15.4c)

This represents another chemically distinct group, with pharmacological properties and potency very similar to morphine but with a longer duration of action and less sedation. Methadone is bound to proteins in various tissues and accumulates with repeated administration. Slow release from these binding sites when administration of the drug is discontinued results in a milder abstinence syndrome than occurs with morphine and other opioid analgesics. Because of this, methadone has been used for treating morphine and heroin addicts.

DEXTROPROPOXYPHENE (Figure 15.4d)

Propoxyphene exists in two isomeric forms, the analgesic action residing in the dextrorotatory isomer, although laevopropoxyphene has some antitussive activity. It is structurally related to methadone but resembles codeine in its actions, although it is less potent. It is therefore used for the relief of mild pain and is effective by the oral route. It is also used in combination with other analgesics such as paracetamol or aspirin (see below).

PENTAZOCINE (Figure 15.5a)

This is a benzomorphan derivative which was synthesized in attempts to find analgesic drugs without abuse potential. It has both opioid agonist and also weak antagonist actions. In small doses its actions are very similar to those of morphine, but as the dose is increased there is not a corresponding increase in the effects. Thus, respiratory depression is not marked even with large doses. However, hallucinations and psychotic-like behaviour can occur. Pentazocine is used mainly for the treatment of moderate pain.

BUPRENORPHINE (Figure 15.5b)

A semisynthetic derivative of thebaine, buprenorphine is a relatively new analgesic which appears to have both agonist and antagonist properties. Its properties are similar to those of morphine but it has a longer duration of action and can be administered parenterally and by the sublingual route. Buprenorphine is unique among the opioid analgesics in that its effects are not fully reversed by the opioid antagonist, naloxone.

(a)

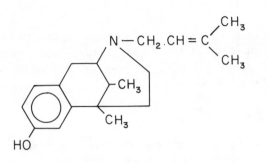

(b)

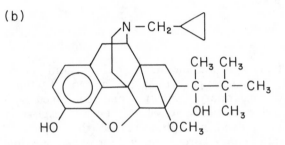

(c)

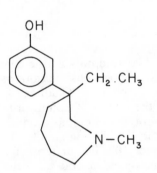

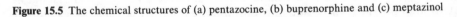

Figure 15.5 The chemical structures of (a) pentazocine, (b) buprenorphine and (c) meptazinol

MEPTAZINOL (Figure 15.5c)

This is another relatively new opioid analgesic with agonist and antagonist properties. It is less potent than morphine but it is claimed that there is a reduced incidence of respiratory depression. However, nausea and vomiting can occur.

Opioid antagonists

These drugs have no overt actions of their own but reverse the actions of opioid agonists and are therefore useful in treating the effects of overdose, particularly respiratory depression.

Naloxone (Figure 15.6a)

This is a synthetic substance which is a pure competitive opioid antagonist and is effective at all three subtypes of opiate receptor (see Chapter 10). Given on its own it is virtually devoid of activity, but it promptly reverses the actions of opioid agonists such as morphine and related analgesics.

Naltrexone (Figure 15.6b)

This is similar to naloxone in its actions but is more potent, has a longer duration of action and, unlike naloxone, is effective by the oral route. It has been used to block the euphoric effects of opioids in addicts.

Nalorphine (Figure 15.6c)

This is structurally related to morphine and was the first opioid antagonist to be discovered, but it is not a pure antagonist and appears to have some agonist actions. Thus, nalorphine can produce mild respiratory depression and, combined with small doses of morphine and related compounds, it will deepen the respiratory depression they produce. On the other hand, nalorphine reduces the respiratory depression produced by large doses of the opioid drugs. Nalorphine was at one time used to treat overdose with opioid drugs but has now been replaced by naloxone.

The mechanism of action of opioid analgesics

Opioid agonists and antagonists have their own receptors in the central nervous system, i.e. opioid receptors at which the endogenous neurotransmitters are peptides, either leu- or met-enkephalin or β-endorphin (see Chapter 10). Actions on these receptors mediate most, if not all, of the effects of opioid drugs, including analgesia. However, there are at least three subtypes of opioid receptors which can be distinguished both pharmacologically and in the binding affinity of opioid drugs (these are described in more detail in Chapter 10). The actions of a number of opioid agonists and antagonists, including the opioid peptides, on the three main receptor subtypes, μ-, δ- and κ- are summarized in Table 15.1. Thus the analgesic drugs that are opioid agonists, such as morphine, pethidine, codeine and fentanyl, act mainly on μ-receptors, which mediate supraspinal analgesia, respiratory depression, miosis, euphoria and physical dependence. They also have some effects on κ-receptors which mediate spinal analgesia, sedation and miosis, and slight effects on δ-receptors which are also thought to be involved in sedation. Pentazocine, which has mixed agonist–antagonist actions, has its main agonist activity at κ-receptors and possibly some agonist activity on δ-receptors but it is an antagonist at μ-receptors. The opioid antagonist naloxone is a competitive antagonist at all three receptor subtypes, but is more potent at μ- than at κ- or δ-receptors. Of the opioid peptides, met- and leu-enkephalin are most active at δ-receptors, with some activity at μ-receptors where met-enkephalin is more potent than leu-; they are inactive at κ-receptors. β-Endorphin also has greater activity at μ- and δ-receptors, while dynorphin is more active at κ- than at μ- or δ-receptors.

   The opioid peptides and their receptors are present in those regions of the central nervous system known to be involved in the transmission of pain. For example, μ-

(a)

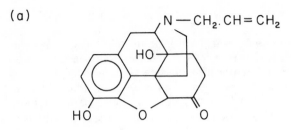

(b)

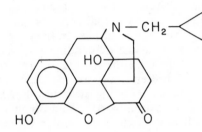

(c)

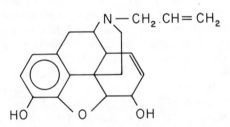

Figure 15.6 The chemical structures of (a) naloxone, (b) naltrexone and (c) nalorphine

Table 15.1 Actions of drugs and peptides at opioid receptors

Compound	Action	Receptor subtype		
		μ	δ	κ
Morphine	Agonist	+++	+	++
Codeine	Agonist	+	+	+
Pethidine	Agonist	++	+	+
Fentanyl	Agonist	++++	++	++
Met-enkephalin	Agonist	++	+++	0
Leu-enkephalin	Agonist	+	+++	0
Naloxone	Antagonist	+++	++	++
Nalorphine	Mixed	Ant	pAg	pAg
Pentazocine	Mixed	Ant	Ag	Ag
Buprenorphine	Mixed	pAg	–	–

Ag = agonist; Ant = competitive antagonist; pAg = partial agonist. The
potency is represented by the number of +; 0, inactive; –, not known

receptors are present on the terminals of primary afferent fibres in the dorsal horn of the spinal cord which release substance P. These presynaptic receptors are activated by enkephalin which is released from the terminals of interneurones (see Chapter 10 and Figure 10.22). This action reduces the release of substance P from the primary afferent terminals, so reducing the transmission of pain. Morphine and related analgesic drugs act on the same receptors, thus mimicking the effects of enkephalin; this is thought to be the basis for the reduction of the sensation of pain. The precise role of κ-receptors, which mediate analgesia in the spinal cord to a greater degree than μ-receptors, is not clear.

Opioids and opioid receptors are also present in the brain stem, in the periaqueductal grey matter and the dorsal raphe nucleus nuclei (Figure 15.1). The action of morphine and of other analgesic drugs on opioid receptors in the brain stem helps to explain the modulation of the perception of pain in the CNS by these drugs. An action in this region will also activate the descending pathway which projects to the dorsal horn, probably to the enkephalinergic interneurones, so influencing the transmission of pain. The presence of opioid receptors in the medulla explains some of the other central effects of analgesic drugs. For example, the respiratory depression and the antitussive action are due to a direct action on the relevant centres in the brain stem. However, while depression of respiration appears to be mediated by μ-receptors, it seems likely that these are distinct from the μ-receptors which mediate analgesia. Thus, the receptors responsible for producing analgesia have been designated μ_1- and those associated with respiratory depression, μ_2-. A selective μ_1-agonist, if such a compound could be developed, might produce analgesia without depression of respiration. It must not be forgotten, however, that both δ- and κ-receptors are also involved in respiratory depression. The nausea and vomiting produced by opioid analgesics is due to an action on the vomiting centre in the medulla (see Chapter 20) and the miosis is due to an excitant action on the nucleus of the oculomotor nerve. The pupillary effects of morphine vary in different species, miosis occurring in dog and man and mydriasis in the cat and monkey.

The mechanism by which euphoria is produced by analgesic drugs is not clear, although δ-receptors in the hippocampus have been suggested as being responsible. The ability of opioid analgesics to produce euphoria varies and some drugs, in large doses, produce dysphoria which is characterized by anxiety. The mechanism for this is not known. The peripheral actions of morphine, e.g. on the GI tract, are due mainly to a local action. Thus morphine acts presynaptically to reduce the release of acetylcholine and this action can account, at least in part, for the effect on smooth muscle. However, the participation of a central mechanism cannot be ruled out because the injection of small quantities of morphine into the cerebral ventricles has been shown to reduce peristaltic movements.

The modulation of the release of other neurotransmitters by the presynaptic action of opioid peptides and drugs has already been referred to. The presence of opioid receptors in tissues containing other transmitters suggests the possibility of other sites for interaction. The locus coeruleus contains noradrenergic neurones and opioid receptors, activation of which inhibits noradrenergic activity and an interaction with histamine has also been demonstrated.

At the cellular level, morphine has been shown to increase the intracellular concentration of calcium, thereby increasing potassium conductance, resulting in hyperpolarization of the cell. Whether the decreased membrane excitability which ensues would be sufficient to reduce the release of transmitter from presynaptic terminals is not known. Opioid drugs also alter the levels of cyclic AMP in the brain by inhibiting the activity of adenylate cyclase. Thus, the level of cyclic AMP is reduced and the stimulant action of catecholamines and prostaglandins on the formation of cyclic AMP is blocked. This action is more likely to be associated with a postsynaptic than a presynaptic action and it has been found that μ-receptors, rather than δ-receptors, are coupled to adenylate cyclase. Mechanisms of this type could be involved in the development of tolerance and dependence (see below).

The clinical uses of opioid drugs

Most of these have already been discussed under the relevant drugs. Thus, morphine, heroin, pethidine, buprenorphine and meptazinol are used for the relief of severe pain. Methadone and levorphanol are also effective against severe pain but are less sedative and longer acting. Codeine, pentazocine and dextropropoxyphene are less potent and are used to treat mild to moderate pain. Mixtures of opium alkaloids, such as papaveretum which is a mixture of morphine, codeine, noscapine and papaverine, are sometimes used but probably have no advantage over morphine alone. Before the invention of the hypodermic needle, a hydroalcoholic solution or tincture of opium, known as laudanum, was used for oral administration. Another tincture of opium with camphor added was paregoric, which was used for the treatment of diarrhoea; morphine, mixed with kaolin, can still be used for this purpose. Morphine was at one time also a constituent of cough mixtures but other antitussive drugs, such as codeine or noscapine, are preferred as they are less likely to result in misuse.

The main adverse and side-effects of the opioid analgesics have already been referred to. These include nausea and vomiting, sedation, depression of respiration, constipation, tolerance and dependence leading to addiction. In addition, urinary retention, bronchoconstriction due to the release of histamine, and hypotension can sometimes occur. The sedation is not always undesirable but can be avoided by using a less sedative drug such as methadone or levorphanol. Alternatively, it has been claimed that the combination of an opioid with a small dose of amphetamine may augment the analgesia while reducing the sedation. The nausea and vomiting can be avoided by combining the analgesic with an anti-emetic drug. Respiratory depression appears with therapeutic doses of morphine and this drug is contra-indicated in cases of impaired pulmonary function. The respiratory depression can be serious in acute overdose or poisoning. The patient is likely to be asleep or stuporous or, if the overdose is large, in coma. The triad of symptoms, namely, coma, pin-point pupils and depressed respiration, is characteristic of opiate poisoning. The opioid antagonist naloxone, given subcutaneously, intramuscularly or intravenously, rapidly reverses the respiratory depression; it is short acting but the injection may be repeated or naloxone may be given by continuous intravenous infusion. The partial agonist nalorphine was at one time used to treat opiate overdose but it can cause further depression of respiration, because of its agonist activity, if the poisoning is due to drugs other than opioids, i.e. barbiturates or alcohol, or to a mixture of drugs. As naloxone has no agonist activity, it is the drug of choice. Large doses of pethidine can result in excitatory symptoms such as tremors, muscle twitches, dilated pupils, hyperactive reflexes and even convulsions. These effects are due to the formation of the metabolite norpethidine, which is excitatory and will accumulate after the ingestion of large doses of pethidine. The excitant effects of pethidine overdose are reversed by naloxone.

Tolerance to and dependence on opioid drugs

Tolerance

In many cases, when a drug is taken repeatedly it becomes progressively less effective and the dose has to be increased in order to maintain the desired effect. This is known as the development of tolerance to the drug and is due to adaptive changes taking place. These changes may occur at the level of the receptor, e.g. up- or down-regulation, or they may be due to increased metabolism of the drug due to enzyme induction, or to increased activity of compensatory reflex mechanisms, i.e. feedback mechanisms. When tolerance has developed to the effects of one drug but is also present for other drugs, usually with similar pharmacological properties, this is known as cross-tolerance and can be due to the drugs acting on the same receptor.

Dependence

If, after tolerance has developed to the effects of a drug, its administration is stopped, i.e. the drug is withdrawn, there may be no untoward effects. However, with many drugs unpleasant withdrawal symptoms occur, in which case the drug has produced dependence. The pattern of withdrawal symptoms is known as the abstinence syndrome. When the symptoms of withdrawal are clearly attributable to physiological changes, as is the case with the opioid analgesics (see below), the dependence is physical. There are drugs that do not cause physical dependence but produce a compulsion to continue using the drug. This phenomenon is known as psychological dependence and, as it is particularly relevant to drug abuse, it is discussed in more detail in Chapter 18.

All the opioid analgesic drugs produce tolerance and physical dependence to a greater or lesser extent. Tolerance occurs to most of the pharmacological effects of morphine, including the analgesia, respiratory depression and euphoria. However, there is less tolerance to certain effects, e.g. miosis and constipation. Thus, addicts consuming large amounts of morphine or heroin may show little respiratory depression but marked pupillary constriction. Tolerance develops more quickly when large doses are given at frequent intervals. In humans, with normal therapeutic doses, although the development of tolerance will begin after the first dose, it usually does not become clinically apparent until after 2–3 weeks. In experimental animals, signs of tolerance can be detected within 24 h. Tolerance is marked with the μ-agonist analgesics and is less marked with agonist–antagonist drugs; it does not occur at all with pure antagonists.

Withdrawal signs appear within 8–12 h of the last dose of morphine or heroin and the effects peak at 36–48 h, after which they subside and have usually disappeared within 5 days, although some may persist for months. The abstinence syndrome consists initially of lachrymation, rhinorrhoea (running eyes and nose), sweating and yawning. After this there is a period of restlessness and additional symptoms appear, including mydriasis, anorexia, gooseflesh, nausea, diarrhoea and insomnia. The restlessness may be accompanied by feelings of anxiety and hostility. The abstinence syndrome can be interrupted by the administration of a suitable dose of morphine or heroin, or by a different opioid analgesic, as these show cross-tolerance. However, administration of the antagonist naloxone to a subject who is physically dependent on an opioid drug will precipitate the abstinence syndrome in an explosive form. This occurs within 5 minutes of the administration of the antagonist, peaking at 10–20 min and largely subsiding after about an hour.

Although the abstinence syndrome which appears following withdrawal of an opioid analgesic such as morphine or heroin is extremely unpleasant, it is not usually life-threatening as is the case with barbiturate drugs (see Chapter 11).

All the opioid analgesics show tolerance, physical dependence and also cross-tolerance, but there is some variation between the different drugs. Thus, the effects of codeine, although qualitatively similar to those of morphine, are considerably less intense and tolerance and dependence rarely occur. Pethidine, also being less potent than morphine, produces less tolerance and dependence and, as it is shorter acting, the withdrawal syndrome subsides more quickly, usually within 24 h. On the other hand, in the case of methadone the abstinence syndrome may take longer to develop and it subsides more slowly, e.g. taking up to 2 weeks. It is also less intense and therefore less unpleasant. For this reason, methadone has been used to treat addicts by substituting methadone for morphine or heroin and withdrawing the drug by gradually reducing the dose consumed. An advantage of this treatment is that the methadone can be given in a single daily dose, by mouth.

The opioids, as they are lipid soluble, readily pass through the placenta into the fetus and babies born to mothers who are addicted can show withdrawal symptoms unless treated. In the fetus, the abstinence syndrome can be fatal. In addition, respiratory depression can be greater in the newborn than in the adult if morphine is administered to a pregnant woman before delivery.

The mechanisms through which tolerance and dependence are produced by the opioid analgesics are not known. However, tolerance to morphine has been demonstrated in isolated tissue preparations in vitro and it is therefore thought that the mechanism is probably related to changes at the level of the receptor rather than in the activity of metabolizing enzymes, for example. Morphine has been shown to produce changes in the activity of the enzyme adenylate cyclase in cell cultures, resulting in the formation of altered amounts of the second messenger, cyclic AMP. This provides a possible basis for mechanisms of tolerance and dependence.

Non-opioid analgesics

These drugs, also known as non-narcotic analgesics, of which aspirin is the prototype, have important actions other than being weak analgesics. Thus they are antipyretic and many of them also have an anti-inflammatory action. In fact, the latter is an important application for this group of drugs, which are also known as non-steroidal anti-inflammatory drugs (or NSAIDs). Their analgesic action is relatively weak and they are ineffective for the relief of severe pain, even when given in large doses. They are therefore used to treat mild pain such as headache, toothache and the pain of dysmenorrhoea.

Salicylates and related substances

Aspirin is acetylsalicylic acid (Figure 15.7a) and is a synthetic salicylate. Naturally occurring salicylates with analgesic and antipyretic properties are salicin, present in the bark of the willow tree, and methylsalicylate (Figure 15.7b), which is found in oil of wintergreen. They are all derivatives of salicylic acid (Figure 15.7c). Other derivatives which are used as analgesics are sodium salicylate (Figure 15.7d) and diflunisal (Figure 15.7e).

(a)

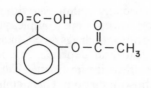

(c)

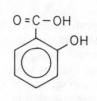

(b)

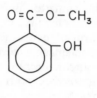

(d)

(e)

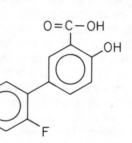

Figure 15.7 The chemical structures of (a) aspirin, (b) methylsalicylate, (c) salicylic acid, (d) sodium salicylate and (e) diflunisal

Aspirin is the drug of choice for relieving moderate pain such as headache, toothache and musculoskeletal pain in adults, but it is not recommended in children and teenagers because of a possible link between aspirin and Reye's syndrome. Aspirin is also antipyretic and anti-inflammatory. It is insoluble but the sodium and calcium salts are soluble. As it is a weak acid, aspirin is relatively unionized in the stomach and this facilitates absorption (see Chapter 2). However, absorption tends to be slow because of the low solubility and takes place mainly in the small intestine. In the blood, aspirin is deacetylated by esterases, yielding salicylate. The drug is metabolized in the liver, partly by conjugation to salicyl-glycine (salicyluric acid) and partly by conjugation to glucuronides, while 10–25% is excreted unchanged.

Aspirin produces a number of unwanted effects, the principal one being gastric erosion which results in bleeding and epigastric discomfort. This is due to a direct irritant action on the gastric mucosa and is more likely to occur with the consumption of tablets than with soluble forms of the drug and can be minimized by consuming aspirin after food. Some increase in faecal blood is thought to occur in most people who take aspirin but occasionally major gastric bleeding occurs. Salicylates, because of their effects on the GI tract, are contra-indicated in patients with peptic ulcers. Aspirin also causes metabolic changes by the uncoupling of oxidative phosphorylation, resulting in increased oxygen consumption and increased production of carbon dioxide which stimulates the respiratory centre. However, the metabolic effects are more likely to occur with large doses.

Poisoning with aspirin is not uncommon, especially in children, due to accidental ingestion. There is likely to be tinnitus (ringing in the ears), dizziness, deafness and confusion. In addition, stimulation of the respiratory centre produces hyperventilation, resulting in respiratory alkalosis and a disturbance of acid–base balance, and this results in metabolic acidosis. Hyperpyrexia, extreme thirst, sweating, nausea and vomiting, resulting in dehydration, are also common. Ultimately, coma and respiratory depression occur. Treatment of poisoning is by preventing further absorption of the drug by provoking emesis and/or gastric lavage and correcting the acid–base disturbance, dehydration and hypothermia, while maintaining adequate renal function.

Aspirin also interacts with a number of other drugs, for example, with oral anticoagulants, by displacing them from binding to plasma proteins. It also interferes with the action of uricosuric agents, such as probenecid.

Aspirin is the most commonly used salicylate; sodium salicylate is less potent but otherwise similar in its actions. Methylsalicylate is toxic if ingested and is used only for topical application, as an ointment or liniment. Salicylic acid is highly irritant and is used only externally, e.g. for the removal of warts. Diflunisal is used as an analgesic and is claimed to produce less intense gastrointestinal effects than aspirin and also less severe toxic effects, e.g. acid–base imbalance. However, it has less antipyretic activity.

Paracetamol (Figure 15.8a)

This drug, which is known in the United States as acetaminophen, is a derivative of the dye aniline. The drugs in this group were at one time known as 'coal tar' analgesics. Another related compound is phenacetin (Figure 15.8b), which was popular at one time as a weak analgesic and antipyretic. However, phenacetin is metabolized to paracetamol and p-phenetidine and, as the latter is toxic, this drug is no longer used. Paracetamol is an effective analgesic and antipyretic, although it lacks an anti-inflammatory action; it is widely used as an alternative to aspirin, especially in children. It is well absorbed after oral administration and is metabolized in the liver to the glucuronide which is then excreted. However, toxic doses cause necrosis of the liver, which may not be immediately apparent, and the therapy for overdose is less satisfactory than that for aspirin. The drug is contraindicated if there is any hepatic impairment.

Benorylate is an ester of aspirin and paracetamol, which is metabolized in the liver to release both active constituents. Gastrointestinal effects and bleeding are

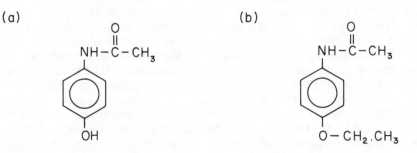

Figure 15.8 The chemical structures of (a) paracetamol and (b) phenacetin

less than with aspirin and the hepatotoxicity in overdose is less than with paracetamol.

Other non-opiate analgesics

There are a number of other weak analgesic drugs, some of which are used mainly for the treatment of inflammation, in which case their analgesic action is also beneficial. This group includes ibuprofen (Figure 15.9a), fenoprofen (Figure 15.9b) and naproxen (Figure 15.9c), all of which are derivatives of propionic acid. Their properties are comparable to those of aspirin and they are used in the treatment of rheumatoid arthritis, osteoarthitis and related conditions. As analgesics they are effective for the relief of pain resulting from injury to soft tissues and for certain types of postoperative pain. Ibuprofen and naproxen are more effective than aspirin in the relief of pain from dysmenorrhoea. Gastrointestinal irritation and bleeding occur, but less frequently than with aspirin.

Mefenamic acid (Figure 15.9d), is a derivative of anthranilic acid; it is an analgesic drug which is also antipyretic and has some anti-inflammatory activity. However, it is toxic and can cause severe diarrhoea and gastric ulceration and bleeding, as well as haematological changes. Its usefulness as an analgesic is therefore limited and it is used only where other analgesic drugs are ineffective.

The mechanism of action of non-opioid analgesics

The non-steroidal anti-inflammatory drugs inhibit the enzyme cyclo-oxygenase, which is involved in the synthesis of prostaglandins (see Chapter 10) and this action is accepted as being responsible for the anti-inflammatory action. The analgesic action may also be related to inhibition of prostaglandin synthesis, as prostaglandins PGE_1 and PGE_2 are known to sensitize peripheral pain receptors to pain-producing substances, such as bradykinin and histamine, although the prostaglandins do not themselves produce pain. The intravenous infusion of prostaglandins has also been found to cause headache and vascular pain. Thus, it seems likely that a major part of the analgesic action of aspirin-like drugs is produced peripherally. This is consistent with the lack of marked central effects, e.g. euphoria, of these drugs. It is also consistent with the fact that there is a definite 'ceiling' to the analgesic effect and increasing the dose above this level does not increase the analgesia further. However, a central component to the analgesic effects of these drugs cannot be ruled out. Finally, the antipyretic action can also be related to inhibition of prostaglandin synthesis, as bacterial endotoxins are believed to stimulate the release of an endogenous pyrogen which passes from the general circulation into the nervous system. The resulting increase in temperature is a consequence of the release of prostaglandins in the hypothalamus. In fact, injection of prostaglandin PGE_2 into the hypothalamus has been shown to induce fever, and women who are given prostaglandins to induce abortion frequently develop a fever.

Thus, the inhibition of the synthesis of prostaglandins by the non-opioid analgesics can explain their analgesic, antipyretic and anti-inflammatory actions. It can also explain some of the other actions of these drugs, e.g. on platelet aggregation, together with certain side-effects, such as gastric irritation, because prostaglandins released from the gastric mucosa inhibit the secretion of acid in the stomach and promote the secretion of mucus in the intestine. Thus, a reduction in the secretion of prostaglandins in the GI tract will result in increased secretion of

(a)

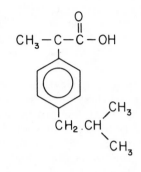

(b)

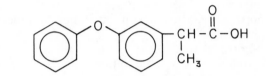

(c)

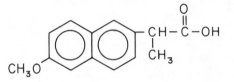

(d)

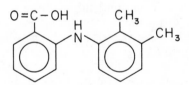

Figure 15.9 The chemical structures of (a) ibuprofen, (b) fenoprofen, (c) naproxen and (d) mefenamic acid

acid and a reduction in the quantity of mucus which protects the intestinal walls. However, there is not, at present, any explanation for the variations in the properties of these drugs. For example, paracetamol is a potent inhibitor of the enzyme cyclo-oxygenase *in vivo* and has good analgesic and antipyretic actions, but is a weak anti-inflammatory drug. An explanation which has been proposed is that paracetamol might be a more effective inhibitor of cyclo-oxygenase in the central nervous system than peripherally.

Chapter 16

Central stimulant drugs

A wide variety of substances, of which some are naturally occurring and others are synthetic, can cause stimulation of the CNS, although very few have any therapeutic use. Some drugs produce central stimulation at toxic levels while others may cause mild stimulation as a side-effect. However, only those drugs which produce central stimulation as their primary action are considered here. The manifestations of CNS stimulation include increased alertness, changes in mood or affect, and even convulsions. Central stimulant drugs can be divided into two main categories according to the type of effect which they produce and their mechanism of action: these are (1) psychomotor stimulants which cause increased alertness and changes in mood; (2) analeptics, which may also increase alertness but are convulsant drugs.

Psychomotor stimulants

The main effect of these drugs is to produce increased alertness but they may also cause changes in mood, e.g. increased nervousness and anxiety, and also euphoria. In animals they cause increased locomotor activity and, in large doses, 'stereotyped' behaviour. The principal members of this group are sympathomimetics (e.g. amphetamine and cocaine), which readily penetrate the blood–brain barrier and therefore produce their main effect on the brain, although they also have peripheral actions (see Chapter 8).

Amphetamine

This is a phenylethylamine (Figure 16.1a) which is optically active and exists in two isomeric forms, dextro- and laevo- or (+)- and (−)-. The racemic mixture, r- or (±)-amphetamine, is also known as 'benzedrine'. Taken by mouth in a dose of 5–10 mg, it is rapidly absorbed and crosses the blood–brain barrier, producing a stimulant effect which is characterized by increased alertness and a feeling of well-being (euphoria); there may also be a feeling of increased energy, and suppression of appetite occurs. Amphetamine was at one time widely used for its central stimulant action and for its anorectic (appetite-suppressant) effect. It was also the principal ingredient in nasal inhalers, used for the relief of nasal congestion, due to its peripheral vasoconstrictor action. However, because it is easy to extract the drug (some 300 mg), inhalers containing amphetamine are no longer marketed. There is no clear-cut evidence that amphetamine can improve performance, either mental or

(a)

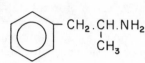

(b)

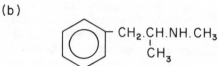

(c)

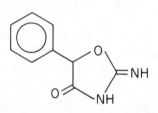

(d)

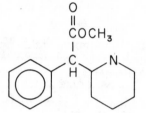

Figure 16.1 The structures of (a) amphetamine, (b) methamphetamine, (c) methylphenidate and (d) pemoline

physical, apart from the indirect effect due to the retardation of fatigue and lethargy. In fact, performance, especially of exacting tasks, can be adversely affected as a result of overconfidence due to the euphoria. In some people there is increased anxiety and irritability when the effect of the drug wears off, and depression can also occur. The peripheral effects include increased blood pressure; however, with repeated administration, the peripheral effects of amphetamine show rapid tachyphylaxis so that only the central effects remain. These may also show tolerance, so that with prolonged use the dose has to be increased in order to maintain an effect. However, with prolonged use of amphetamine, severe depression can ensue when administration of the drug is stopped.

In animals, small doses of amphetamine cause increased locomotor activity and grooming and there may be an increase in aggressive behaviour. Large doses of amphetamine cause the appearance of 'stereotyped' behaviour in which the animal performs repeated purposeless movements, such as chewing, licking or rearing, or it adopts an abnormal posture for long periods.

D- or (+)-Amphetamine, also known as dexedrine, has similar effects to those of r-amphetamine but is more potent centrally, whereas L- or (−)-amphetamine is slightly more potent peripherally. Methylamphetamine (methamphetamine, Figure

16.1b) is a closely related drug with effects similar to those of amphetamine. It is converted to amphetamine in the liver.

The amphetamines are drugs of abuse (see Chapter 18). For this reason, and because they have very limited therapeutic usefulness and can cause dependence leading to addiction, they are now regarded as dangerous drugs with very limited availability. Furthermore, it is known that the consumption of amphetamine over a long period, or in large doses, can result in the appearance of a psychotic-like state resembling paranoid schizophrenia, and this 'amphetamine psychosis' may not be reversed when the drug is withdrawn (see Chapter 12). Amphetamine is mainly excreted unchanged in the urine, the rate of excretion being increased if the urine is acidified.

The mechanism of action of amphetamine

Peripherally, amphetamine is an indirectly acting sympathomimetic amine, being taken up into the presynaptic terminals of sympathetic nerves and producing its stimulant action by displacing the transmitter noradrenaline from the intra-neuronal storage sites. A similar mechanism operates in the central nervous system; however, in the CNS, dopamine as well as noradrenaline is released from nerve terminals. Amphetamine has some other actions: it blocks the re-uptake of catecholamines and it has some agonist activity at receptors for dopamine and 5-hydroxytryptamine. In large doses it inhibits the enzyme monoamine oxidase, and it also acts as an antagonist at α-adrenoceptors.

Nevertheless, the presynaptic release of noradrenaline and dopamine in the brain explains most of the behavioural effects of the drug. For example, the increased alertness produced by amphetamine can be explained in terms of the release of noradrenaline from the terminals of neurones of the ascending pathway which arises from the locus coeruleus nucleus in the brain stem, and which is known to be involved in arousal responses (see Chapter 10). These noradrenergic terminals are widely distributed throughout the cerebral cortex, where the alerting effect of amphetamine is manifested. The euphoria, on the other hand, is probably mediated by the release of noradrenaline from terminals in the limbic system. In addition, descending noradrenergic pathways in the spinal cord are known to influence peripheral muscular activity and a stimulant action on this pathway can explain the feeling of increased muscular energy produced by amphetamine. Finally, the release of dopamine from presynaptic terminals of dopaminergic fibres explains the 'stereotyped' behaviour produced by large doses of amphetamine in animals and the 'amphetamine-psychosis' in humans, as dopamine is known to be involved in psychotic illness (see Chapter 12). In fact, small doses of amphetamine have been found to exacerbate the symptoms of schizophrenia. Even the anorectic action of amphetamine (see Chapter 20) can be attributed to the release of noradrenaline, because the latter substance is known to be involved in 'rewarding' activities.

Methylphenidate (Ritalin, Figure 16.1c)

This drug has effects similar to those of amphetamine although its mechanism of action more closely resembles that of cocaine (see below). It is less potent as a stimulant than amphetamine but also has less tendency to produce anorexia.

Pemoline (Figure 16.1d)

This is a mild stimulant that is structurally unlike amphetamine and also lacks an anorectic action. It has been used to combat fatigue and debility in elderly patients, as it has fewer side-effects than other central stimulants such as amphetamine (see Chapter 20).

Cocaine

This is a local anaesthetic drug (see Chapter 9) which, because of its central stimulant effect, is also a drug of abuse. It occurs naturally in the leaves of the shrub *Erythroxylon coca*, which is indigenous to South America, where the leaves are chewed for the central stimulant action. There is initially a feeling of well-being and euphoria, which may be accompanied by increased talkativeness, restlessness and excitement. The sensation of fatigue is diminished and, with small doses of cocaine, this can lead to an increased capacity for muscular work. However, as the dose is increased, tremors and convulsive movements occur, eventually leading to tonic–clonic convulsions. The stimulant action on the medulla results in stimulation of respiration, which becomes rapid and shallow. The vasomotor and vomiting centres may also be stimulated, resulting in a rise in blood pressure and emesis. The stimulation is followed by depression, and depression of the medullary centres results in respiratory failure which is the usual cause of death from overdose. Small doses of cocaine slow the heart as a result of central vagal stimulation, whereas larger doses cause tachycardia which is probably due both to stimulation of the medullary sympathetic centres and peripheral stimulation of noradrenergic transmission. Large doses of cocaine, administered intravenously, have a direct toxic action on the heart muscle and are likely to cause death from cardiac failure.

Cocaine is a drug of abuse because of its psychomotor stimulant action (see Chapter 18); it also produces dependence and is addictive. Because of this and also its toxicity, the use of cocaine as a local anaesthetic is mainly restricted to surface anaesthesia.

The mechanism of action of cocaine

It is well established that the peripheral actions of cocaine are due to blockade of the re-uptake of noradrenaline into the nerve terminals of the sympathetic system, so potentiating the action of the neurotransmitter (see Chapter 8). Cocaine also, although to a lesser degree, potentiates the actions of circulating adrenaline. The stimulant effects of cocaine on the CNS are due to a similar action, i.e. blocking the re-uptake of the monoamines noradrenaline and dopamine. Although the mechanisms of action of cocaine and amphetamine are different, their central effects are very similar. However, cocaine does not produce stereotyped behaviour in animals, nor does it induce psychotic-like symptoms in man. Thus, in the case of cocaine, the blockade of the re-uptake of noradrenaline is probably more important than that of dopamine.

Methylxanthines

The three most important alkaloids derived from xanthine are caffeine (Figure 16.2a), theophylline (Figure 16.2b) and theobromine (Figure 16.2c). They all occur

(a)

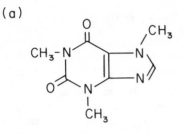

(b)

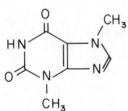

(c)

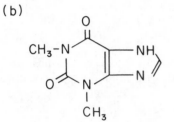

Figure 16.2 The structures of (a) caffeine, (b) theophylline and (c) theobromine

naturally, being found in various plants from which beverages are made. They are therefore present in drinks such as tea, coffee and cocoa, and also cola-flavoured drinks. Coffee contains caffeine almost exclusively, while tea contains slightly less caffeine and a little theophylline, and cocoa contains theobromine and some caffeine. These substances have a number of pharmacological actions: they stimulate the CNS; they act on the kidney to cause diuresis; they stimulate cardiac muscle, and they relax smooth muscle, particularly bronchial muscle. All three xanthine derivatives have these actions but vary in potency.

Caffeine and theophylline are both potent CNS stimulants, whereas theobromine is relatively inactive in this respect. The ingestion of beverages containing methylxanthines such as caffeine and theophylline results in a reduction in drowsiness and fatigue, with improved concentration and a clearer flow of thought. There may also be a reduction in reaction time. These effects are produced by between 85 and 250 mg of caffeine, the amount present in 1–3 cups of coffee. However, it has been found that tasks involving delicate muscular coordination and accurate timing may be affected adversely. Insomnia is likely to occur with these doses and the consumption of larger doses is likely to result in nervousness, restlessness and tremors. Compared with amphetamine, the methylxanthines do not produce euphoria or stereotyped behaviour, nor do they produce psychotic-like symptoms in large doses. They do not cause as much locomotor stimulation as does amphetamine, but they do stimulate the respiratory centre in the medulla and this action has been utilized clinically (see below).

The mechanism of action of methylxanthines

All three methylxanthines inhibit the enzyme phosphodiesterase, which is responsible for the breakdown of cyclic AMP. Thus, in those systems where cyclic AMP is a second messenger (see Chapters 3 and 10), the effects of the transmitters will be potentiated and prolonged, and it has been demonstrated that inhibitors of phosphodiesterase potentiate responses in the autonomic nervous system which are mediated by β_1- and β_2-adrenoceptors. Such an action by the methylxanthines can readily explain the cardiac stimulation and bronchodilation which they produce. This hypothesis is now regarded with suspicion as it has been found that the concentrations of methylxanthines needed to produce appreciable inhibition of phosphodiesterases are much greater than would be expected to occur *in vivo*. However, the methylxanthines have also been found to be antagonists of adenosine at purinergic P_1 receptors and receptors for adenosine have been found in the heart, where adenosine decreases the force of contraction, and in the bronchi, where it causes bronchoconstriction. Thus an antagonist action by the methylxanthines at adenosine receptors is a more likely mechanism of action. The methylxanthines have other actions, including effects on the translocation of calcium ions intracellularly and the potentiation of inhibitors of the synthesis of prostaglandins; it is possible that either or both of these mechanisms may contribute to their effects.

Analeptics

These are central nervous system stimulants that are also convulsant drugs. Although there is a large number of substances in this category, only a few have been used therapeutically, mainly as respiratory stimulants. However, some are important for experimental purposes as they can be used in the analysis of inhibitory processes in the CNS. Their actions are mainly on the brain stem and spinal cord, where they increase reflex excitability and stimulate the respiratory and vasomotor centres. Compared with the psychomotor stimulants, they appear to have little effect on mental function.

Strychnine (Figure 16.3a)

This is the principal alkaloid found in the seeds of the tree *Strychnos nux-vomica*, which grows in India. It has been used for centuries as a pesticide, mainly as rat poison. Strychnine is a potent convulsant drug, increasing neuronal excitability in the CNS by blocking inhibition. The convulsant action is manifested mainly on the spinal cord, where strychnine is an antagonist at receptors for glycine, the inhibitory neurotransmitter in the spinal cord (see Chapter 10). Thus, the blocking of the postsynaptic action of glycine, released from the terminals of Renshaw cells on motor neurones in the spinal cord, can explain the convulsant action of strychnine. Because of this predominant action on the spinal cord, the convulsions induced by strychnine have features which are not shown by other convulsant drugs which act on the brain. In the early stages there is increased reflex excitability and any sensory stimulus may produce violent extensor spasms. Ultimately, all the

(a)

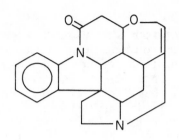

(b)

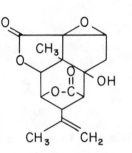

(c)

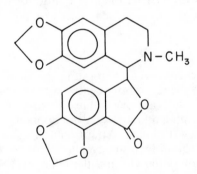

(d)

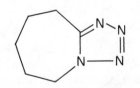

Figure 16.3 The structures of (a) strychnine, (b) picrotoxin, (c) bicuculline and (d) pentylenetetrazol

voluntary muscles of the body are in full contraction and the hyperextension or opisthotonus results in a characteristic posture in which the back is arched and only the crown of the head and the heels are touching the ground. As the action of strychnine is mainly confined to the spinal cord, the patient may remain conscious and fully aware of sensory stimuli. Death results from asphyxia due to impaired respiration.

Picrotoxin (Figure 16.3b)

This too, is a naturally occurring substance which is found in the berries of the climbing shrub, *Anamirta cocculus*, which is indigenous to the East Indies. The active principle in picrotoxin is picrotoxinin. It differs from strychnine in that its action is not restricted to any one part of the CNS. Picrotoxin is also an antagonist at receptors for γ-aminobutyric acid (GABA), but is not a competitive antagonist. Picrotoxin blocks both presynaptic and postsynaptic inhibition mediated by GABA in the CNS, probably by a direct action on chloride channels (see Chapter 10).

Bicuculline (Figure 16.3c)

This is also a plant alkaloid. It is a competitive GABA antagonist and is selective for $GABA_A$ receptors which control chloride permeability (see Chapter 10). The pattern of convulsions produced by bicuculline is similar to that of picrotoxin.

Pentylenetetrazol (Figure 16.3d)

This is a synthetic compound that has been widely used, particularly for the screening of anticonvulsant drugs, because the convulsions it produces are thought to resemble those which occur in epileptic attacks (see Chapter 14). It acts mainly on the brain, probably by interfering with GABA-mediated inhibition, but the exact mechanism of action is not known.

Other analeptics

A number of other analeptic drugs have been used as respiratory stimulants as they were thought to have a selective action on the respiratory centre in the medulla. The main ones are nikethamide (Figure 16.4a), amiphenazole (Figure 16.4b) and doxapram (Figure 16.4c). They all have stimulant actions on the brain and, because of their action on the medullary centre, they stimulate respiration and cause a rise in blood pressure. These effects occur at doses which are smaller than those which produce convulsions, but the safety margin is narrow and the effect on respiration may be transient. Amiphenazole and doxapram are claimed to have larger safety margins but they both have undesirable side-effects (see below). The mechanism of action of these drugs is not known but it is thought that they may act by enhancing excitation in the brain rather than by blocking inhibition.

The clinical uses of central stimulant drugs

The former uses of amphetamine as a central stimulant, for the treatment of obesity and as a nasal decongestant, have already been discussed. Because of the dangers associated with its use, amphetamine and related substances now have few therapeutic applications. However, amphetamine is still used in the treatment of narcolepsy, a condition in which the patient falls asleep during the daytime for no apparent reason. Both amphetamine and methylphenidate have also been found to be useful in the treatment of hyperkinetic children who are, paradoxically, calmed by these drugs. Except for the limited use of cocaine in local surface anaesthesia, it

(a)

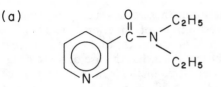

(b)

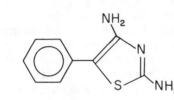

(c)

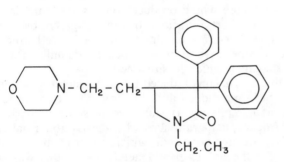

Figure 16.4 The structures of (a) nikethamide, (b) amiphenazole and (c) doxapram

has no other applications, apart from sometimes being included in elixirs of analgesics for the relief of terminal pain.

In addition to their wide consumption in beverages, the methylxanthines have some uses. Aminophylline, a combination of theophylline and ethylenediamine, is more water soluble than theophylline and is used as a bronchodilator for the relief of asthma. However, the high incidence of side-effects, such as tachycardia, palpitations, nausea and other gastrointestinal disturbances, as well as insomnia, nervousness and tremor, have restricted its usefulness. Sustained-release preparations of aminophylline and theophylline can be used for the treatment of chronic asthma and usually show a reduced incidence of side-effects.

Caffeine is used therapeutically for counteracting the respiratory depression induced by barbiturates or opioid drugs, especially in overdose. Caffeine is also frequently combined with preparations of analgesics such as aspirin. The reason for this is not clear, as caffeine does not contribute to the analgesic or anti-inflammatory actions. Although caffeine has relatively few side-effects and is also safe in overdose, it could aggravate the gastric irritation caused by aspirin. In combination with an ergot derivative, such as ergotamine, caffeine has been used in the treatment of migraine. It is believed that the ability of caffeine to produce contraction of the cerebral blood vessels may improve the therapeutic response.

The analeptic drugs were at one time popular as respiratory stimulants for the treatment of barbiturate overdose, particularly if the patient was in coma or suffering from respiratory failure. For example, picrotoxin was used for treating barbiturate poisoning, but it is now recognized that these drugs have very limited application. Although they produce some restoration of function, the effect is usually very short-lived and the narrow margin of safety means that there is a great risk of producing convulsions. In fact, it has been shown that the use of these drugs does not reduce mortality and alternative, conservative methods of management of comatose patients have proved to be safer and more effective. The reduced use of barbiturate drugs (Chapter 11) has diminished the need for the treatment of barbiturate poisoning. Of the analeptic drugs available, only two – nikethamide and doxapram – have any clinical use. Nikethamide is the drug of choice to arouse patients with carbon dioxide narcosis. It is given by slow intravenous injection but has a short duration of action. However, repeat injections can be given. The side-effects of nikethamide include sweating, nausea, restlessness and tremor and, if the dose is too large, convulsions followed by CNS depression can occur. Doxapram, which is claimed to have a wider margin of safety, i.e. between the doses causing stimulation of respiration and those which produce convulsions, can also be used and, although the effect is of short duration, it can be given by continuous intravenous infusion. The side-effects are similar to those of nikethamide. Doxapram is also used to relieve postoperative respiratory depression unless this is due to the use of opiate analgesics, against which it is ineffective.

The similarity between the convulsions induced by pentylenetetrazol and epileptic convulsions has already been mentioned and this drug was at one time thought to be useful in the diagnosis of epilepsy. It was used in subconvulsive doses in patients in whom the electroencephalogram showed no gross abnormal signs but who were suffering from fits, perhaps nocturnal, which might or might not be due to epilepsy. The rationale for the use of pentylenetetrazol in this way was that epileptic patients had a lower seizure threshold than non-epileptics and that a subconvulsive dose of pentylenetetrazol, injected intravenously, would produce an abnormality in the EEG of the suspected epileptic, without inducing a convulsion. However, the test has never become popular, probably because there are more satisfactory and less invasive ways of diagnosing epilepsy.

As strychnine is a naturally occurring substance and has also been used as a rat poison, cases of strychnine poisoning, especially in children, are not uncommon. There have also been cases of strychnine being used to adulterate the heroin used by drug addicts. This is, of course, extremely dangerous as the lethal dose of strychnine, taken orally, is of the order of 100 mg but it is much more toxic if injected intravenously. It is therefore possible that some deaths of addicts, which have been attributed to heroin overdose, might have been caused by the contamination of heroin with strychnine. In children, the fatal dose of strychnine can be as low as 15 mg. The early symptoms consist of stiffness of the face and neck muscles, followed by heightened reflex excitability so that any sensory stimulus may produce a violent response. Finally, there may be a full tetanic convulsion, as described above. The primary objective in treating strychnine poisoning is to prevent the convulsions and to support respiration. Preventing the patient from receiving external sensory stimuli can also be effective. Barbiturates will block the convulsions due to strychnine but the benzodiazepine diazepam is now the drug of choice. It is injected intravenously in a dose of up to 10 mg and may be repeated if necessary. If adequate respiratory ventilation is not restored, mechanical assistance will be needed.

Chapter 17

Drugs used in the treatment of affective disorders

The affective disorders are mental states in which the main abnormality is a change in mood, either depression or mania, and other symptoms are secondary to this. The illness is usually phasic and there is a return to full normality during periods of remission. The classification of affective disorders is the subject of much debate but it is generally recognized that there are two main types, bipolar and unipolar. In bipolar affective disorder, or manic-depressive psychosis, there is an oscillation between depression and mania, with bouts of normality between the episodes. Unipolar illness, or recurrent or endogenous depression, consists only of depression, of unknown origin, but again there may be periods of normality. Another type of unipolar illness has been recognized, known as 'reactive' depression. This is depression which is related to environmental circumstances, e.g. bereavement, changes in financial circumstances, etc. and is not normally treatable with drugs. Both manic-depressive psychosis and endogenous depression are amenable to drug treatment, although other methods, such as electroconvulsive therapy (ECT), are also effective.

Mania is characterized by euphoria, a feeling of increased well-being and an excess of enthusiasm and energy. Patients with mania are expansive and talkative; their speech is rapid and discursive and they often flit from one subject to another. In 'hypomania', the overactivity increases to the point where the patient is in continuous restless movement and activity, and his speech becomes so distracted that it is difficult to follow. The euphoria may be replaced by outbursts of rage and there can be sexual overactivity. The depressive phases of manic-depressive psychosis and endogenous depression are clinically indistinguishable. The mood can range from mild sadness to profound melancholia with feelings of guilt, anxiety and apprehension. There is a loss of 'drive' which results in a lack of interest in food, sex and work, and disturbances of sleep frequently occur. Affective disorders are not uncommon, approximately 2% of the population suffering at some time during their life, and genetic factors are believed to play a significant part. An important distinction between bipolar and unipolar illness is that different drugs are effective in their treatment.

Antidepressant drugs

Three main classes of drugs are used to treat endogenous depression: (1) tricyclic antidepressants; (2) monoamine oxidase inhibitors and (3) the so-called 'second generation' or 'atypical' antidepressants, derived mainly from the tricyclics. In addition, centrally acting sympathomimetic stimulants, such as amphetamine (Chapter 16), were at one time used to relieve acute depressive states but the use of such drugs is now discouraged because of the risks of addiction and of inducing a state of psychosis. In addition, when the euphoric effects of amphetamine wear off, there is usually a rebound depression which could therefore exacerbate the original condition.

Tricyclic antidepressants

These are currently the most widely used antidepressant drugs. Chemically, they are dibenzazepines and are related to the phenothiazines, the main structural difference being the presence of an ethylene group in the central ring in place of the sulphur atom. The first drug of this type to be synthesized was imipramine (Figure 17.1a) which was tested as a possible neuroleptic. However, imipramine was relatively ineffective as a neuroleptic but was found to have an antidepressant action, and it became the forerunner of a series of drugs with similar structures (Figures 17.1 and

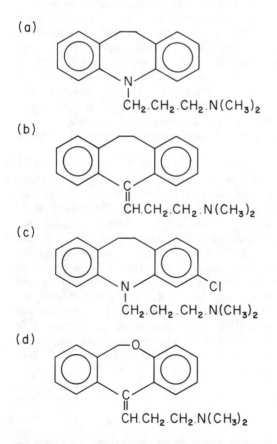

Figure 17.1 The chemical structures of some tricyclic antidepressant drugs which are tertiary amines: (a) imipramine, (b) amitriptyline, (c) clomipramine and (d) doxepin

(a)

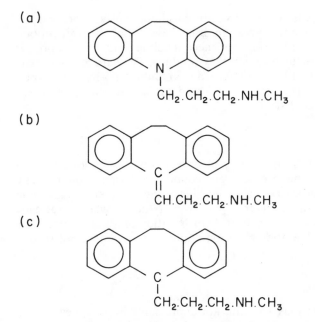

CH$_2$.CH$_2$.CH$_2$.NH.CH$_3$

(b)

C
||
CH.CH$_2$.CH$_2$.NH.CH$_3$

(c)

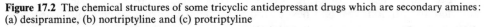

C
|
CH$_2$.CH$_2$.CH$_2$.NH.CH$_3$

Figure 17.2 The chemical structures of some tricyclic antidepressant drugs which are secondary amines: (a) desipramine, (b) nortriptyline and (c) protriptyline

17.2). The main difference between the drugs shown in Figures 17.1 and 17.2 is in the aliphatic side-chains on the nitrogen or carbon atom in the central ring. Thus, imipramine (Figure 17.1a), amitriptyline (Figure 17.1b), clomipramine (Figure 17.1c) and doxepin (Figure 17.1d) are tertiary amines, while desipramine (Figure 17.2a), nortriptyline (Figure 17.2b) and protriptyline (Figure 17.2c) are secondary amines. All the drugs in this group have no substitution on either of the outer rings, except for clomipramine, which therefore most closely resembles the phenothiazines. They all have similar actions, although there are some differences in side-effects (see below). However, the tertiary amines are rapidly demethylated in the body to the corresponding secondary amines, which are themselves active. Thus, imipramine is demethylated to desipramine, and amitriptyline to nortriptyline.

Mechanism of action

The main action of the tricyclic antidepressant drugs is to block the re-uptake of noradrenaline and 5-hydroxytryptamine into their respective nerve terminals in the brain. This results in increased amounts of these neurotransmitters being available at the synapse and, hence, increased noradrenergic and serotoninergic activity in the brain. In most cases the re-uptake of dopamine is only slightly affected. The discovery of this action aroused considerable interest as it was consistent with the 'amine theory of depression' and it was thought to be the basis of the therapeutic action of the drugs. However, the theory has had to be modified, mainly because of differences in the time course of the pharmacological and therapeutic actions (see below). The tricyclics do not affect the synthesis or storage of amine neurotransmitters but some appear to increase release by acting as antagonists at presynaptic α_2-adrenoceptors. All the tricyclic antidepressant drugs have anticholinergic properties, antagonizing the muscarinic actions of acetylcholine and this action is responsible for many of the side-effects which they produce. They are also sedative, an action which is probably related to the increased availability of 5-hydroxytryptamine. The sedative action is not necessarily a disadvantage as many depressed patients suffer from disturbances of sleep.

Pharmacokinetics

The tricyclic antidepressant drugs are rapidly absorbed from the gastrointestinal tract after oral administration and are strongly bound to plasma proteins. The unbound drug is rapidly distributed to other tissues, including the liver, kidney, lung and brain. Metabolism occurs in the liver; apart from N-demethylation (already mentioned) which produces active metabolites, hydroxylation produces metabolites which become more water soluble after glucuronidation and are therefore readily excreted.

Clinical uses of tricyclic antidepressants

The differences between the various tricyclic antidepressant drugs appear to be slight as far as their therapeutic effects are concerned. Depressed patients who are agitated and anxious respond best to the more sedative drugs, such as amitriptyline, while withdrawn and apathetic patients will derive most benefit from less sedative compounds, such as imipramine. A characteristic feature of all these drugs is that the therapeutic action is slow in onset and may take up to 2–3 weeks to reach maximum effectiveness. Furthermore, not all depressed patients respond to treatment with tricyclic antidepressants.

   The most common side-effects, apart from sedation, are those related to the anticholinergic actions of the drugs. These are atropine-like effects which include dry mouth and blurred vision, which are relatively unimportant, and also urinary retention and paralytic ileus, which may require intervention. Cardiovascular effects, such as hypotension and tachycardia, are frequent and disturbances of cardiac rhythm may appear. Acute overdose, which can occur accidently or deliberately, results in confusion and excitement, which may lead to convulsions, followed by coma and respiratory depression. Severe cardiac arrhythmias are likely, leading to heart block and death; these drugs are therefore contra-indicated in patients with heart disease. The anticholinesterase drug physostigmine has been used to relieve some of the acute toxic symptoms by offsetting the antimuscarinic effects. Tolerance to the anticholinergic side-effects usually develops and they can often be avoided by starting treatment with a small dose which is then gradually increased.

Monoamine oxidase inhibitors

These drugs, although discovered before the tricyclics, are less widely used because they are more toxic and interact with other drugs and with constituents of diet. They are used mainly in patients who do not respond to treatment with tricyclic antidepressants. The antidepressant action of monoamine oxidase inhibitors was discovered when it was observed that patients being treated for tuberculosis with

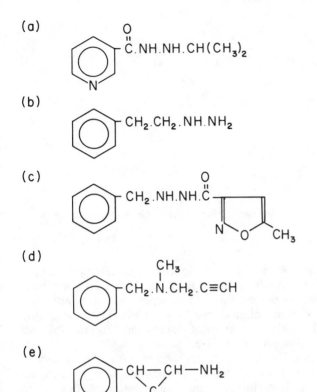

(a)

(b)

(c)

(d)

(e)

Figure 17.3 The chemical structures of monoamine oxidase inhibitors: (a) iproniazid, (b) phenelzine, (c) isocarboxazid, (d) pargyline and (e) tranylcypromine

iproniazid showed elevation of mood. However, iproniazid (Figure 17.3a), which is a hydrazine derivative, is very toxic and, in the search for less toxic antidepressant drugs, various other inhibitors of monoamine oxidase have been synthesized. Some, e.g. phenelzine (Figure 17.3b) and isocarboxazid (Figure 17.3c), are also hydrazines but others, e.g. pargyline (Figure 17.3d) and tranylcypromine (Figure 17.3e), more closely resemble amphetamine (Chapter 16, Figure 16.1a) in chemical structure.

The pharmacology of the monoamine oxidase inhibitors has been described in Chapter 8 and only those aspects relevant to the treatment of depression will be discussed here. The enzyme monoamine oxidase (MAO) is present in most tissues and exists in two forms, MAO_A and MAO_B, which are distinguished on the basis of substrate specificity, MAO_A inactivating preferentially noradrenaline and 5-hydroxytryptamine, while MAO_B has a substrate preference for phenylethylamine. Both subtypes of enzyme metabolize dopamine. Inhibitors which are selective for these subtypes have been developed, e.g. clorgyline (Figure 17.4a), which selectively inhibits MAO_A and selegiline (also known as deprenyl; Figure 17.4b), which shows a preference for MAO_B. As MAO_B is the major form of the enzyme in the human brain, it might be expected that selegiline, which is selective for MAO_B, would be an effective antidepressant. However, this does not appear to be the case

(a)

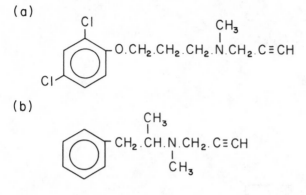

(b)

Figure 17.4 The chemical structures of the selective monoamine oxidase inhibitors: (a) clorgyline and (b) selegiline

and selegiline, when given in doses which selectively inhibit MAO_B, is not effective in relieving depression, although when administered in larger doses that affect both MAO_A and MAO_B, it is. Selegiline is not used as an antidepressant drug, although it is used in the treatment of Parkinson's disease (see Chapter 19). The monoamine oxidase inhibitors that are used for the treatment of depression (Figure 17.3) are non-selective for the subtypes of monoamine oxidase.

The wide distribution of monoamine oxidase in the body accounts for many of the side-effects produced by the inhibitors (see below). Also, apart from showing no selectivity for MAO_A or MAO_B, they inhibit other enzymes, including those involved in the metabolism of other drugs and this accounts for many of the interactions that occur.

Mechanism of action

The enzyme monoamine oxidase is localized to the outer membranes of the mitochondria that are present in nerve terminals containing noradrenaline, dopamine and 5-hydroxytryptamine. The enzyme inactivates the amine neurotransmitters by oxidative deamination, thus regulating the intraneuronal concentration of the transmitter. The blocking of this action by inhibitors of monoamine oxidase results in an increased content of these neurotransmitters in the terminals. The effect is greater for noradrenaline and 5-hydroxytryptamine than it is for dopamine. The increase is in the cytoplasmic concentration of transmitter rather than the vesicular stores; thus, the amount released by nerve stimulation is not appreciably altered. However, spontaneous release is increased and also that produced by indirectly acting sympathomimetic amines, such as amphetamine and tyramine. Similar changes occur in peripheral tissues and result in increased plasma levels of the monoamines. Apart from being involved in the metabolism of endogenous amines, monoamine oxidase in the wall of the gut and in the liver is also responsible for the inactivation of ingested amines, which might otherwise produce unwanted effects. The blocking of this action can have serious consequences (see below).

The monoamine oxidase inhibitors are structurally not dissimilar to the normal substrates of the enzyme and it is thought that the inhibitory action of the hydrazine group is due to the formation of covalent bonds between the inhibitor and enzyme, resulting in a non-competitive and long-lasting inhibition. As a consequence of this, recovery of the enzyme after inhibition can take several weeks.

Clinical use of monoamine oxidase inhibitors

Although widely used in the treatment of depression before the discovery of the tricyclics, the monoamine oxidase inhibitors are now used only in depression which is refractory to other forms of treatment. In addition, because of the persistent effects of monoamine oxidase inhibitors, it is easier to use them after treatment with tricyclics has been unsuccessful, rather than vice versa. Depressed patients with phobias, hypochondria or hysterical features are thought to respond best to these drugs. As with the tricyclic antidepressants, the therapeutic effects are delayed and may take up to 3 weeks to appear and a further 1–2 weeks to become maximal, in spite of the biochemical effects being produced immediately. Whereas the tricyclics are often given initially in a small dose, which is then gradually increased in order to allow tolerance to develop to the sedative effects, the monoamine oxidase inhibitors are administered in a full dose initially, the dose being gradually reduced after beneficial effects have been obtained, until an optimal maintenance dose has been established. In the case of tranylcypromine there is an initial stimulant effect, probably attributable to its close relationship to amphetamine; this can result in insomnia and other side-effects.

The side-effects produced by the monoamine oxidase inhibitors are mainly due to the inhibition of the enzyme at various sites outside the CNS. Thus, hepatotoxicity may develop, although the incidence is low. Tremors, insomnia and agitation, and even delirium and hallucinations, can result from overstimulation of the CNS. Atropine-like side-effects, such as dry mouth, blurred vision and urinary retention, can occur but are less troublesome than those observed with the tricyclics. Sleep disturbances, manifested by the blocking of REM sleep (see Chapter 11), are not uncommon and the REM sleep 'rebounds' when the drug is discontinued. Postural hypotension is a fairly frequent side-effect and is perhaps surprising in view of the increased levels of catecholamines which occur. A possible explanation for this is that, because of inhibition of monoamine oxidase, other routes for the degradation of monoamines, which are normally of lesser importance, become the main routes of metabolism. Thus substances which are normally minor metabolites, such as tyramine and octopamine, may be formed. It is known that octopamine can be taken up by noradrenaline-containing nerve terminals and can be released as a 'false' transmitter, thus reducing noradrenergic transmission and hence sympathetic activity (see Chapter 8).

Of considerable importance is the interaction between the effects of the inhibitors of monoamine oxidase and certain constituents of diet. Many commonly consumed foods, such as cheese, red wine, yeast extracts, broad beans, etc, contain large quantities of tyramine which is normally innocuous because it is rapidly metabolized by monoamine oxidase present in the gut and liver. With the enzyme inhibited, the tyramine passes into the systemic circulation and releases noradrenaline from sympathetic nerve terminals. This can cause severe hypertension which may be dangerous. A throbbing headache is an early warning of a hypertensive crisis and patients being treated with monoamine oxidase inhibitors are advised to avoid food and drink containing large amounts of tyramine. Certain proprietary medicines, such as cough mixtures and nasal decongestants, may also contain sympathomimetics and these can cause a dangerous rise in blood pressure in patients taking monoamine oxidase inhibitors.

There are also interactions with various drugs, e.g. CNS depressants, opioid analgesics, anticholinergic drugs and hypotensive agents, which are normally demethylated by monoamine oxidase. In some cases this is simply an enhancement of the action of the drug but in the case of pethidine, for example, symptoms which are not associated with overdose, e.g. restlessness, hyperpyrexia and coma, appear. It is thought that this is due to the formation of an abnormal metabolite because the usual pathway for demethylation is blocked. Interactions between monoamine oxidase inhibitors and tricyclic antidepressants can also be dangerous, although attempts have been made to increase therapeutic efficacy by using such combinations. In fact, it is recommended that at least 14 days should elapse between the cessation of therapy with a monoamine oxidase inhibitor and the administration of a tricyclic antidepressant. However, as indicated above, the reverse order for these drugs is to be preferred.

'Second generation' antidepressants

These are also known as 'atypical' antidepressants and form a heterogeneous group of drugs, most of which were developed in an attempt to (1) increase the speed of onset of action and (2) reduce the incidence of side-effects. Many are derived from the tricyclics but there are also some compounds which are unrelated to the tricyclics.

Mianserin

This is a tetracylic compound (Figure 17.5a) which does not block the re-uptake of either noradrenaline or 5-hydroxytryptamine and does not inhibit monoamine oxidase. It has less marked anticholinergic actions than the tricyclic antidepressants, therefore having weaker cardiovascular effects. Its mechanism of action is uncertain but it is known to block presynaptic α_2-adrenoceptors on noradrenergic nerve terminals, which would have the effect of increasing the release of noradrenaline by reducing feedback inhibition (see Chapter 8). The onset of the therapeutic action of mianserin appears to be shorter than that of the tricyclics, being of the order of 1–2 weeks.

Iprindole (Figure 17.5b)

This has a tricyclic structure but is quite different pharmacologically to the typical tricyclic antidepressants. It has no effect on the uptake of monoamine neurotransmitters, does not inhibit monoamine oxidase, nor does it have an action on presynaptic α_2-receptors as does mianserin. However, it does cause the 'down regulation' of β-adrenoceptors in brain and it is currently thought that this may provide the basis for its therapeutic action as it is a very effective drug and has relatively few side-effects.

Maprotiline

This also has a tricyclic structure (Figure 17.5c), but differs from the typical tricyclic drugs. It blocks the re-uptake of noradrenaline but not that of 5-hydroxytryptamine (see Figure 17.7). Anticholinergic side-effects occur less fre-

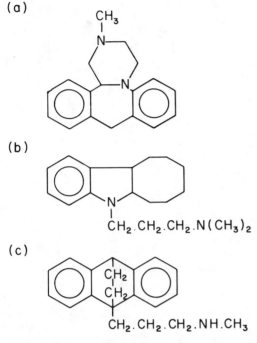

(a)

(b)

$CH_2.CH_2.CH_2.N(CH_3)_2$

(c)

$CH_2.CH_2.CH_2.NH.CH_3$

Figure 17.5 The chemical structures of some 'atypical' antidepressant drugs: (a) mianserin, (b) iprindole and (c) maprotiline

quently with maprotiline but rashes are common and convulsions can occur with large doses.

Nomifensine **(Figure 17.6a)**

This is similar to maprotiline in that it blocks the re-uptake of noradrenaline and not that of 5-hydroxytryptamine (Figure 17.7), but it also blocks the re-uptake of dopamine.

Viloxazine **(Figure 17.6b)**

This is structurally unrelated to other known antidepressant drugs. Like maprotiline, it blocks the re-uptake of noradrenaline. It is claimed to have fewer and milder side-effects than the 'typical' antidepressants and a more rapid onset of action. However, nausea and headaches can occur.

Zemelidine **(Figure 17.6c)**

This is an example of an antidepressant drug which selectively inhibits the re-uptake of 5-hydroxytryptamine, with little or no effect on the re-uptake of noradrenaline (Figure 17.7). It has also been found to decrease the density of β-adrenoceptors.

Other drugs in this group include trazodone, fluoxetine, citalopram and bupropion, all of which resemble the drugs described above.

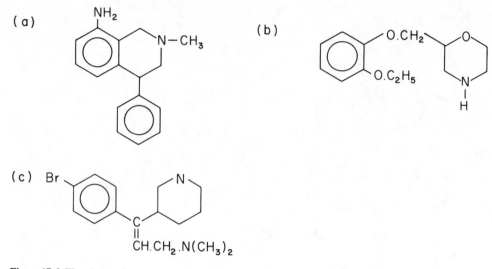

Figure 17.6 The chemical structures of 'atypical' antidepressant drugs: (a) nomifensine, (b) viloxazine and (c) zemelidine

The monoamine theory of depression

This theory had its origins partly in knowledge of the pharmacological properties of drugs which are effective in relieving depression and of those which can induce a state of mental depression resembling endogenous depression, and partly through biochemical studies in patients suffering from depression. Thus, reserpine, which causes a depletion of both catecholamines and 5-hydroxytryptamine in the brain by releasing them from intracellular stores (see Chapter 12), produces mental depression. This was noticed in patients being treated with large doses of reserpine to relieve hypertension, some 15% of whom became psychotically depressed. On the other hand, drugs which release amine neurotransmitters, e.g. amphetamine, elevate mood, and drugs used to treat depression increase the availability of monoamines by blocking either their re-uptake (tricyclics) or their metabolism (monoamine oxidase inhibitors). It seemed, therefore, that depression might be due to reduced levels or reduced activity of monoamines in the brain. Originally, the theory was formulated in terms of noradrenaline, but 5-hydroxytryptamine was also found to be involved when reduced levels of the metabolite of 5-hydroxytryptamine, 5-hydroxyindole acetic acid, were found in the cerebrospinal fluid of patients suffering from depression, indicating either reduced levels or reduced turnover of 5-hydroxytryptamine in depression. Following this finding, attempts were made to treat depressed patients with the administration of large quantities of the precursor of 5-hydroxytryptamine, L-tryptophan (see Chapter 10), but the results have been equivocal. It therefore seemed that both noradrenaline and 5-hydroxytryptamine were involved in depression. The relative potencies of antidepressant drugs in blocking the re-uptake of noradrenaline and 5-hydroxytryptamine are shown in Figure 17.7. Drugs such as citalopram, which affect the uptake of 5-hydroxytrypta-

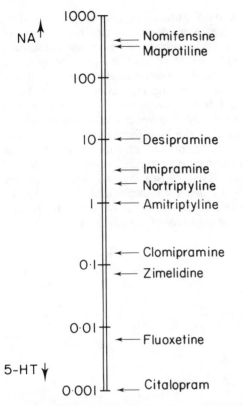

Figure 17.7 The relative potencies of various antidepressant drugs as inhibitors of the uptake of noradrenaline (NA) or 5-hydroxytryptamine (5-HT) (redrawn from Iversen and Mackay, 1979)

mine exclusively, are just as effective as antidepressants as those which affect only the re-uptake of noradrenaline, e.g. maprotiline and nomifensine.

The major problem with the theory outlined above was that, although the biochemical and pharmacological effects of the drugs used to treat depression were immediate, the therapeutic action was delayed and took 2–3 weeks to manifest itself. Various explanations have been put forward to account for this delay but none are plausible. A second argument against the theory that treatment with antidepressant drugs was simply restoring the levels or availability of monoamines in the brain arose from the discovery that some of the new antidepressant drugs did not block the re-uptake of monoamines, nor did they inhibit monoamine oxidase. Because of the long delay in the appearance of the therapeutic effects of the antidepressant drugs, attention has been directed towards the possibility that long-term adaptive changes might be responsible, i.e. that the therapeutic action might be related to secondary, adaptive changes, rather than to the primary pharmacological effect of the drug. Studies with long-term chronic administration of antidepressant drugs in animals resulted in a change being found in postsynaptic β-receptors in the brain. This change was a reduction in the activity of noradrenaline-sensitive adenylate cyclase in response to a given stimulus. This adaptive change had a time course similar to the time course for the onset of the therapeutic action. Furthermore, the effect was produced by all known antidepressant drugs, including iprindole which does not affect the re-uptake of monoamines nor the activity of monoamine oxidase and also, suprisingly, by the non-drug treatment for depression, electroconvulsive therapy (ECT). This type of long-term adaptive change in receptor activity, which results in hypoactivity, has been called 'down-regulation' and the opposite change, producing hyperactivity, 'up-regulation'. The reduced response or hypoactivity of β-receptors has been interpreted as being due to a reduction in the number of β-adrenoceptors and the results of binding studies support this view. However, it seems likely that the long-term changes may come about through the drug initially blocking presynaptic α_2-adrenoceptors. As these inhibit the release of noradrenaline from the nerve terminals, their blockade will result in increased release of transmitter. This causes overstimulation of the postsynaptic β-receptors, which will eventually become desensitized (Figure 17.8).

Although this hypothesis is applicable to all known antidepressant drugs, and also to ECT, it does not, in its present form, involve 5-hydroxytryptamine. In

(a)

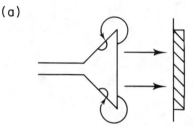

(b)

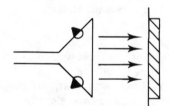

(c)

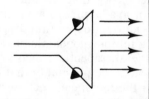

Desensitization
(reduced
response)

Figure 17.8 Diagrammatic representation of the 'down-regulation' of postsynaptic β-receptors. (a) Normal state: the released transmitter (noradrenaline) feeds back on to presynaptic α_2-receptors to regulate further release; the postsynaptic β-receptor shows normal sensitivity. (b) The presynaptic α_2-receptors are blocked by the drug (▲) and this results in increased release of transmitter. (c) The postsynaptic β-receptor becomes desensitized as the result of increased activation by the transmitter and produces a reduced response

contrast to the effects on adrenoceptors, long-term treatment with antidepressant drugs has not been found to produce any consistent changes in receptors for 5-hydroxytryptamine in the brain, although some antidepressant drugs, e.g. imipramine, have been found to bind to receptors of the 5-HT$_2$ type. It is possible that there is an interaction between the two systems, the one modulating the other, as there is some evidence that the action of the antidepressant drugs in down-regulating β-receptors is dependent on the integrity of 5-hydroxytryptamine-containing terminals in the cerebral cortex. However, it is generally believed that the antidepressant drugs exert their therapeutic action in the limbic system of the brain.

The treatment of manic-depressive psychosis

One clear way of distinguishing unipolar affective disorders (depression) from bipolar disorders (manic-depressive psychosis) is that the drugs used in their treatment are completely different. The most effective treatment for manic-depressive illness is lithium, which controls the manic phase and, when used prophylactically, prevents the swings of mood, thus controlling the depressive as well as the manic phases of the illness. It has no effect on unipolar depression. Taken orally, lithium salts are rapidly absorbed from the gut and enter most peripheral organs, although it may take up to 24 h for the peak level to be reached in the brain. The therapeutic index is low and toxic effects readily appear; it is therefore usual to monitor the plasma concentrations, which should be between 0.6 and 1.2 mM. Overdose (with plasma concentrations over 1.5 mM) may be fatal and the toxic effects are numerous. They include neurological effects such as tremor, ataxia, nausea, dizziness, convulsions, and finally coma and death; endocrine effects, which include hypothyroidism; and renal effects, including polyuria which can lead to disturbances of electrolyte balance. As 95% of the lithium is excreted through the kidneys, long-term renal damage can occur and it is essential to monitor the renal function of patients on long-term treatment with lithium. There can also be gastrointestinal side-effects, such as nausea and vomiting, and also cardiovascular effects, including ECG changes. The toxic effects of lithium are exacerbated by sodium depletion; thus, concurrent use of sodium-depleting diuretics such as thiazides should be avoided. Prolonged treatment with lithium may result in permanent damage to the renal tubules, even when therapeutic levels have been maintained.

Mechanism of action

Lithium is a monovalent cation and will readily substitute for sodium and potassium, as well as for magnesium and calcium, although the degree of substitution varies with the cation and the conditions. The mechanism of action is not known but it is thought that the ability of lithium to substitute for sodium is important. Thus, lithium ions can penetrate neuronal membranes through the voltage-sensitive channels that are responsible for the generation of the action potential. However, although lithium and sodium ions compete for the enzyme Na$^+$-K$^+$ ATPase, lithium is not pumped out as quickly as sodium and therefore tends to accumulate inside the cell. This leads to partial loss of intracellular potassium and also to partial depolarization. One of the actions of lithium is therefore to reduce the excitability of nervous tissue by slowing the rate of repolarization. It also affects other processes which are sodium-dependent: for example, the uptake of choline is slowed by lithium and the synthesis and release of acetylcholine are reduced.

Lithium also has effects on other neurotransmitter systems in the brain: for example, it has been found to prevent the development of supersensitivity of dopamine receptors in the striatum after the chronic administration of neuroleptic drugs. Lithium has been shown to reduce the release of 5-hydroxytryptamine in the hippocampus by an action on 5-HT autoreceptors and also to decrease the density of 5-HT_1 receptors in the hippocampus. In addition, it inhibits the adenylate cyclase system which is linked to postsynaptic β-adrenoceptors. Many other actions of lithium have been described, for example on transmission mediated by γ-aminobutyric acid. It is therefore difficult to pin-point any single action which could explain the therapeutic effects. However, the prevention of the development of supersensitivity of dopamine receptors is consistent with the anti-mania action and the effect on postsynaptic β-receptors is consistent with an antidepressant action. However, other actions such as those on 5-HT and on transmission mediated by γ-aminobutyric acid in the brain may also be important.

Chapter 18

Psychotomimetic drugs and drugs of abuse

Psychotomimetic drugs produce effects in normal, healthy subjects which resemble the symptoms of naturally occurring psychosis, e.g. hallucinations and disturbances of thought, mood and behaviour, but which disappear when the effect of the drug wears off. They are also known as hallucinogenic or psychodelic drugs. Many drugs, such as amphetamine, atropine and cocaine, have psychotomimetic side-effects if taken in large doses or over prolonged periods. However, the primary action of these drugs, when they are used in smaller doses, is not psychotomimetic and the term 'psychotomimetic' is confined here to those drugs, the main action of which is to produce effects resembling psychotic states. However, the resemblance between the effects produced by psychotomimetic drugs in healthy subjects and the symptoms which occur naturally in psychotic patients is not always complete. For example, the drugs are said to be hallucinogenic but they do not necessarily produce hallucinations in the true sense, i.e. sensory experiences which arise in the absence of environmental stimulation, but rather distortions of existing images, whether visual, auditory, tactile, etc. Because the sensations are subjective, they vary considerably between different individuals and are therefore difficult to define precisely.

Drugs which are psychotomimetic vary considerably in their chemical structure and pharmacological properties. However, they can be divided into the following groups: (1) phenylethylamine derivatives; (2) indolealkylamines; (3) anticholinergics (atropine-like drugs); (4) miscellaneous. Many are naturally occurring and have a long tradition of use for religious or social purposes.

The classification of psychotomimetic drugs

Phenylethylamine derivatives

Mescaline

This is 3,4,5-trimethoxyphenylethylamine (Figure 18.1a) and is structurally related to amphetamine (Chapter 16, Figure 16.1a). It is naturally occurring and is probably one of the oldest psychotomimetic drugs known, having been in use for centuries. Mescaline is one of the many alkaloids present in the peyote cactus, a plant which is indigenous to Mexico and the Southern United States. The term 'peyote' is in fact derived from the Aztec word 'peyotl' which means 'divine messenger'. The Mexican Indians used 'mescal buttons' which are the dried tops cut

(a)

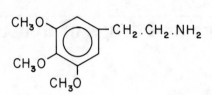

(b)

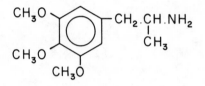

(c)

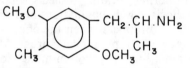

(d)

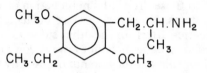

(e)

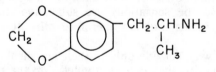

(f)

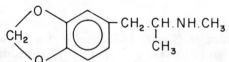

(g)

Figure 18.1 The chemical structures of phenylethylamine psychotomimetic drugs: (a) 3,4,5-trimethoxy-phenylethylamine (mescaline); (b) trimethoxyamphetamine (TMA); (c) 2,5-dimethoxy-4-methyl-amphetamine (DOM); (d) 2,5-dimethoxy-4-ethylamphetamine (DOET); (e) 3,4-methylene-dioxy-amphetamine (MDA); (f) 5-methoxy-3,4-methylenedioxyamphetamine (MMDA); (g) 3,4-methylene-dioxy-methylamphetamine (MDMA)

from the peyote cactus, having the appearance of mushroom-like discs. Much has been written about mescaline and its effects, some of which have been described by Aldous Huxley in his book *The Doors of Perception*.

Mescaline is not a very potent drug and oral doses of the order of 250–500 mg are required. The early effects (i.e. during the first 1–2 h) may be unpleasant and include nausea, tremors and perspiration, due to autonomic stimulation, but these effects wear off and are eventually replaced by a hallucinatory dream-like state which can last for up to 12 h. Mescaline does not appear to have become popular as a drug of abuse, possibly because of the long delay before its effects become apparent and also because the early effects are unpleasant. The long latency suggests that a metabolite of mescaline may be active and the known metabolites, *N*-acetylmescaline and 3,4,5-trimethoxyphenylacetic acid, have been found to possess psychotomimetic activity. The mechanism of action of mescaline is unknown, although it has been suggested that it is the same as that of LSD 25 (see below). Structure–activity studies of analogues of mescaline have shown that the methoxy-substitution in position 5 is essential for psychotomimetic activity.

Other phenylethylamines

Many other psychotomimetic compounds structurally related to amphetamine have been made, many illicitly. They include trimethoxyamphetamine (TMA, Figure 18.1b), which is α-methyl mescaline and is about ten times more potent than mescaline as a psychotomimetic but is less stimulant than amphetamine. Another derivative is 2,5-dimethoxy-4-methylamphetamine (Figure 18.1c, also known as DOM and as 'STP' for serenity, tranquillity and peace), which has similar effects to those of mescaline but is 40–50 times more potent, being effective in doses of the order of 10 mg by mouth. A related compound is 2,5-dimethoxy-4-ethylamphetamine (DOET, Figure 18.1d). Other similar drugs are 3,4-methylenedioxyamphetamine (MDA, also known as the 'love pill'; Figure 18.1e), 5-methoxy-3,4-methylenedioxyamphetamine (MMDA, Figure 18.1f) and 3,4-methylenedioxymethylamphetamine (MDMA, dubbed 'ecstasy'; Figure 18.1g), all of which are psychotomimetic, although very little else is known about them, except that some are reported to produce enhanced self-awareness rather than hallucinations.

Indolealkylamines

D-*Lysergic acid diethylamide* (*LSD 25 or LSD*, Figure 18.2a)

This compound was first synthesized in 1938 but its psychotomimetic properties were not known until it was accidentally ingested by the Swiss chemist Hoffmann in 1943, the effects being subsequently confirmed in a number of trials. It is now the 'prototype' psychotomimetic drug, being the most potent and producing fewer side-effects than the other psychotomimetic drugs. In fact, it is probably the most potent drug known to act on the central nervous system, being effective in humans in doses of 50 μg or less (see Table 18.1), and electrophysiological effects in experimental animals have been detected with doses as small as 1.0 μg/kg. It is a semisynthetic drug and is related to ergot which is produced in wheat by the fungus *Claviceps purpurea*, together with a number of related substances, e.g. lysergic acid. Reports of the effects of LSD 25 in humans tend to be anecdotal and the effects have to be experienced to be fully appreciated. Essentially, they consist of heightened aware-

(a)

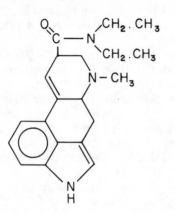

(b)

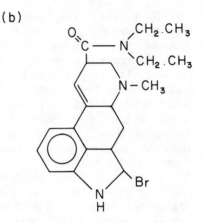

Figure 18.2 The chemical structure of (a) the indolealkylamine psychotomimetic drug D-lysergic acid diethylamide (LSD 25) and (b) the non-psychotomimetic derivative, brom-LSD

Table 18.1 Approximate minimal doses of some drugs of abuse

Drug	Route	Dose (μg)
Ethyl alcohol	oral	7 000 000–20 000 000
Cocaine	s.c.	80 000–3 000 000
Mescaline	oral	10 000–20 000
Morphine	s.c.	5 000–10 000
Atropine	s.c.	3 000–10 000
Methamphetamine	oral	1 500–3 000
LSD	oral	30–50

(s.c. = subcutaneous)

ness, depersonalization and fluctuating mood changes. Visual hallucinations and distortions of body image are common. Trance-like states can also occur. The drug seems to exaggerate any underlying trends in normal subjects: thus someone who is mildly obsessional becomes more so and any tendency towards paranoia becomes exaggerated.

D-Lysergic acid diethylamide is a drug of abuse (see below). The behavioural effects show tolerance although there is no physical dependence and withdrawal symptoms are not seen when administration of the drug is discontinued. Toxicity is low and untoward effects, which can sometimes result in death, are due to judgement being distorted, rather than to a direct effect of the drug. Thus, a mistaken belief in the ability to fly while intoxicated with LSD 25 can have disastrous consequences! Panic reactions ('bad trips') also occur.

N,N-Dimethyltryptamine (DMT, Figure 18.3a)

This substance is present in South American snuff. Although its effects are similar to those of LSD, it is much less effective when taken by mouth, but it is active when given intravenously or intramuscularly. Thus, a dose of 1.0 mg produces a brief but intense LSD-like experience. It is usually taken as snuff or smoked.

(a)

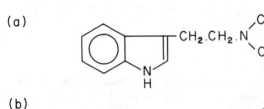

(b)

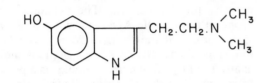

(c)

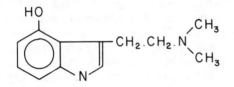

(d)

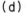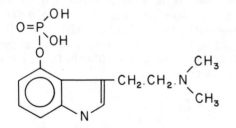

Figure 18.3 The chemical structures of (a) N,N-dimethyltryptamine (DMT), (b) 5-hydroxy-N,N-dimethyltryptamine (bufotenin), (c) 4-hydroxy-N,N-dimethyltryptamine (psilocyn) and (d) 4-phosphoryl-N,N-dimethyltryptamine (psilocybin)

Bufotenin

This is 5-hydroxy-N,N-dimethyltryptamine (Figure 18.3b) and is widely distributed in plants as well as being found in the skin of toads of the genus *Bufo*; it is also present in South American snuff. It is very weak as a psychotomimetic, being about

1000 times less potent than LSD even when given intravenously, and the effects are transient. As well as hallucinations however, it produces severe autonomic effects.

Psilocyn and psilocybin

Psilocyn is 4-hydroxy-N,N-dimethyltryptamine (Figure 18.3c) and psilocybin is 4-phosphoryl-N,N-dimethyltryptamine (Figure 18.3d); they are both present in Mexican mushrooms of the species *Psilocybe semilanceata* (also known as 'magic mushrooms' and 'Liberty cap'). Their effects are similar to those of LSD but they are much less potent, oral doses of the order of 8 mg being needed.

Anticholinergic psychotomimetic drugs

Large doses of belladonna alkaloids, such as atropine and hyoscine (scopolamine), can produce hallucinations, confusion and amnesia and the plants from which they are derived have been used for centuries for their effects. The belladonna plant (*Atropa belladonna*), was used in Europe in the Middle Ages as a witch's brew and the dried leaves of *Hyocyamus muticus* (black henbane), which grows in the Middle East, were smoked for their hallucinogenic effects. *Hyocyamus niger* (henbane) was widely cultivated in Europe and was also used by the Ancient Greeks as a poison to produce a state of dementia. Some recently developed anticholinergic drugs are more potent as psychotomimetics. These are piperidyl benzilate esters, a large number of which have been synthesized. An example is Ditran (or JB 329, Figure 18.4), which is a mixture of two esters. The peripheral effects of Ditran are similar to those of atropine but its actions on the CNS are stimulatory. It causes feelings of apprehension, disorientation in time and space, depersonalization and sensory disturbances and hallucinations, followed by confusion, emotional disturbances and paranoid feelings. There is also a period of amnesia and some subjects show a marked elevation of mood, characterized by euphoria and increased initiative and activity, after the psychotomimetic effects have disappeared. Ditran was therefore tested as a possible treatment for depression but has never been widely used. The effects of the psychotomimetic anticholinergic drugs differ from those of the phenylethylamine derivatives and the indolealkylamines in that they produce amnesia, intellectual impairment and confusion; it is thought that their mechanism of action in the CNS is different (see below).

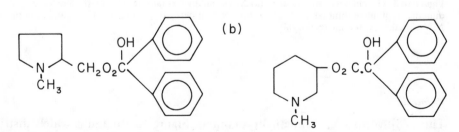

Figure 18.4 The chemical structures of the glycolate esters in Ditran, which consists of a mixture of 70% of (a) and 30% of (b)

Miscellaneous psychotomimetic drugs

Harmala alkaloids

Both harmine (Figure 18.5a) and its 3,4-dihydro derivative, harmaline (Figure 18.5b) are β-carbolines and are psychotomimetic. They are inhibitors of monoamine oxidase and antagonists of 5-hydroxytryptamine. Very little is known about these compounds but, as they can be formed from endogenous tryptamines, they may play a part in disturbances of mental function.

Phencyclidine (Figure 18.5c)

This is related to ketamine which is used as a dissociative anaesthetic (see Chapter 11 and Figure 11.3c). In fact, phencyclidine was developed as a potential anaesthetic agent and was marketed under the name 'Sernyl'. However, it was withdrawn because of the psychotomimetic effects, particularly hallucinations, which appeared during recovery. Nevertheless, it is used for veterinary anaesthesia. It has atropine-like activity, causing mydriasis and dry mouth and, like ketamine, is a potent analgesic. Phencyclidine is a drug of abuse, being known as 'angel dust'. It is potent (doses of 5–20 mg are effective), is active regardless of the route of administration (oral, injection or smoking) and is relatively easy to synthesize. Its main effect is to produce a distortion of body image, detachment from the environment and vivid dreaming. There seems to be a loss of ability to integrate sensory information, especially tactile and proprioceptive, which may account for some of these effects as well as contributing to the analgesia. There may also be euphoria, but anxiety and depression can occur. Because of its atropine-like activity, phencyclidine is sometimes classified with the anticholinergic psychotomimetics. However, its central effects do not appear to be related to a central anticholinergic action (see below). Phencyclidine appears to be more toxic than most other psychotomimetic drugs. In overdose it can cause motor seizures and coma. Deaths resulting from respiratory depression and cardiac arrest have occurred.

(a)

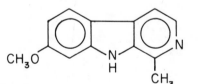

(b)

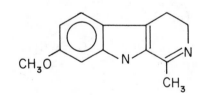

(c)

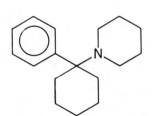

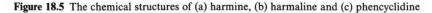

Figure 18.5 The chemical structures of (a) harmine, (b) harmaline and (c) phencyclidine

Myristicin (Figure 18.6a)

This substance is present in the dried seeds of the nutmeg tree (*Myristica fragrans*) which grows in Indonesia and it is known that the consumption of large amounts of nutmeg can produce psychotomimetic effects, including hallucinations, distortions of perception and drowsiness. Unpleasant effects, such as dry mouth, tachycardia, flushing of the face, anxiety and agitation can also occur and can lead to death. The myristicin molecule contains an analogue of mescaline and it is possible that the psychotomimetic effects may be due to mescaline being formed as a metabolite.

Agonists of γ-aminobutyric acid

The mushroom *Amanita muscaria* (fly agaric) contains a number of pharmacologically active alkaloids, including muscarine, ibotenic acid (Figure 18.6b), and muscimol (Figure 18.6c), the latter two substances being potent agonists at GABA receptors. Both are psychotomimetic and are thought to account for the effects of the intact mushroom, dried preparations of which are consumed in parts of Asia. The effects resemble those of alcohol, with drowsiness, euphoria, dizziness and ataxia leading to a delirious state with visual and auditory disturbances, confusion and agitation. The effects last for several hours and are often followed by sedation and sleep. In Europe, *Amanita muscaria* is regarded as being poisonous and is used as an insecticide.

(a)

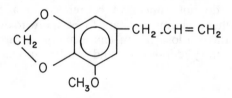

(b)

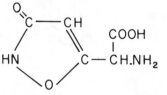

(c)

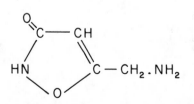

Figure 18.6 The chemical structures of (a) myristicin, (b) ibotenic acid and (c) muscimol

The mechanism of action of psychotomimetic drugs

Of the psychotomimetic drugs described above, D-lysergic acid diethylamide is not only the most potent but has been the most widely studied. Because of its structural similarity to the endogenous indoleamine 5-hydroxytryptamine, it was thought that LSD might act on 5-HT receptors in the CNS. Moreover, LSD was found to act peripherally as an antagonist to 5-HT and it was suggested that a similar action in the CNS might be responsible for the psychotomimetic effects. However, the 2-bromo-derivative of LSD (or brom-LSD, Figure 18.2b) is also a 5-HT antagonist peripherally, but is not a psychotomimetic. Nevertheless, antagonist actions of LSD, which are selective for 5-HT receptors and are not shown by brom-LSD, have been found on neurones in the brain stem in regions which are involved in the filtering and integration of sensory information. Such actions could well account for the sensory disturbances, e.g. hallucinations, produced by this drug. The indolealkylamine psychotomimetics, including LSD, have been found to have an inhibitory action on the firing of 5-HT-containing neurones in the raphe nucleus and this effect is produced by a preferential agonist action at 5-HT autoreceptors. These receptors are likely to be of the 5-HT_1-subtype (see Chapter 10); however, LSD has been shown to bind with an equal affinity to both 5-HT_1 and 5-HT_2 receptors, the latter being postsynaptic. The inhibitory action on neurones of the raphe nucleus has been found not only with LSD and related psychotomimetic drugs, such as psilocybin, psilocyn and dimethyltryptamine, but also with lisuride, a substance which is structurally similar to LSD, but which is not psychotomimetic. This finding throws some doubt on the theory that inhibition of the activity of raphe neurones is responsible for the psychotomimetic effects of LSD and related drugs. A third possibility is related to the finding that 5-HT can have a facilitatory action on certain motor neurones in the CNS and that this facilitatory action is enhanced by small doses of LSD. This effect is also produced by mescaline, which does not act on raphe neurones in the same way as LSD. As cross-tolerance between LSD and mescaline has been demonstrated in a number of species, it has been suggested that the two drugs share a common site of action. Nevertheless, it is difficult to relate an enhancement of 5-HT-induced facilitation of motor neurones to the perceptual changes produced by psychotomimetic drugs; similar effects on sensory pathways need to be demonstrated in order to lend credibility to this hypothesis. Thus, the precise mechanism through which LSD and related drugs produce their psychotomimetic effects remains uncertain.

The facts that mescaline is structurally related to amphetamine and that amphetamine, consumed in large doses and/or over prolonged periods, can induce a psychotic-like state in normal individuals (see Chapters 12 and 16) point to a common mechanism of action for these two drugs. The main pharmacological action of amphetamine is to release noradrenaline and dopamine from presynaptic nerve terminals, and dopamine has been implicated in psychotic states. Thus, an amphetamine-like action by mescaline, i.e. releasing dopamine presynaptically, could account for its psychotomimetic activity. However, there is little evidence either for or against this hypothesis and the fact that mescaline and LSD show cross-tolerance suggests that the theory is improbable.

The psychotomimetic effects of the anticholinergic drugs can be blocked by anticholinesterase drugs, such as physostigmine, which prevent the breakdown of acetylcholine. This clearly links their psychotomimetic effects with cholinergic mechanisms in the brain.

Phencyclidine interacts with a number of neurotransmitter systems: for example, it inhibits the re-uptake of noradrenaline, dopamine and 5-hydroxytryptamine. However, the effects of phencyclidine are not blocked by either antagonists or agonists of these neurotransmitters, nor are they mimicked. Binding studies have shown that independent binding sites for phencyclidine are present in the brain. These have been designated as σ-receptors and were at one time considered to be a fourth subtype of opiate receptor. However, as the effects of phencyclidine and of other drugs which act at σ-receptors are not blocked by the opioid antagonists, such as naloxone, these receptors are now regarded as non-opiate. They are present in the highest concentration in the hippocampus and frontal cortex, with a moderate density in the cerebellum. No endogenous ligand has been found for the σ-receptor and it is not certain whether this receptor mediates the psychotomimetic effects of phencyclidine, although the opiate analgesic pentazocine (Chapter 15) can produce dysphoria and psychotomimetic effects which are thought to be mediated by σ-receptors. Phencyclidine is also an antagonist at the N-methyl-D-aspartate subtype of glutamate receptor (see Chapter 10 and Figure 10.11c). It seems likely, however, that the receptor for N-methyl-D-aspartate and the σ-receptor are not identical but that the two receptors interact allosterically. As phencyclidine mimics many of the symptoms of schizophrenia, it was thought that a drug which acted as a competitive antagonist at the σ-receptor might be a good antipsychotic agent. So far, this search for a new class of antipsychotic drugs has not proved fruitful. However, some drugs which act at N-methyl-D-aspartate receptors appear to have a 'neuroprotective' function (see Chapter 20).

The uses of psychotomimetic drugs

The psychotomimetic drugs as such do not have any therapeutic application, although LSD was at one time used as an adjunct to psychotherapy and in the treatment of addiction to opioids and alcoholism. It has also been used to produce a state of tranquillity in terminal cancer and to reduce the amount of opiate analgesic needed. There is no clear evidence, however, that the drug has any major beneficial effects and, because it became a drug of abuse, its use for such purposes was discouraged and eventually abandoned. The state produced by LSD in otherwise normal individuals has been described as a 'model psychosis' because the symptoms produced so closely resemble those in naturally occurring psychotic states, such as schizophrenia, and it lacks the unpleasant effects of mescaline. It was even suggested at one time that all psychiatrists should undergo the experience of taking LSD in order to appreciate more fully the mental state of their patients. This idea is almost certainly false*. There is no certainty, either, that the 'model psychosis' can be used for the analysis of underlying mechanisms, because there is no reason to

---

* As a participant in what was probably one of the first controlled trials of the effects of LSD in normal subjects, the writer can confirm from personal experience that, although there were marked sensory disturbances, including those of body image, there was never any loss of insight. This was also reported by the other subjects; they were always aware that they were taking part in an experiment. Whether this was related to the small doses of LSD which were used, it is difficult to say. The study was carried out by a group of psychiatrists most of whom were also the experimental subjects and the results were published in 1953.

believe that the mechanisms through which the drug produces its effects are the same as those responsible for the symptoms of schizophrenia.

Drugs of abuse

The term 'abuse' refers to the self administration of a drug for non-medical purposes. Usually the purpose is pleasure seeking, the abatement of anxiety or alterations in states of consciousness; often, excessive amounts of the drug are consumed. The definition of abuse is a social one because in some societies the use of drugs for non-medical purposes, e.g. religious experiences, is tolerated and in the Western world, the acute abuse of alcohol is largely tolerated whereas chronic abuse is not. Also tolerated are the abuse of tobacco, probably the greatest cause of preventable deaths, and the abuse of methylxanthines.

Many of the psychotomimetic drugs described above are also drugs of abuse, e.g. LSD, the phenylethylamines and phencyclidine. In addition, there are a number of drugs of abuse which, although they have marked effects on mental function, are not truly psychotomimetics. This group includes cocaine, amphetamine, cannabinols, organic solvents and gases. Finally, there are drugs such as the opiate analgesics, barbiturates, alcohol and nicotine (tobacco).

Cocaine and amphetamine

The pharmacological actions of cocaine are described in Chapters 8 and 16, and its use as a local anaesthetic in Chapter 9. The actions of amphetamine are described in Chapter 16. Both drugs produce euphoria and a sense of increased energy and alertness; the reported subjective effects are indistinguishable and the acute toxic syndromes are similar. It might seem, therefore, that the differences in the mechanisms of action of these two drugs do not influence the abuse potential. However, after intravenous administration the effects of cocaine are very brief, lasting for only a few minutes, whereas those of methamphetamine may last for hours. Amphetamine and related substances are usually taken either by mouth or intravenously, whereas the commonest route for cocaine is intranasal, i.e. sniffing or 'snorting', although it is also smoked. The vasoconstriction produced by cocaine often leads to necrosis and ultimately, perforation of the nasal septum. Tolerance develops to some of the central effects of amphetamine, particularly the euphoria, and the chronic user will have to increase the dose in order to obtain the desired effect. However, the toxic syndrome does not show tolerance. Tolerance to the central effects of cocaine is much less likely to occur. Both amphetamine and cocaine produce dependence with long-term use, withdrawal resulting in a craving for the drug, prolonged sleep, general fatigue, lassitude, depression and extreme hunger (hyperphagia). This suggests that both psychological and physical dependence are produced by these drugs. Fatalities are more likely to occur with cocaine, due to its action on the heart. The effects of acute overdose with amphetamine can be treated with chlorpromazine or diazepam to control convulsions, together with acidification of the urine to increase excretion. Diazepam is also used for overdose with cocaine but a β-blocker, such as propranolol, may also be needed.

Cannabinoids

The most important substance here is cannabis or marihuana, which occurs naturally in the flowering top of the hemp plant *Cannabis sativa*, which grows in many parts of the world. The use of the drug goes back to antiquity and many different names have been given to the extracts of the plant, which may be prepared in different ways. For example, in Africa the preparation for smoking is 'dagga', while in India the corresponding preparation, made from dried flowering tops of cultivated plants, is 'ganja'. A less potent preparation, made only from dried leaves and used in India for making tea, is 'bhang'. On the other hand, the most potent form, consisting of dried blocks of the resin which exudes from the tops of the plants, is known as 'hashish' in the Middle East and N. Africa and 'charas' in the Far East. The plant will grow in almost any climate but the drug cannabis is present in larger amounts in warm climates. Both the male and female plants contain cannabinoids.

The active principle in cannabis is Δ^9-tetrahydrocannabinol (Δ^9-THC, Figure 18.7). Many related substances occur naturally or have been synthesized but are either inactive or show only weak activity. Δ^9-Tetrahydrocannabinol is sometimes classified with the psychotomimetic drugs but it is not a true psychotomimetic, at least according to the definition at the beginning of this chapter.

The main pharmacological effects of Δ^9-THC are on the CNS and the cardiovascular system. Because it is highly lipid soluble, Δ^9-THC rapidly enters the CNS. The consumption of an oral dose of 20 mg or the smoking of one or two marihuana cigarettes, each containing 2.5– 5 mg, results in a change in mood, characterized by euphoria and a sense of relaxation accompanied by sleepiness, especially if the subject is alone. The perception of visual and auditory stimuli is enhanced and time perception is altered so that time appears to pass much more slowly. Short-term memory is impaired and the ability to carry out tasks requiring successive steps to reach a specific goal is impeded. This phenomenon is known as 'temporal disintegration'. These effects persist for 4–8 hours. Larger doses can induce hallucinations, delusions and feelings of paranoia. Thinking may become confused and disorganized and depersonalization may occur. The euphoria may be replaced by anxiety, which can reach panic proportions.

The main cardiovascular effects are an increase in heart rate, which is dose related, and peripheral vasodilatation. The latter results in swelling of the small conjunctival blood vessels and the appearance of bloodshot eyes (or 'red eye'), a feature which is common in cannabis smokers. Irritation of the throat and coughing

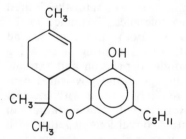

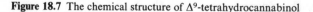

Figure 18.7 The chemical structure of Δ^9-tetrahydrocannabinol

is common in habitual cannabis smokers, together with increased hunger and frequency of micturition. Long-term effects include bronchitis and asthma, together with personality changes. Chromosomal damage has been reported and also interference with the functioning of the immune system. Impotence and temporary sterility can occur in men and teratogenic effects on the fetus in pregnant women. Tolerance to Δ^9-THC develops slowly and there is no evidence of dependence. The mechanism of action is unknown.

Strangely, although most of the effects of cannabis are undesirable, there are some potential therapeutic applications. For example, although adverse effects on pulmonary function result from chronic smoking, the acute response to Δ^9-THC is a significant and long-lasting bronchodilatation, to which little tolerance develops. Used in an aerosol, Δ^9-THC has been found to produce good bronchodilatation without tachycardia or appreciable central effects; a derivative of Δ^9-THC which lacked central effects would therefore be of value in the treatment of asthma. Secondly, Δ^9-THC has an anti-emetic action which is especially effective against the nausea and vomiting caused by chemotherapeutic agents used in the treatment of cancer. In fact, a synthetic derivative of Δ^9-THC, nabilone (see Chapter 20), has been used to reduce the nausea caused by cancer chemotherapy or irradiation therapy in cases where other anti-emetics have proved to be ineffective, the tachycardia being prevented with a β-blocker. A third area of potential usefulness is in the treatment of glaucoma (see Chapter 7) as Δ^9-THC and related cannabinoids have been found to reduce intra-ocular pressure. Another potential area of usefulness is in the treatment of hypertension due to peripheral vasodilatation. Cannabinoids have also been shown to possess anticonvulsant and analgesic properties. So far, apart from the anti-emetic drug nabilone, none of these possible therapeutic uses has been fully explored or new drugs, related to Δ^9-THC but without its central effects, produced.

Solvents and gases

The range of substances in this category is impressive and increasing almost daily. It includes anaesthetic gases, such as nitrous oxide, ether and chloroform, although access to these is necessarily difficult. Industrial solvents, such as paint thinners and strippers, and typewriter-correcting fluid, are used by the so-called 'glue sniffers' (the structures of some of these substances are shown in Figure 18.8). Alkyl nitrites, butyl, isobutyl and amyl, which are used medically as vasodilators, are abused for their aphrodisiac effects. Finally, some of the inert gases which are used as propellants in aerosols, e.g. Freon (Figure 18.9), are also abused. The problems of abuse of these substances is exacerbated by the availability of a wide range of preparations in which they can be found and by their cheapness. The inhalation of these substances results in a quick intoxication of short duration, with enhancement of mood. The effects reported are light-headedness, a pleasant exhilaration, euphoria and excitement. These effects may be followed by ataxia, slurred speech, disorientation and loss of consciousness. Often the substance is inhaled from a plastic bag and fatalities frequently occur.

The toxicity of such a miscellaneous group of substances varies considerably and the cause of death is not always clear. Inhalation of volatile material from a plastic bag will result in an extremely high concentration of the vapour, as well as hypoxia. Fluorinated hydrocarbons (e.g. aerosol propellants) produce cardiac arrhythmias; chlorinated solvents (e.g. carbon tetrachloride and trichlorethylene) depress myo-

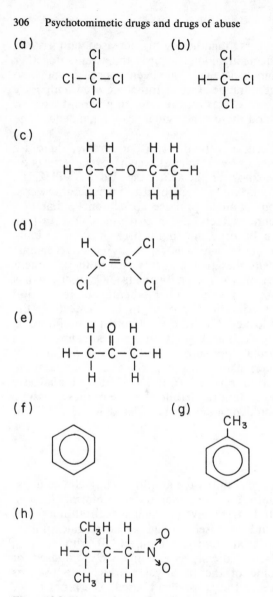

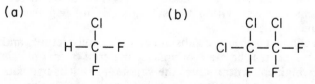

Figure 18.8 The chemical structures of some solvents and gases which are abused: (a) carbon tetrachloride, (b) chloroform, (c) diethyl ether, (d) trichlorethylene, (e) acetone, (f) benzene, (g) toluene and (h) amyl nitrate

Figure 18.9 The chemical structures of two halogenated hydrocarbons which are used as aerosol propellants: (a) chlorodifluoromethane (Freon 22) and (b) trichlorotrifluoroethane (Freon 113)

cardial contractility and sympathetic activity will be increased reflexly. Peripheral neuropathies and progressive fatal neurological deterioration have followed long-term abuse of solvents, and brain damage has been found after the chronic inhalation of aerosol propellants.

Opiate analgesics

The most abused opioid drug is heroin, probably because of its high lipid solubility which results in rapid penetration into the brain and also because of its availability, although morphine and, to a lesser extent, codeine and dextropropoxyphene are also abused. The precise reasons for the abuse of opioid drugs is not clear. One possibility is that use of the drug begins in the context of medical treatment; however, this group appears to constitute a very small proportion of the population of opioid drug abusers. The second possibility relates to experimental or 'recreational' use of drugs, which progresses to more intensive use. This group mainly involves adolescents and young adults, with males far outnumbering females. The euphoria which these drugs produce, together with the analgesia, provide the initial attraction, and the rapidity with which tolerance and dependence develop ensures their continued use. Surprisingly, the user's first experience with an opioid drug may be unpleasant, with nausea and vomiting being the prevalent features; however, many repeat the experience after a suitable interval, which may be days or weeks. The preferred route of administration of heroin is intravenous and it results in a warm flushing of the skin and sensations in the lower abdomen described by heroin addicts as being similar to a sexual orgasm. This effect lasts for about 45 seconds and is known as a 'rush'. Tolerance develops rapidly when the drug is administered intravenously, particularly as the 'rush' is short-lasting and the addict will repeat the injection frequently and will constantly have to increase the dose. The development of tolerance to and dependence on opioid drugs, and the abstinence syndrome which follows their withdrawal, are described in Chapter 15. The abstinence syndrome can be severe in addicts, particularly addicts on intravenously administered heroin, and slow withdrawal of the drug is essential, combined with rehabilitation. Fatalities among opioid abusers are frequent and may be due to number of causes; death from overdose is likely to be due to depression of respiration. However, infections due to the use of dirty hypodermic needles or syringes for injection, and even contamination of the drug, are not uncommon.

Barbiturates and other sedatives

The pattern of non-medical use of sedative drugs is very varied, ranging from infrequent periods of gross intoxication, lasting for a few days, to prolonged compulsive daily consumption of large quantities of the drug and a preoccupation with securing and maintaining adequate supplies. These drugs are often used by people with emotional disorders and the original contact with the drug may have been through it having been prescribed for insomnia or anxiety. The fact that barbiturates are no longer used to treat these conditions, together with their restricted availability, has probably helped to reduce the abuse of these drugs. However, the benzodiazepines that have largely replaced them, although less dangerous, also have an abuse potential.

The effects sought by the users of sedatives are similar to those of alcohol. However, after the initial disinhibition, which is followed by drowsiness, speech may be slurred and incoordination can occur. Some users may never exhibit signs of intoxication but may, nevertheless, be taking the drugs several times a day. The rapid tolerance and physical dependence which develops with the barbiturates, leading to addiction and an abstinence syndrome when the drug is withdrawn (see Chapter 11), makes these drugs extremely dangerous. The fact that the sedative effect of barbiturates shows tolerance but the depression of respiration does not, can result in death occurring with inadvertent or deliberate overdose, or when used in combination with other respiratory depressants, such as alcohol, because the effects on the medullary respiratory centre are additive. While the benzodiazepines are less dangerous because their toxicity is low, tolerance and dependence can occur and withdrawal of the drug may induce insomnia and rebound anxiety (see Chapter 13).

Most of the sedative drugs show cross-tolerance, indicating the probability of a common mechanism for the development of tolerance; this is important when combinations of drugs are used (see below).

Psychotomimetics

Most of these drugs have been abused at some time. However, the potent semi-synthetic or synthetic compounds like LSD, phencyclidine and the phenylethyl-amines, have proved to be more popular than mescaline and the anticholinergics. The psychotomimetics are often used intermittently, i.e. at intervals of weeks or months, rather than chronically. The behavioural effects of LSD show tolerance and there is cross-tolerance between LSD, mescaline and psilocybin but not between LSD and amphetamine, or between LSD and the anticholinergics or Δ^9-THC. Withdrawal symptoms do not occur and these drugs are relatively non-toxic, although deaths with overdose of phencyclidine have occurred.

Drug combinations

People who abuse sedatives and anti-anxiety agents may also abuse alcohol but are not likely to abuse opiate drugs. On the other hand, opiate addicts may sometimes abuse sedative drugs. Combinations of sedatives and amphetamines have also been used and a mixture of dextro-amphetamine (5 mg) and amylobarbitone (30 mg), sold under the trade name Drinamyl (or 'purple hearts') was popular at one time. The barbiturate was thought to counteract the anxiety produced by the amphetamine without reducing the euphoria and excitement. Those who abuse psychotomimetic drugs rarely also take drugs of other types, although they may use marihuana. On the other hand, many of those who use marihuana, often as the first drug they become involved with, are thought to progress to abuse of heroin. However, this may not be related to the properties of the drugs but to other factors, such as pressure from drug 'pushers'.

Models of drug abuse

Numerous attempts have been made to establish models of 'drug-taking' behaviour in animals in the hope that analysis of the underlying mechanisms might throw some light on how tolerance, dependence and addiction are produced in humans. In fact, animals learn quickly to self administer drugs and, when given continuous access to a drug, show patterns of self administration that are very similar to those shown by human users of the drug. This suggests that there is no underlying predisposition to drug taking and that it is the drug itself which acts as the reinforcement. However, not all centrally acting drugs are self administered in animals although most of the drugs used for non-medical purposes are, namely opiate analgesics, barbiturates, alcohol, CNS stimulants, cocaine, caffeine and phencyclidine, etc. Whether an animal will self administer a drug depends on a number of factors, including, of course, the nature of the drug, but also the route of administration, the size of the dose, the interval between the animal's response and delivery of the drug (schedule of reinforcement) and any previous exposure to drugs. It has been found that drugs can serve as internal stimuli, i.e. that they can have the same function as exteroceptive stimuli. Furthermore, it has been shown that drugs can act as reinforcers, so that positive reinforcement by a drug of the response which led to its administration, e.g. pressing a lever, will lead to self administration of the drug. Negative reinforcement, or an aversive effect of the drug, will result in it not being self administered, an example of such a drug being chlorpromazine. It is currently thought that these effects of drugs are produced through an interaction with conditioning processes. It is hoped that further information about the nature of these processes may throw some light on the mechanisms responsible for drug abuse and on the way in which tolerance and dependence develop.

Chapter 19

Drugs used in the treatment of neurological disorders

The main disease of the peripheral nervous system which can be treated with drugs is myasthenia gravis and it is discussed in Chapter 5. This chapter, therefore, is concerned only with disorders of the central nervous system. These are principally disorders of movement such as Parkinson's disease, Huntington's chorea and spastic conditions.

Parkinson's disease

Parkinsonism is a relatively common disease in those over the age of 55, in which it has an incidence of approximately 1 in 1000. Although the incidence of the disease is fairly constant it appears to be genetically determined. It is a progressive disease which is characterized by (1) muscular rigidity, (2) tremor of the limbs at rest and (3) hypokinesia or akinesia. The rigidity is confined mainly to the muscles of the limbs, trunk and face; it is detected by resistance to passive movement of the limbs and is due to increased muscle tone. The tremor usually starts with 'pill-rolling' movements of the hands and disappears during voluntary movements. The hypokinesia, a decreased frequency of voluntary movements, or akinesia, an inability to initiate voluntary movements, results in those with this disease having difficulty in moving around. It also results in patients with Parkinson's disease having a fast shuffling gait which is difficult for them to start and, once started, is also difficult to stop. It is not known if the main deficit is in planning the movements or in their execution. The akinesia also results in a 'masked' facial expression. In most cases, parkinsonism is idiopathic, i.e. of unknown origin, but it can occur after cerebral ischaemia and also many years after infective encephalitis. The symptoms of Parkinson's disease appear as the side-effects of many neuroleptic drugs (see Chapter 12) and can be relieved with the same drugs that are used to treat idiopathic parkinsonism. Recently, a neurotoxic substance, MPTP (see below) has been found to produce a condition in primates which closely resembles all the features, both pathological and biochemical, of the disease and may well provide a useful model for Parkinson's disease. This discovery has also led to the suggestion that substances similar to MPTP may occur in the environment and that repeated exposure to small quantities of such chemicals, combined with ageing, may be factors in the aetiology of the disease.

The neuropathology of Parkinson's disease

It has long been known that Parkinson's disease is a disorder of the basal ganglia and, before the advent of drug therapy, symptomatic relief was obtained with surgical lesions in this region of the brain. It was also known that 80% of the dopamine content of the brain is found in the basal ganglia and, in 1960, it was discovered that the brains from patients with Parkinson's disease showed, *post mortem*, a deficiency of dopamine in this region. Subsequently, it was found that this deficiency was due to a progressive and selective degeneration of dopamine-containing neurones of the substantia nigra (see Figure 10.5), particularly the pigmented cells of the zona compacta (Figure 19.1a), with the consequent loss of the dopamine-containing nerve terminals which project to the caudate nucleus and putamen (compare Figure 19.1a and b). This pathway is part of the extrapyramidal system which controls movement. The dopamine released from the terminals in the caudate nucleus–putamen complex has an inhibitory action and probably exerts fine control over the activity of the output neurones in this region. Thus, the loss of this control will result in overactivity. This may be why lesions in this area were beneficial to patients with Parkinson's disease.

However, dopamine is not the only neurotransmitter involved. Studies which showed a deficiency of dopamine in the basal ganglia of patients with Parkinson's disease also showed reductions, to a lesser extent, in the content of noradrenaline and 5-hydroxytryptamine, although the loss of noradrenaline-containing neurones is mainly in the locus coeruleus (Figure 10.4). Some changes in other neurotransmitters may be secondary to the degeneration of dopamine-containing neurones. Nevertheless, both acetylcholine and γ-aminobutyric acid (GABA) are known to be involved, as neurones utilizing these neurotransmitters are present in the basal ganglia (Figure 19.1).

Although the precise relationships between the various neurotransmitter systems in the basal ganglia are not clear, it is known that the dopaminergic input to the striatum inhibits the activity of intrinsic cholinergic neurones (Figure 19.1a). In addition, there are GABA-containing neurones which provide a feedback pathway from the striatum to the substantia nigra, as well as intrinsic GABA-containing neurones within the striatum (Figure 19.1a). It is thought that it is mainly the balance between the activity of dopaminergic and cholinergic neurones that is important in Parkinson's disease. Thus, when the dopamine-containing neurones have degenerated below a certain critical level (Figure 19.1b), the inhibitory influence of dopamine is reduced and the excitatory effects of the cholinergic neurones predominate. Before this stage is reached, compensatory mechanisms, e.g. supersensitivity of dopamine receptors, accommodate for the loss of dopaminergic function and prevent the appearance of symptoms. This theory is probably too simplistic and does not allow for the fact that the influence of GABA in the striatum is also reduced, as the levels of glutamate decarboxylase, the enzyme involved in the synthesis of GABA (see Chapter 10), are also diminished in Parkinson's disease. This reduced influence of GABA, which is also inhibitory, would allow further dominance of competing excitatory cholinergic mechanisms. However, the theory is supported by the fact that both replacement therapy to compensate for the deficiency in dopamine and treatment with antagonists of acetylcholine are effective in relieving the symptoms of Parkinson's disease.

The concept that it is the deficit in dopamine which is the principal cause of the symptoms of Parkinson's disease was supported by the discovery that the neuro-

313

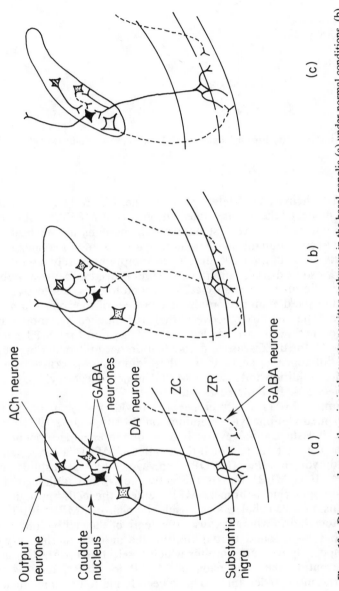

(a)

(b)

(c)

Figure 19.1 Diagram showing the principal neurotransmitter pathways in the basal ganglia (a) under normal conditions, (b) in Parkinson's disease and (c) in Huntington's chorea. In Parkinson's disease (b) the influence of the inhibitory nigrostriatal dopaminergic (DA) pathway on the striatum is diminished due to degeneration of dopamine-containing neurones in the substantia nigra. There is also a reduction in the inhibitory influence of GABA, both in the substantia nigra and also in the striatum. The net result is hyperactivity of the cholinergic (ACh) neurones in the striatum which influence the activity of the output neurones. In Huntington's chorea (c), the degeneration is mainly in the striatum. There is reduced activity of GABA both in the striatum and in the substantia nigra and also of cholinergic neurones in the striatum, while the dopaminergic pathway is not affected. ZC, zona compacta; ZR, zona reticulata (redrawn from Bradford, 1986)

(a)   (b)

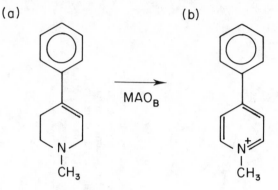

MAO_B

Figure 19.2 The chemical structure of (a) 1-methyl-4-phenyl-1,2,3,6-tetrahydropyridine (MPTP) and (b) its active metabolite MPP+

toxin MPTP (1-methyl-4-phenyl-1,2,3,6-tetrahydropyridine, Figure 19.2a) provided a remarkably accurate model of the disease state. The effects of MPTP, a substance which is available commercially, were first observed in humans as the result of it being produced as a contaminant in the illicit synthesis of an analogue of meperidine. The addicts, some in their 20s, developed symptoms closely resembling those of idiopathic Parkinson's disease, and the condition proved to be irreversible. The drug, which is active in many other species, was found to cause a selective and irreversible destruction of the dopamine-containing neurones of the zona compacta of the substantia nigra. The similarity between the drug-induced symptoms and those of the naturally occurring disease has led to the suggestion that MPTP may provide an accurate model for the disease and may help in our understanding of its aetiology. The main difference appears to be that idiopathic parkinsonism is progressive whereas the condition induced by MPTP is not. Nevertheless, it has been found that the effect of MPTP increases with age.

As it is a tertiary amine, MPTP easily crosses the blood–brain barrier. In the brain it is oxidized to 1-methyl-4-phenyl-pyridinium ion (MPP+, Figure 19.2b) by a two-stage process: the first stage involves the B form of the enzyme monoamine oxidase (i.e. MAO_B, see Chapter 10) in which the non-toxic MPTP is converted to 1-methyl-4-phenyl-2,3-dihydropyridine (MPDP); however, this is unstable and auto-oxidizes to MPP+. It is MPP+ that is the active toxin and, although it is formed outside the dopaminergic neurones, MPP+ enters the cells through the specific uptake mechanism for catecholamines. Inside the neurone, MPP+ is further concentrated in the mitochondria where it causes the death of the cell by inhibiting aerobic glycolysis. It has been found that inhibiting the activity of the enzyme monoamine oxidase, especially with an inhibitor which is selective for MAO_B, such as selegiline, thus preventing the conversion of MPTP to MPP+, reduces the toxicity of MPTP. Furthermore, older animals have been found to be more efficient at converting MPTP to MPP+ and this may correlate with the increased activity of monoamine oxidase with age. The discovery of MPTP has led to the suggestion that Parkinson's disease may be due to the formation and accumulation of a toxic compound, of either endogenous or exogenous origin, within the dopamine-containing neurones of the substantia nigra and that the toxin is formed by the action of monoamine oxidase. The fact that MPTP selectively depletes dopamine in the basal ganglia and produces symptoms closely resembling those of parkinsonism, supports the concept that the defect in dopamine is primarily responsible for the symptoms of the disease.

The treatment of Parkinson's disease

Before the discovery of the dopamine deficiency in Parkinson's disease, antagonists of the muscarinic actions of acetylcholine were used successfully. The drugs of choice are now those which increase the levels of dopamine or are dopamine agonists; nevertheless, anticholinergic drugs still have a role in treatment.

Levodopa

After the discovery that there was a deficiency of dopamine in the basal ganglia of patients with Parkinson's disease, attempts were made to use replacement therapy to restore the levels of dopamine. As dopamine itself does not cross the blood–brain barrier, the amino acid precursor of dopamine, L-3,4-dihydroxyphenylalanine (L-dopa or levodopa, Figure 19.3), was used with immediate success and this drug

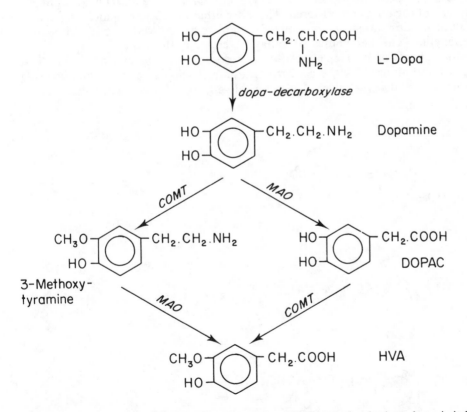

Figure 19.3 The synthesis and metabolism of dopamine. The enzymes involved are shown in italics. L-dopa, L-3,4-dihydroxyphenylalanine; DOPAC, 3,4-dihydroxyphenylacetic acid; HVA, 3-methoxy-4-hydroxyphenylacetic acid; MAO, monoamine oxidase; COMT, catechol-*O*-methyltransferase

is now the first line of treatment in all types of parkinsonism, except that associated with the use of neuroleptic drugs.

Levodopa is well absorbed following oral administration but it has to be given in large doses to be effective. It is converted to dopamine by the enzyme dopa-decarboxylase (see Chapter 8 and Figure 19.3). However, this conversion occurs at the periphery as well as in the CNS and 90–95% of the levodopa given orally is converted to dopamine peripherally. Because the dopamine formed peripherally cannot cross the blood–brain barrier, large doses must be given to allow the accumulation of adequate amounts of levodopa in the brain. In fact, it has been found that only about 1% of the orally consumed dose of levodopa reaches the brain. Alternatively, the concurrent administration of a peripherally acting inhibitor of dopa-decarboxylase, such as carbidopa (Figure 19.4a) or benserazide (Figure 19.4b), will reduce the dose of levodopa needed by preventing the conversion of levodopa to dopamine peripherally. Approximately 75% of patients with Parkinson's disease respond favourably to administration of levodopa and the effects are immediate and sometimes dramatic. Hypokinesia and rigidity usually respond more quickly and more consistently than the tremor; however, the tremor often improves when therapy is maintained. Dopamine is metabolized to yield two main metabolites: 3,4-dihydroxyphenylacetic acid (DOPAC) and 3-methoxy-4-hydroxyphenylacetic acid (or homovanillic acid, HVA) (Figure 19.3); these account for approximately 50% of the dose administered. There are other metabolites which are formed in small quantities and small amounts of dopamine are converted to noradrenaline and adrenaline. The metabolites are rapidly excreted in the urine.

The side-effects of levodopa are generally dose dependent and reversible, and they can be minimized by the concurrent administration of a peripherally acting inhibitor of dopa-decarboxylase. The main side-effects of levodopa are disturbances

(a)

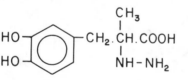

(b)

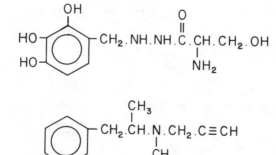

(c)

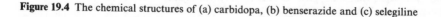

Figure 19.4 The chemical structures of (a) carbidopa, (b) benserazide and (c) selegiline

of the gastrointestinal tract, e.g. anorexia, nausea and vomiting. These effects are thought to be caused by direct stimulation of the chemoreceptor trigger zone of the area postrema of the medulla oblongata by dopamine (see Chapter 20). They may occur in up to 80% of patients treated with levodopa and are most likely to occur if the dose is increased too rapidly; however, these side-effects usually show tolerance and disappear after a few weeks. Orthostatic hypotension also occurs early in therapy in some 30% of patients; again, tolerance develops and the hypotension usually disappears with continued administration of the drug. Its onset can be minimized by starting treatment with small doses and gradually increasing to the therapeutic level. The hypotension is thought to be due to dopamine accumulating in noradrenergic nerve terminals where it acts as a false transmitter, as dopamine is not an effective agonist at α_1-adrenoceptors. Cardiac arrhythmias can also occur, particularly in older patients, although the incidence is low. These are attributed to stimulation of β-receptors in the heart by dopamine.

More serious side-effects which appear with long-term use of levodopa are dyskinesias, or involuntary choreiform movements of the limbs, hands, trunk, face and tongue. They are thought to be due to the development of supersensitivity of dopamine receptors and can be reduced by lowering the dose of levodopa; however, the symptoms of Parkinson's disease may then reappear. This side-effect does not show tolerance but many patients are prepared to accept a degree of dyskinesia if their mobility is improved by treatment with levodopa. Serious mental disturbances occur in about 15% of patients receiving levodopa, the symptoms resembling those of schizophrenia, e.g. delusions, hallucinations, paranoia and mania. This is thought to be due to overstimulation of dopamine receptors (see Chapter 12). Many patients on long-term therapy with levodopa experience vivid dreams or night-mares, delusions and visual hallucinations. If serious psychiatric problems occur, the dose can be reduced or the patient can be given a 'drug holiday' (see below). Occasionally, mania involving inappropriate or excessive sexual behaviour may occur.

The treatment of Parkinson's disease with levodopa is often accompanied by fluc-tuations in the clinical condition. The symptoms of the disease, which previously had been well controlled, may reappear quite suddenly and may last for periods of a few minutes or hours and then remit again. This 'on–off' phenomenon can occur once a day or many times a day and tends to develop after treatment with levodopa has continued for approximately 2 years. There is no satisfactory explanation for the phenomenon although there appears to be a relationship between the 'on–off' effect and the plasma levels of the drug. One approach to the problem has been to divide the daily dose of levodopa into smaller doses which are given more frequently.

Very often, after treatment for 5–6 years, levodopa may begin to lose its effectiveness in controlling the symptoms of Parkinson's disease. This is, perhaps, not surprising because there is a progressive degeneration of neurones, for which the drug does not provide a cure but simply relief from the symptoms. While the progressive loss of dopaminergic neurones provides one explanation for the loss of effectiveness of levodopa after long-term treatment, another possibility is that desensitization of dopamine receptors may occur. This hypothesis has led to the idea of 'drug holidays' in which all medication is withdrawn for a period of some days in order to allow the receptors to 'resensitize', after which the medication can be gradually re-introduced and is often effective at a dose lower than that needed before the 'drug holiday': furthermore, side-effects may be less troublesome.

However, the benefits of 'drug holidays' have not been clearly demonstrated and it is not possible to predict which patients are likely to respond.

Selegiline (Figure 19.4c)

This is an inhibitor of the enzyme monoamine oxidase which is selective for the MAO_B form that predominates in the CNS. Thus, selegiline does not cause potentiation of the peripheral effects of catecholamines resulting in a hypertensive crisis, as do the non-selective monoamine oxidase inhibitors (see Chapter 17). Selegiline is therefore much less dangerous, even when taken concurrently with tyramine-containing foods. However, by inhibiting the action of MAO_B in the brain, selegiline prevents the breakdown of dopamine in the basal ganglia. It has some effect of its own on the symptoms of Parkinson's disease but it is more effective when used as an adjunct to treatment with levodopa. When selegiline is added, the dose of levodopa can be reduced without loss of therapeutic effectiveness and there is evidence that selegiline can prolong the effectiveness of levodopa. Selegiline is particularly effective against the akinesia which develops when the effect of levodopa begins to wear off, the so-called 'end-of-dose' akinesia.

Bromocriptine (Figure 19.5a)

This drug is a dopamine agonist, with a preference for D_2 dopamine receptors. It is a derivative of ergot and is one of a number of dopamine agonists with anti-parkinson activity, such as apomorphine and lergotrile. However, most of the others have serious side-effects and are not used clinically. The therapeutic effects of bromocriptine are very similar to those of levodopa and the side-effects are also very similar. Bromocriptine has no advantages over levodopa and its use is restricted to patients who do not respond well to levodopa. An improved thera-peutic response has been obtained in some patients with a combination of bromocriptine and levodopa, but abnormal involuntary movements and confusional states may occur. Bromocriptine stimulates dopamine receptors in the anterior pituitary and inhibits the release of prolactin. It has other endocrinological effects such as the suppression of lactation and it is used to treat several endocrine disorders.

Amantadine (Figure 19.5b)

This is an antiviral agent that was found by chance to be effective in the treatment of Parkinson's disease. Its mechanism of action is uncertain, but it has been shown to increase the release of dopamine from nerve terminals. It is less potent than levodopa and tolerance to the therapeutic effect develops fairly quickly, often in a matter of weeks; however, amantadine is relatively free from side-effects.

Anticholinergic drugs

These drugs were used successfully for the treatment of Parkinson's disease for many years before the discovery of the involvement of dopamine. They are all antagonists of the muscarinic actions of acetylcholine, and they act centrally to produce their effect by blocking the overactivity of the intrinsic cholinergic neurones in the striatum resulting from reduced inhibitory dopaminergic influence

(a)

(b)

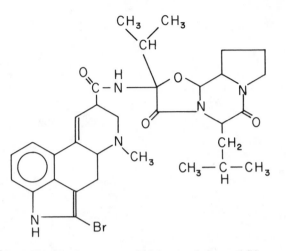

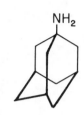

Figure 19.5 The chemical structures of (a) bromocriptine and (b) amantadine

(Figure 19.1). Examples are orphenadrine (Figure 19.6a), benzhexol (Figure 19.6b), benztropine (Figure 19.6c) and procyclidine (Figure 19.6d). At one time the phenothiazine ethopropazine was used as it possessed appreciable anticholinergic activity. The anticholinergic drugs are less effective than levodopa, reducing tremor and rigidity to a greater extent than the hypokinesia, which is often more disabling. The side-effects are those to be expected from acetylcholine antagonists, namely dry mouth, blurred vision, constipation and urinary retention and, when given in large doses, confusion and delirium. The use of these drugs has been largely superseded by levodopa although they may be used as first-line drugs in mild cases of Parkinson's disease, particularly when tremor and rigidity are the main symptoms, and they may be used as an adjunct to therapy with levodopa. The anticholinergic drugs are used to treat the symptoms of Parkinson's disease produced by phenothiazines and other neuroleptic drugs (see Chapter 12). They are effective in relatively small doses, but tardive dyskinesia is not improved and may be made worse.

Thus, of the drugs available, levodopa combined with a peripherally acting dopa-decarboxylase inhibitor, such as carbidopa or benserazide, is the treatment of first choice in idiopathic Parkinson's disease. It is less effective in postencephalitic parkinsonism and should not be used for drug-induced (neuroleptic) extrapyramidal symptoms where the anticholinergic drugs are more effective. Treatment with levodopa is initiated with small doses which are increased gradually. There is an argument for delaying the start of therapy with levodopa because of the limited duration of its effectiveness, and patients with mild symptoms may be treated initially with anticholinergic drugs before eventually being transferred to levodopa as the disease progresses. However, it is more likely that the failure of therapy with levodopa after some years is due to progression of the underlying disease and will therefore occur anyway.

(a)

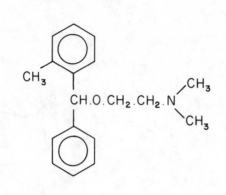

(b)

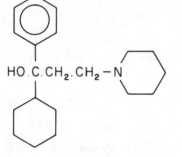

(c)

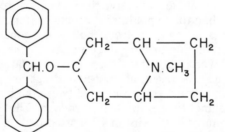

(d)

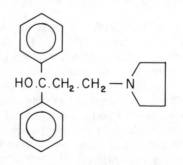

Figure 19.6 The chemical structures of (a) orphenadrine, (b) benzhexol, (c) benztropine and (d) procyclidine

Huntington's chorea

This is an inherited progressive degenerative disease of the brain which is comparatively rare, affecting 1 in 10–20 000 of the population. The onset is delayed, the first symptoms usually appearing in middle life, between the ages of 35 and 45 years, with death occurring some 15 years from onset. The condition is characterized by both mental retardation, leading to dementia, and progressively severe chorea, consisting of involuntary movements of the limbs, head and trunk and impeded speech.

The pathology of Huntington's chorea shows marked atrophy of the basal ganglia and shrinking of the cortex, with enlargement of the ventricles. The caudate and putamen are particularly affected, often being reduced to half their normal size, while the substantia nigra is less affected although there is some atrophy in the zona reticulata (Figure 19.1c). As with Parkinson's disease, there is an imbalance between the activity of dopamine, acetylcholine and GABA systems in the basal ganglia. However, in Huntington's chorea the dopamine content of the striatum is normal or slightly increased, but there is a reduction in the levels of GABA, both in the striatum and in the substantia nigra, which is due to reduced activity of the enzyme glutamic acid decarboxylase (GAD), which synthesizes GABA (see Chapter 10). There is also some reduction in acetylcholine, because of reduced activity of the enzyme choline acetyltransferase, which synthesizes acetylcholine. It is believed that the abnormal involuntary movements are caused by hyperactivity of dopaminergic mechanisms in the basal ganglia, due to the loss of GABA-mediated inhibitory influences both in the striatum and in the substantia nigra (see Figure 19.1). The reduced activity of the cholinergic neurones further shifts the balance between the dopaminergic and cholinergic systems in favour of overactivity of the dopaminergic inhibitory drive. Thus, the neuropathology of Huntington's chorea is in some respects a mirror image of that in Parkinson's disease: dopamine agonists, such as levodopa and bromocriptine, which are effective in Parkinson's disease, exacerbate the symptoms of Huntington's chorea, while dopamine antagonists are effective in reducing the involuntary movements. There is no effective treatment to halt the progression of the disease in Huntington's chorea. Drugs such as tetrabenazine and the neuroleptic pimozide (see Chapter 12, Figures 12.1b and 12.6a), can be used to decrease the choreiform movements. Identification, through the use of recombinant DNA techniques, of the faulty genetic material that is associated with this disease is more likely to be successful than the development of new drugs, as the aetiology of the disease is probably much more complex than outlined above. For example, the activity of 5-hydroxytryptamine has been found to be changed and decreases in peptide neurotransmitters, including substance P, enkephalins, angiotensin and cholecystokinin, have been found at post-mortem examination in the brains of patients with Huntington's chorea.

Spastic conditions

Spasticity can result from lesions at various levels of the central nervous system. It may consist of hyperexcitability of stretch reflexes or an increase in muscle tone which may be both painful and disabling. Weakness of the muscles can occur and there may be loss of dexterity. The causes can be birth injury, cerebral vascular disease or lesions of the spinal cord. The mechanisms are poorly understood but dysfunction of descending pathways in the spinal cord (corticospinal, vestibulo-spinal and reticulospinal) which control the activity of motor neurones, appears to be involved. Spasticity can be controlled either with drugs acting on the central nervous system or by drugs which act directly on skeletal muscle, e.g. dantrolene (see Chapter 5). The main drugs used to control muscle tone through a central action are the benzodiazepine diazepam, and baclofen.

Diazepam

This drug, the structure of which is shown in Figure 13.1b (Chapter 13), has a muscle-relaxant action that is manifested at the level of the spinal cord, as it is effective in patients with spinal cord lesions. However, it produces sedation at the doses required to reduce muscle tone. The action of diazepam is on primary afferents in the spinal cord, resulting in an increased level of presynaptic inhibition of muscle tone.

Baclofen (p-chlorophenyl GABA, Figure 19.7)

This is a derivative of γ-aminobutyric acid which penetrates the blood–brain barrier. The mechanism of action is not fully known but it depresses both mono- and polysynaptic reflexes in the spinal cord. These effects resemble those of GABA which is released by interneurones in the spinal cord and depolarizes the axon terminals of primary afferent fibres, resulting in presynaptic inhibition of motor neurones (see Chapter 10 and Figure 10.16). However, whereas these actions of GABA are blocked by bicuculline, those of baclofen are not. Furthermore, baclofen does not cause depolarization of primary afferent nerve terminals. The effects of baclofen are therefore probably exerted by an agonist action at $GABA_B$ receptors (see Chapter 10).

$$HOOC.CH_2.CH.CH_2.NH_2$$

Figure 19.7 The chemical structure of baclofen

Baclofen is rapidly absorbed after oral administration and has a half-life in plasma of 3–4 hours. It is excreted largely unchanged by the kidneys. It is used mainly for treating spasticity associated with multiple sclerosis or other diseases of the spinal cord and also spasticity due to trauma. The use of baclofen may be limited by its adverse effects, which include drowsiness, fatigue, nausea, vomiting and confusion. However, these can be minimized by initiating treatment with a small dose, which is then gradually increased. Overdose can result in coma, respiratory depression and seizures and an increase in the frequency of seizures has been observed in epileptic patients. Abrupt withdrawal of baclofen after chronic treatment can cause auditory and visual hallucinations, anxiety and tachycardia.

Chapter 20

Miscellaneous centrally acting drugs

The drugs discussed in this chapter do not fit into any of the categories of the preceding chapters but all produce their effects through an action on the central nervous system, even though the effects may be manifested peripherally. They include anti-emetics, antitussives, anorectic drugs, drugs which improve cognitive function and, finally, drugs with a new type of action which is best described as 'neuroprotective'.

Anti-emetic drugs

Vomiting or emesis has been described as the forceful expulsion of the gastrointestinal contents through the mouth. It is usually preceded by signs of autonomic stimulation, including salivation, pallor, sweating, dilatation of the pupils and nausea. The act of vomiting consists of a complex series of coordinated activities involving the muscles of the gastrointestinal tract and the respiratory and abdominal muscles. Although vomiting is normally preceded by nausea, it can occur in the absence of nausea and the feeling of nausea is not invariably followed by vomiting. Nevertheless, the drugs used in the treatment of vomiting (anti-emetics) are also effective against nausea and the two phenomena have similar origins. When the movements of vomiting take place without the expulsion of the gastric contents, this is known as retching.

Vomiting can arise through a variety of circumstances and physical, chemical or psychological stimuli can initiate the vomiting reflex. It can result from the ingestion of toxic or irritant substances, in which case the vomiting has a protective function and will be self limiting, i.e. ceasing when the offending material has been removed. Vomiting may also occur as a symptom of disease, as the side-effect of a drug, after exposure to ionizing radiation and during recovery from general anaesthesia; it may also occur as a complication in pregnancy. Vomiting is also a common and distressing component of motion or travel sickness.

The complex movements which comprise the vomiting reflex are coordinated by a region of the medulla oblongata known as the vomiting centre, which is located close to those centres in the brain stem which control cardiovascular, respiratory and other autonomic functions (Figure 20.1). It is thought that the close proximity of the vomiting centre to these autonomic centres accounts for the salivation, sweating, pallor, etc. which accompany vomiting. Closely associated with the vomiting centre is the chemoreceptor trigger zone which consists of a group of cells

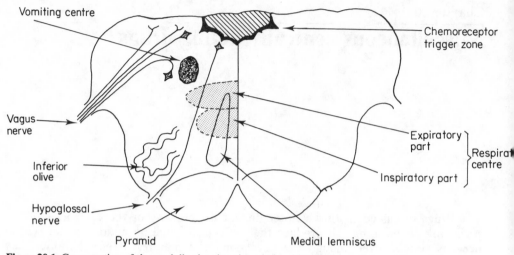

Figure 20.1 Cross-section of the medulla showing the relationship of the vomiting centre and the chemoreceptor trigger zone on the floor of the fourth ventricle, to other important structures in this region of the brain stem (redrawn from Crossland, 1980)

on the floor of the fourth ventricle, in a region known as the area postrema (Figure 20.1). This region, which is sensitive to chemical stimuli and is the site of action of many emetic and anti-emetic drugs (see below), is the primary site through which the vomiting centre is activated. Thus, many substances which cause vomiting after entry into the bloodstream stimulate the trigger zone, which then activates the vomiting centre (Figure 20.2). The chemoreceptor trigger zone is also believed to be

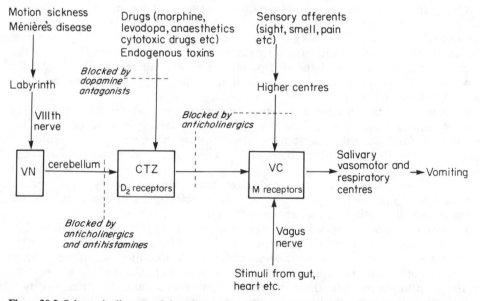

Figure 20.2 Schematic diagram of the control of vomiting, showing influences on both the vomiting centre (VC) and the chemoreceptor trigger zone (CTZ). VN, vestibular nuclei

involved in the vomiting associated with disease states and with radiation sickness. In Menière's disease, spontaneous bursts of activity occur in the semicircular canals and in the sensory nerves leading from them, resulting in dizziness (vertigo), loss of balance, nausea and vomiting. The chemoreceptor trigger zone is also involved in motion sickness. Motion sickness is caused by certain kinds of movements which result in abnormal stimulation of the labyrinth which, in turn, sends impulses via the vestibular nuclei and the cerebellum to the chemoreceptor trigger zone which then activates the vomiting centre (Figure 20.2).

The chemoreceptor trigger zone contains dopamine receptors which are of the D_2 subtype. However, acetylcholine and histamine are also involved, as drugs acting on these neurotransmitter systems can influence the activity of this region. Other neurotransmitters, such as γ-aminobutyric acid and glutamic acid, may also be involved. The main indication as to the nature of the receptors involved comes from the pharmacological properties of the drugs which produce vomiting or have anti-emetic actions.

Emetic drugs

Some drugs, e.g. cardiac glycosides, levodopa and opiates, may cause vomiting as an unwanted side-effect. However, emetic drugs are those which cause vomiting as their main action.

Apomorphine (Figure 20.3)

This is a derivative of morphine and is a dopamine agonist which acts directly on the dopamine receptors in the chemoreceptor trigger zone, as it has been shown to induce vomiting when injected directly into the fourth ventricle. It is not used to induce emesis in poisoning, although sub-emetic doses of apomorphine have been utilized in aversion therapy to interrupt the pattern of drug dependence by producing reflex vomiting. For example, in alcoholics, conditioning with apomorphine so that a sensation of nausea occurs every time alcohol is consumed has been found to be effective; however, such methods have not become popular for treating alcoholism.

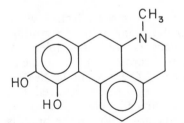

Figure 20.3 The chemical structure of apomorphine

Pilocarpine (see Chapter 7, Figure 7.3a)

This drug is a muscarinic cholinergic agonist which penetrates the blood–brain barrier. It produces its effects by stimulating the frontal lobe of the cerebellum, the impulses generated there passing directly to the vomiting centre (see Figure 20.2).

Thus, the chemoreceptor trigger zone is not involved in the emetic action of pilocarpine.

The therapeutic use of emetic drugs is limited mainly to the treatment of orally ingested poisons. However, this procedure is useful only if (1) the patient is conscious, (2) the poison is non-corrosive and (3) a substantial amount of the poison remains in the stomach. The substance normally used is ipecacuanha, which is a naturally occurring extract of the dried roots of the plant *Cephaëlis ipecacuanha* which is indigenous to Central America and Brazil. Ipecacuanha has an irritant action on the gut and also stimulates the chemoreceptor trigger zone.

Anti-emetic drugs

There are four main types: anticholinergics, antihistamines, dopamine antagonists and cannabinoids. They are used to treat different conditions.

Anticholinergics

These are muscarinic cholinergic antagonists. Hyoscine (see Chapter 7 and Figure 7.5b) is the most important. It readily enters the central nervous system and is very effective in the prophylactic treatment of motion sickness. It is less effective when given after sickness has occurred and is ineffective against the emesis induced by apomorphine. It gives good results when administered orally, although side-effects such as drowsiness, dry mouth, blurred vision and urinary retention may occur. A method of transdermal administration, through a self-adhesive skin patch, may provide continuous low-level release of the drug in a dose sufficient to be anti-emetic without producing marked side-effects. Atropine and other muscarinic antagonists are much less effective as anti-emetics.

The precise mechanism of action is not clear but the fact that hyoscine is effective against motion sickness suggests that it blocks impulses from the vestibular system; it may act on the same pathway through which pilocarpine produces emesis.

Antihistamines

These, like hyoscine, also relieve motion sickness and are more effective when given prophylactically, but they do not act against apomorphine-induced vomiting. They are less effective than hyoscine but the side-effects are better tolerated. Examples are cyclizine (Figure 20.4a), dimenhydrinate (Figure 20.4b) and promethazine (Figure 20.4c), the latter being a phenothiazine. There seem to be few differences between the various antihistamines although cyclizine is less sedative than dimenhydrinate and promethazine. These drugs are all antagonists at H_1 histamine receptors (see Chapter 10) but their mechanism of action in the brain is not known.

Dopamine antagonists

A number of phenothiazines (see Chapter 12) possess anti-emetic actions. For example, chlorpromazine and trifluoperazine, as well as being used as antipsychotic drugs, are used as anti-emetics. On the other hand, thiethylperazine (Figure 20.5a)

(a)

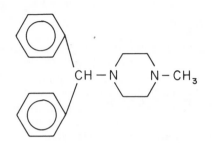

(b)

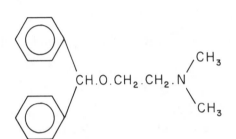

(c)

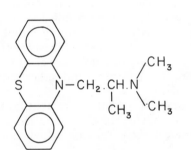

Figure 20.4 The chemical structures of (a) cyclizine, (b) dimenhydrinate and (c) promethazine

is used only as an anti-emetic. Other neuroleptics, such as the butyrophenones haloperidol and droperidol (see Chapter 12), have potent anti-emetic actions although the side-effects can limit their usefulness. Other examples of non-phenothiazine anti-emetic drugs are metoclopramide (Figure 20.5b) and domperidone (Figure 20.5c). All these drugs are dopamine antagonists and they act on the D_2 dopamine receptors in the area postrema, blocking the influence of the chemoreceptor trigger zone on the vomiting centre. They all block apomorphine-induced vomiting: metoclopramide, for example, is 35 times more potent than chlorpromazine in blocking apomorphine-induced vomiting in the dog. These drugs are less effective against vomiting associated with disturbances of labyrinthine function. The side-effects are mainly those associated with the neuroleptic drugs, i.e. sedation, hypotension and extrapyramidal symptoms. However, with the butyrophenones, restlessness and agitation can occur. As well as their central anti-emetic effects, metoclopramide and domperidone have peripheral actions. For example, metoclopramide increases the motility of the stomach and the intestine

(a)

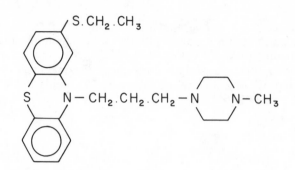

(b)

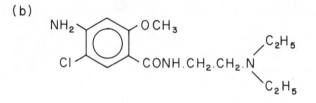

(c)

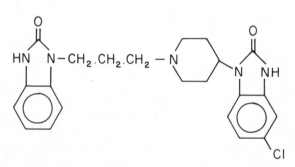

Figure 20.5 The chemical structures of (a) thiethylperazine, (b) metoclopramide and (c) domperidone

and this adds to its anti-emetic effect. This drug also causes relaxation of the oesophagus and acceleration of gastric emptying by increasing gastric peristalsis and relaxing the pylorus. Some of these actions of metoclopramide are utilized to facilitate diagnostic procedures. Domperidone also has peripheral effects and increases the motility of the gut. It has been shown that domperidone does not penetrate the blood–brain barrier particularly well and, therefore, its anti-emetic effect may be due mainly to peripheral actions. However, the area postrema on the floor of the fourth ventricle is functionally outside the blood–brain barrier and so drugs which do not penetrate the blood–brain barrier can still act on the chemoreceptor trigger zone. Side-effects, attributable to actions on the basal ganglia, occur less frequently with domperidone than with the other centrally acting dopamine antagonists, probably because of its poor penetration into the brain.

Cannabinoids

A synthetic derivative of tetrahydrocannabinol (see Chapter 18), nabilone, has been found to be an effective anti-emetic. It appears to act on the chemoreceptor trigger zone as it blocks apomorphine-induced vomiting in the cat. It is well absorbed after oral administration but side-effects, especially drowsiness, dizziness and dry mouth, are common and repeated use of nabilone must be avoided because of the risk of neurotoxic effects (see Chapter 18).

Clinical uses of anti-emetic drugs

Some of these have been discussed above. Hyoscine, or one of the antihistamines, is used for the prophylactic treatment of motion sickness, although such drugs are less effective if vomiting has already occurred. The dopamine antagonists, phenothiazines, metoclopramide and domperidone are ineffective in motion sickness. The exception is promethazine, which is a phenothiazine, but its anti-emetic action is related to its antihistaminergic rather than its antidopaminergic properties. Hyoscine and the antihistamines may cause drowsiness but this is not always undesirable. The vertigo and nausea associated with Menière's disease is difficult to treat but hyoscine, antihistamines and the phenothiazines have been used. The nausea and vomiting that occurs during the first trimester of pregnancy usually only persists for a few weeks and the use of anti-emetic drugs is to be avoided because of the risk of teratogenic effects. In some cases the nausea and vomiting may be incapacitating, in which case an antihistamine drug, or the phenothiazine promethazine, is used.

The nausea and vomiting associated with disease, exposure to radiation, analgesic and anaesthetic drugs and cancer chemotherapy is best treated with antidopamine drugs, which are less effective against motion sickness and disorders of the labyrinthine system. These drugs can be used in small doses for prophylactic treatment but larger doses are required if vomiting has already occurred. Domperidone, used for the relief of nausea and vomiting due to treatment with cytotoxic drugs, has the advantage over the phenothiazines and metoclopramide in that it produces fewer central side-effects. This drug can also be used to control vomiting induced by levodopa and bromocriptine in the treatment of Parkinson's disease. Finally, the cannabinoid nabilone has been reported to be effective in the relief of nausea and vomiting associated with therapy using cytotoxic drugs.

Antitussive drugs

The cough is a reflex mechanism that is partly under voluntary control and serves to clear the respiratory passages of foreign material and excess secretions. It is, therefore, a protective mechanism and should not be suppressed indiscriminately. There are, however, situations in which the cough does not serve any useful purpose but may prevent rest and sleep. In such a situation the cough reflex may be suppressed with a drug. In theory, it should be possible to interrupt any part of the cough reflex; however, most of the antitussive drugs in use suppress coughing by a central action. It seems likely that there is a 'cough centre' in the medulla but this has not been precisely defined.

The drugs that are most effective in suppressing coughing are the opiate

(a)

(b)

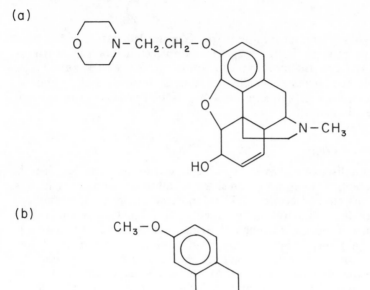

Figure 20.6 The chemical structures of (a) pholcodine and (b) dextromethorphan

analgesics, one of the most widely used being codeine (Chapter 15, Figure 15.2b). Others are pholcodine (Figure 20.6a), dextromethorphan (Figure 20.6b) and noscapine. The dose of codeine required for the antitussive action is less than that needed to produce analgesia; nevertheless, constipation can occur as a side-effect. Pholcodine has similar effects but is thought to be less likely to produce dependence at the dose level required for suppressing coughing. Dextromethorphan is interesting because it is related to levorphanol (Chapter 15, Figure 15.3b), being the dextro-isomer of the methyl ether of levorphanol. It has no analgesic action and is not addictive but is similar in potency to codeine as an antitussive. However, in large doses, dextromethorphan can cause drowsiness and gastrointestinal disturbances. Noscapine is a naturally occurring alkaloid that is present in the opium poppy (see Chapter 15); it seems to have no central effects other than the antitussive action. These antitussive drugs are frequently used in 'over-the-counter' cough preparations, often in combination with other active ingredients.

The more potent opiate analgesics, such as morphine and methadone, are used for their antitussive action to suppress distressing coughing in terminal lung cancer.

Expectorants stimulate the secretory activity of the respiratory tract, causing the mucous to become less viscous. They are thought to be beneficial in alleviating a dry, irritant, unproductive cough, by increasing secretion of mucus lubricating the air passages and so making the cough more 'productive'. Emetic drugs, such as ipecacuanha, in sub-emetic doses, are used for this purpose but there are doubts about their effectiveness as expectorants.

(a)

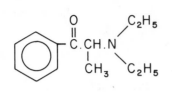

(b)

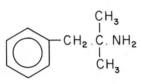

(c)

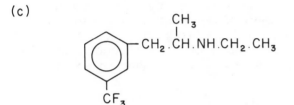

(d)

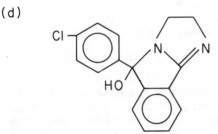

Figure 20.7 The chemical structures of (a) diethylpropion, (b) phentermine, (c) fenfluramine and (d) mazindol

Anorectic drugs

The psychomotor stimulant drugs, such as amphetamine and dextro-amphetamine (Chapter 16), are effective in suppressing appetite, so reducing food intake, and they have been used in the treatment of obesity. However, the stimulant action, together with the dangers of addiction, have led to these drugs being withdrawn for this purpose and others, with less central stimulant action, have been developed.

Diethylpropion (Figure 20.7a)

Although diethylpropion has a weaker central stimulant action than amphetamine, its peripheral effects resemble those of amphetamine (see Chapter 16), although cardiovascular effects are less marked. However, dependence has been reported and insomnia can occur.

Phentermine (Figure 20.7b)

The actions of this substance resemble those of diethylpropion. It has been claimed that this drug produces fewer side-effects than either amphetamine or dexamphetamine and that it is less likely to be abused. Nevertheless, dependence has been reported with phentermine.

Fenfluramine (Figure 20.7c)

This is a phenylethylamine and therefore chemically related to the amphetamines. However, it has a depressant rather than a stimulant action on the CNS and can cause drowsiness. This can be an advantage where the obesity is accompanied by anxiety, but it can affect the performance of tasks such as driving and the drug should not be used if there is any history of depression. Gastrointestinal disturbances can also occur. Tolerance to the actions of fenfluramine may develop and rebound depression can occur if administration is discontinued abruptly; therefore, fenfluramine is best used for short periods and should be withdrawn gradually.

Mazindol (Figure 20.7d)

This drug differs chemically from the other anorectic agents as it is an imidazoline derivative. Mazindol is a weaker CNS stimulant than amphetamine but is more potent as an anorectic than the drugs described above. However, it does cause cardiovascular stimulation and tolerance develops to the anorectic effect.

The mechanism of action of anorectic drugs

The principal pharmacological action of amphetamine is to release the endogenous catecholamines noradrenaline and dopamine from presynaptic nerve terminals and there is reason to believe that this mechanism is involved in the anorectic action. Thus, interruption of the noradrenergic pathway to the hypothalamus in the rat reduces the anorectic effect of amphetamine, as does pretreatment with the neurotoxin 6-hydroxydopamine, and the enzyme inhibitor α-methyl-p-tyrosine, both of which reduce the levels of catecholamines in the brain (see Chapter 10). In addition, the anorectic action of amphetamine can be reduced by pretreatment with dopamine antagonists such as pimozide and haloperidol (see Chapter 12). Thus, the presynaptic release of both dopamine and noradrenaline appears to be involved in the anorectic action of amphetamine, whereas 5-hydroxytryptamine does not seem to be involved, because neither antagonists of 5-HT, nor reduction in the levels of 5-HT produced by lesions of the raphe nuclei, nor pretreatment with the neurotoxin 5,6-dihydroxytryptamine, modify the anorectic effect of amphetamine. On the other hand, the anorectic action of fenfluramine is not modified by depletion of catecholamines or by dopamine antagonists, but is reduced by pretreatment with antagonists of 5-HT, e.g. methysergide, or by depletion of 5-HT in the brain. In fact, fenfluramine has been shown to block the re-uptake of 5-HT into nerve endings and to stimulate release. Mazindol appears to combine these actions, as it not only blocks the re-uptake and stimulates the release of catecholamines but it has the same actions for 5-HT, i.e. blocking re-uptake and stimulating release. It therefore appears that anorexia can be attributable to enhancement of the actions of dopamine and noradrenaline as neurotransmitters in the brain, or of the actions of 5-hydroxytryptamine, or both. The dual action of mazindol may account for its greater potency as an anorectic drug. However, metabolic effects may also be involved: for example, fenfluramine increases the uptake of glucose by muscle and the mobilization and metabolism of fat. How much this peripheral action contributes to the anorectic effect of fenfluramine is not known.

Effects of drugs on memory

One of the features of deteriorating intellectual function brought about by such conditions as degenerative neuronal disease or cerebral atherosclerosis in the elderly is a loss of cognitive function and, particularly, loss of memory. The use of drugs for ameliorating disturbances of memory in elderly or demented patients is controversial. On the whole, the drugs used are not very effective and doubts have been expressed as to whether they are effective at all. However, with the increasing age of the population, this is an area which ought not to be ignored.

It is generally believed that the processes of learning and memory are related to synaptic mechanisms in the brain and that recent or short-term memory is probably encoded in neuronal circuits, whereas long-term, established memories are stored in some more permanent form, e.g. in proteins. There is evidence to support this hypothesis from the fact that recent memory is more labile than long-term memory. Thus, a blow to the head, whiplash injury to the neck, or electric shock, such as electroconvulsive therapy, can produce retrograde amnesia in which there is loss of only recent events. The control of protein synthesis by ribonucleic acid (RNA) is thought to be important in the laying down of permanent memory traces; certainly, inhibitors of protein synthesis have been found to impair learning and memory, although the claim that learned responses can be transferred from one animal to another by the transfer of tissue containing the appropriate proteins is highly dubious. If memory traces are associated with synaptic activity, then drugs which affect synaptic transmission should have effects on memory and this is, in fact, the case.

Cholinergic drugs

It has long been known that drugs that affect neurotransmission mediated by acetylcholine in the brain can affect memory in both animals and man. For example, atropine in large doses is known to cause loss of memory, and hyoscine (scopolamine) produces a state of temporary amnesia. Both these drugs are antagonists of the muscarinic actions of acetylcholine (see Chapters 7 and 10). In animals the administration of physostigmine, an inhibitor of cholinesterase which crosses the blood–brain barrier and will therefore increase the level of acetylcholine in the brain, has been shown to improve the performance of tasks which involve learning and memory and to antagonize the adverse effects of hyoscine on memory.

In man, probably the best evidence for the involvement of cholinergic mechanisms in memory processes comes from the neuropathology of Alzheimer's disease. This disease affects some 5% of the population over 65 years of age and is the principal cause of senile dementia. When Alzheimer's disease occurs earlier, i.e. in people in their 50s, it is responsible for the condition known as presenile dementia. The onset of senile dementia is generally characterized by cognitive deficits, such as an impairment in recent memory. Post-mortem examination of the brains of patients suffering from Alzheimer's disease has shown reduced activity of choline acetyltransferase, the enzyme which synthesizes acetylcholine (see Chapter 5), in the cerebral cortex and hippocampus. This is due to the degeneration of nerve terminals and is characterized anatomically by the appearance of neurofibrillary tangles and neuritic plaques. This degeneration of nerve terminals in the cortex and hippocampus is a consequence of the degeneration of neuronal cell bodies in the nucleus basalis (see Chapter 10, Figure 10.2), which send their axons to the cerebral cortex. Attempts to restore the deficit in cholinergic transmission have so far proved unsuccessful. Thus, administration, in large amounts, of the precursor of acetylcholine, choline, or its dietary source, lecithin, to demented patients has not proved particularly successful. One explanation for this is that there may be an inadequate number of surviving neurones to cope with the deficiency in the transmitter. Some improvement in the mental state of demented patients has been obtained with physostigmine; however, the usefulness of this drug in man is limited by its short duration of action and its toxic effects.

Stimulant drugs

Psychomotor stimulant drugs, such as amphetamine and methylphenidate (Chapter 16), have been used to counteract deteriorating intellectual function in the elderly, but the effects produced are probably due to the stimulant action of the drugs counteracting lethargy and withdrawal, rather than to specific effects on memory. The dangers of using these drugs outweigh their possible usefulness (see Chapter 16). However, pemoline (Figure 20.8a), which is structurally similar to methylphenidate, is claimed to have minimal cardiovascular effects.

(a)

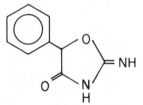

(b)

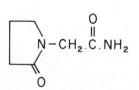

Figure 20.8 The chemical structures of (a) pemoline and (b) piracetam

Peptides

Certain endogenous peptides, such as adrenocorticotrophic hormone (ACTH) which is present in the anterior pituitary, have been shown to have effects on learning and memory in animals. However, ACTH has been found to increase arousal and the effects on learning and memory may therefore be indirect. Vasopressin, a peptide present in the posterior pituitary, has been shown to have effects similar to those of ACTH on learning and memory but, in the case of vasopressin, they are of longer duration and can last for several days. There is no evidence that vasopressin has any beneficial effect in Alzheimer's disease, although its use in memory disorders resulting from trauma has been proposed. However, the use of this substance is highly controversial and it is possible that any apparent beneficial effects may be due to peripheral autonomic actions and therefore, like those of ACTH, indirect.

No-otropic drugs

This name has been coined to describe drugs which have been developed for their cognition-enhancing effects. There are a number of them, most being related to piracetam (Figure 20.8b), which was the first no-otropic drug to be described. Piracetam is a derivative of γ-aminobutyric acid and has been shown, both in animals and man, to increase the transfer of information from one cerebral hemisphere to the other. The significance of this action is not clear but if the inter-hemispheric transfer, via the corpus callosum, involves facilitation of synaptic transmission, then a similar action at other sites in the brain might account for the effect on cognitive function. It is not certain whether the relationship to γ-aminobutyric acid is important for the pharmacological actions of piracetam, as this drug has been found to facilitate cholinergic mechanisms, at least peripherally.

Improvements in mood, alertness and memory in the elderly have also been observed with vasodilators, and derivatives of vincamine have been found to improve cerebral blood flow, thus increasing oxygen availability to the brain and stimulating cerebral metabolism.

In spite of considerable research interest in this area, the use of drugs to improve impaired memory is not widespread, probably because none of the drugs at present available is particularly effective. It seems unlikely that where deterioration of function is due to degenerative neuronal disease, adequate compensation can be made by replacement therapy with drugs or by stimulating the remaining functional neurones, although both seem to work in the case of Parkinson's disease. Possible hope for the future in the case of degenerative diseases, such as Alzheimer's disease and Parkinson's disease, lies in the development of drugs which arrest the degenerative process (see below) or the transplant of fetal neuronal tissue to replace the missing neurotransmitters.

Neuroprotective agents

These provide a relatively new type of action which is currently represented by one drug, (+)-5-methyl-10,11-dihydro-5H-dibenzo[a,d]cyclo-hepten-5,10-imine maleate (MK-801, Figure 20.9). This is an antagonist of the N-methyl-D-aspartate type of excitatory amino acid receptor (see Chapter 10) which not only blocks the

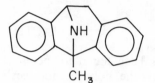

Figure 20.9 The chemical structure of MK-801

depolarization produced by *N*-methyl-D-aspartate and related agonists such as quinolinic acid, but also prevents their neurotoxic action. Thus, pretreatment with MK-801 has been shown to give complete protection from the neuronal degeneration produced by either *N*-methyl-D-aspartate or quinolinic acid. Excessive release of excitatory neurotransmitters has been shown to occur in epilepsy, hypoxia and ischaemia, leading to the degeneration of nerve cells by an action involving *N*-methyl-D-aspartate receptors and an increased concentration of calcium intracellularly. In an animal model of ischaemia, MK-801 prevented appreciable neuronal degeneration from occurring, even when given after the ischaemia. It is possible that drugs with this kind of action may be useful in the treatment of strokes and degenerative disorders of the nervous system.

References to sources of illustrations

D. Anderson (1987) In: *Epilepsy: Progress in Treatment* (eds M. Dam, S. I. Johannessen, B. Nilsson and M. Sillanpää) pp. 1–9. John Wiley, Chichester

J. Anson, ed. (1966) *Morris' Human Anatomy* (12th edn) McGraw-Hill, New York

R. Birks, H. E. Huxley and B. Katz (1960) *Journal of Physiology* **150**, 134–144

W. C. Bowman and M. J. Rand (1980) *Textbook of Pharmacology* (2nd edn) Blackwell, Oxford

H. F. Bradford (1986) *Chemical Neurobiology* W. H. Freeman, New York

J. R. Cooper, F. E. Bloom and R. H. Roth (1986) *The Biochemical Basis of Neuropharmacology* Oxford University Press, Oxford

E. Costa (1988) *Life of Science* **42**, 1407–1417

I. Creese, D. I. Burt and S. H. Snyder (1978) *Science* **192**, 481–483

J. Crossland (1980) *Lewis's Pharmacology* (5th edn) Churchill Livingstone, Edinburgh

A. C. Cuello and M. V. Sofroniew (1985) In: *Neurotransmitters in Action* (ed. D. Bousfield) pp. 309–318. Elsevier, Amsterdam

W. C. Dement and N. Kleitman (1957) *Electroencephalography and Clinical Neurophysiology* **9**, 673–690

R. M. Eccles and B. Libet (1961) *Journal of Physiology* **157**, 484–503

T. Hökfelt, K. Fuxe, M. Goldstein and O. Johansson (1974) *Brain Research* **66**, 235–261

L. L. Iversen and A. V. P. McKay (1979) In: *Psychopharmacology of Affective Disorders* (eds E. S. Paykel and A. Coppen) pp. 60–90. Oxford University Press, Oxford

S. Konishi, A. Tsunoo, N. Yanihara and M. Otsuka (1980) *Biomedical Research* **1**, 528–536

Z. L. Kruk and C. J. Pycock (1983) *Neurotransmitters and Drugs* (2nd edn) Croom Helm, London

W. Penfield and H. Jasper (1954) *Epilepsy and the Functional Anatomy of the Human Brain* Little, Brown, Boston

J. H. Pincus and G. Tucker (1974) *Behavioural Neurology* Oxford University Press, Oxford

S. J. Singer and G. L. Nicolson (1972) The Fluid Mosaic Model of the Structure of Cell Membranes. *Science* **175**, 720–731

T. E. Starzl, G. W. Taylor and H. W. Magoun (1951) *Journal of Neurophysiology* **14**, 479

U. Ungerstedt (1971) *Acta physiologica scandinavica*, Supplement 367, 49–67

Further reading

General

A. G. Gilman, L. S. Goodman, T. W. Rall and F. Murad (eds) (1985) *The Pharmacological Basis of Therapeutics* (7th edn) Macmillan, London

H. P. Rang and M. M. Dale (1987) *Pharmacology* Churchill Livingstone, Edinburgh

Selected topics

Chapter 1

T. P. Kenakin (1987) *Pharmacologic Analysis of Drug–Receptor Interaction* Raven Press, New York

R. B. Barlow (1980) *Quantitative Aspects of Chemical Pharmacology* Croom Helm, London

Chapter 2

A. Goldstein, L. Aranow and S. M. Kalman (1974) *Principles of Drug Action* (2nd edn), Chapters 2 and 3. Wiley, Chichester

J. W. Lamble (ed.) (1983) *Drug Metabolism and Distribution* Elsevier, Amsterdam

Chapter 3

J. C. Eccles (1964) *The Physiology of Synapses* Academic Press, New York

B. Katz (1966) *Nerve, Muscle and Synapse* McGraw-Hill, New York

Chapters 4 and 5

W. C. Bowman (1980) *Pharmacology of Neuromuscular Function* John Wright, Bristol

E. Zaimis (ed.) (1976). Neuromuscular Junction. *Handbook of Experimental Pharmacology*, **42,** Springer-Verlag, Berlin

D. A. Kharkevich (ed.) (1986) New Neuromuscular Blocking Agents *Handbook of Experimental Pharmacology*, **79,** Springer-Verlag, Berlin

Chapter 6

C. A. Keele, E. Neil and N. Joels (1982) *Samson Wright's Applied Physiology* (13th edn). Part VII. Oxford Medical Publications, Oxford

Chapters 7 and 8

M. D. Day (1979) *Autonomic Pharmacology* Churchill Livingstone, Edinburgh

D. A. Kharkevich, (ed.) (1980) Pharmacology of Ganglionic Transmission *Handbook of Experimental Pharmacology*, **53**, Springer-Verlag, Berlin

L. Szekeres (ed.) (1980) Adrenergic Activators and Inhibitors *Handbook of Experimental Pharmacology*, **54**, Parts I and II. Springer-Verlag, Berlin

Chapter 9

G. R. Strichartz (ed.) (1985) Local Anaesthetics *Handbook of Experimental Pharmacology*, **74**, Springer-Verlag, Berlin

Chapter 10

J. R. Cooper, F. E. Bloom and R. H. Roth (1986) *The Biochemical Basis of Neuropharmacology* (5th edn) OUP, Oxford

H. F. Bradford (1985) *Chemical Neurobiology, An Introduction to Neurochemistry* W. H. Freeman, New York

J. W. Lamble (ed.) (1981) *Towards an Understanding of Receptors* Elsevier, Amsterdam

J. W. Lamble and A. C. Abbott (eds) (1984) *Receptors Again* Elsevier, Amsterdam

D. Bousfield (ed.) (1985) *Neurotransmitters in Action* Elsevier, Amsterdam

Chapter 11

M. D. Vickers, H. Schnieden and F. G. Wood-Smith (1984) *Drugs in Anaesthetic Practice* Butterworth, London

F. Hoffmeister and G. Stille (eds) (1982) Psychotropic Agents Part III *Handbook of Experimental Pharmacology*, **55**, Chapters 9, 10, 11, 12 and 14. Springer-Verlag, Berlin

Chapter 12

P. B. Bradley and S. R. Hirsch (eds) (1986) *The Psychopharmacology and Treatment of Schizophrenia* Oxford

Heather Ashton (1986) *Brain Disorders and Psychotropic Drugs* Part V. Oxford University Press, Oxford

F. Hoffmeister and G. Stille (eds) (1980) Psychotropic Agents, Part III *Handbook of Experimental Pharmacology*, **55**, Chapters 1 to 15. Springer-Verlag, Berlin

Chapter 13

F. Hoffmeister and G. Stille (eds) (1981) Psychotropic Agents, Part II *Handbook of Experimental Pharmacology*, **55**, Chapters 1 to 8. Springer-Verlag, Berlin

Heather Ashton (1986) *Brain System Disorders and Psychotropic Drugs* Part I. Oxford University Press, Oxford

Chapter 14

H. H. Frey and D. Janz (eds) (1985) Antiepileptic Drugs *Handbook of Experimental Pharmacology*, **74**, Springer-Verlag, Berlin

D. M. Woodbury, J. K. Penry and C. E. Pippenger (eds) (1982) *Antiepileptic Drugs* Raven Press, New York

P. C. Jobe and H. E. Laird (eds) (1987) *Neurotransmitters and Epilepsy* Humana Press, New Jersey

Chapter 15

M. J. Kuhar and G. W. Pasternak (eds) (1984) *Analgesics: Neurochemical, Behavioural and Clinical Perspectives*. Raven Press, New York

J. Hughes, H. O. J. Collier, M. J. Rance and M. B. Tyers (eds) (1984) *Opioids, Past, Present and Future* Taylor and Francis, London

G. W. Pasternak (ed.) (1988) *The Opiate Receptors* Humana Press, New Jersey

Chapter 16

F. Hoffmeister and G. Stille (eds) (1981) Psychotropic Agents, Part II *Handbook of Experimental Pharmacology*, **55**, Chapters 14, 15 and 16. Springer-Verlag, Berlin

F. Hoffmeister and G. Stille (eds) (1982) Psychotropic Agents, Part III *Handbook of Experimental Pharmacology*, **55**, Chapter 17. Springer-Verlag, Berlin

Chapter 17

Heather Ashton (1987) *Brain System Disorders and Psychotropic Drugs* Part IV. Oxford University Press, Oxford

W. G. Dewhurst and G. B. Baker (eds.) (1985) *Pharmacotherapy of Affective Disorders. Theory and Practice* Croom Helm, Beckenham

E. S. Paykel (ed.) (1982) *Handbook of Affective Disorders* Churchill Livingstone, Edinburgh

Antidepressants and Receptor Function. Ciba Foundation 123, Wiley, Chichester, 1986

Chapter 18

F. Hoffmeister and G. Stille (eds) (1982) Psychotropic Agents, Part III *Handbook of Experimental Pharmacology*, **55**, Chapters 1 to 8. Springer-Verlag, Berlin

B. L. Jacobs (ed.) (1984) *Hallucinogens: Neurochemical, Behavioural and Clinical Perspectives*. Raven Press, New York

Chapter 19

C. D. Marsden and S. Fahn (eds) (1982) *Movement Disorders* Butterworth, London

A. N. Davison and R. H. S. Thompson (eds.) (1981) *The Molecular Basis of Neuropathology* Arnold, London

S. P. Markey, N. Castagnoli, A. J. Trevor and I. J. Kopin (eds.) (1986) *MPTP: A Neurotoxin Producing a Parkinsonian Syndrome* Academic Press, New York

Chapter 20

H. L. Borison and S. C. Wang (1953) Physiology and Pharmacology of Vomiting *Pharmacological Reviews*, **5**, 193–230

Heather Ashton (1987) *Brain System Disorders and Psychotropic Drugs*. Part III. Oxford University Press, Oxford

Index